D0068831

Understanding Suicide's Allure

Understanding Suicide's Allure

Steps to Save Lives by Healing Psychological Scars

Stanley Krippner, Linda Riebel,
Debbie Joffe Ellis, and Daryl S. Paulson

Foreword by Harris L. Friedman, PhD

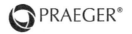

PRAEGER®

An Imprint of ABC-CLIO, LLC

Santa Barbara, California • Denver, Colorado

Library of Congress Cataloging-in-Publication Data

Names: Krippner, Stanley, 1932- author. | Riebel, Linda, author. |
    Joffe-Ellis, Debbie, 1956- author. | Paulson, Daryl S., 1947- author.
Title: Understanding suicide's allure : steps to save lives by healing
    psychological scars / Stanley Krippner, Linda Riebel, Debbie Joffe
    Ellis, and Daryl S. Paulson ; foreword by Harris L. Friedman, PhD.
Description: Santa Barbara : ABC-CLIO, 2021. | Includes bibliographical
    references and index.
Identifiers: LCCN 2020031231 (print) | LCCN 2020031232 (ebook) | ISBN
    9781440862540 (hardcover) | ISBN 9781440862557 (ebook)
Subjects: LCSH: Suicide—Psychological aspects. | Suicidal behavior. |
    Suicidal behavior—Prevention.
Classification: LCC HV6545 .K675 2021 (print) | LCC HV6545 (ebook) | DDC
    616.85/8445—dc23
LC record available at https://lccn.loc.gov/2020031231
LC ebook record available at https://lccn.loc.gov/2020031232

ISBN: 978-1-4408-6254-0 (print)
        978-1-4408-6255-7 (ebook)

25 24 23 22 21   1 2 3 4 5

This book is also available as an eBook.

Praeger
An Imprint of ABC-CLIO, LLC

ABC-CLIO, LLC
147 Castilian Drive
Santa Barbara, California 93117
www.abc-clio.com

This book is printed on acid-free paper ∞

Manufactured in the United States of America

This book discusses treatments (including types of medication and mental health therapies), diagnostic tests for various symptoms and mental health disorders, and organizations. The authors have made every effort to present accurate and up-to-date information. However, the information in this book is not intended to recommend or endorse particular treatments or organizations, or substitute for the care or medical advice of a qualified health professional, or used to alter any medical therapy without a medical doctor's advice. Specific situations may require specific therapeutic approaches not included in this book. For those reasons, we recommend that readers follow the advice of qualified health care professionals directly involved in their care. Readers who suspect they may have specific medical problems should consult a physician about any suggestions made in this book.

Contents

Foreword   ix

Acknowledgments   xi

To the Reader   xiii

When the Crisis Is Global: Coronavirus and PTSD   xv

Section I	**The Allure of Suicide**	1
Chapter 1	Who Is Attracted by the Allure of Suicide?	3
Chapter 2	Suicide Is Complicated	10
Chapter 3	The Pioneer of Suicidology and What He Found	16
Chapter 4	Suicide among Minorities	21
Chapter 5	The Most Beautiful Alluring Demon I Have Ever Known	28
	Those Who Survived: William Styron	34
Chapter 6	Dreams, Nightmares, and Suicide	36
Chapter 7	Mental Illness and Suicide	42
Chapter 8	Teenage Suicides	48
Chapter 9	Physician-Assisted Suicide	52
	Those Who Survived: Colin Wilson	57

Section II   **Suicide in the Military**   59

Chapter 10   Daryl Paulson's Story   61

Chapter 11   Hard-Earned Insights from Combat Experience   67

Chapter 12   The Parking Lot Suicides   73

Chapter 13   An Integrative Treatment of PTSD   77

                  Those Who Survived: Jimmy Stewart   84

Section III   **Sexual Assault and Suicide**   85

Chapter 14   Two Cases of Sexual Assault   87

Chapter 15   Sexual Assault Can Lead to Suicide   93

Chapter 16   Sexual Assault in Churches and Faith Groups   98

Chapter 17   Sexual Assault in the Military   104

Section IV   **Bullying**   109

Chapter 18   How Bruno Was Bullied to Death   111

Chapter 19   Bullying and the Vulnerable   115

Chapter 20   Bullies, Victims, and Bystanders   120

Chapter 21   Preventing Bullying   126

Section V   **Depression, Anxiety, and PTSD**   131

Chapter 22   The Three Dangers   133

Chapter 23   Treating Depression   139

Chapter 24   Deconstructing Anxiety: A New Way of Dealing
                  with Suicidality   143

Chapter 25   Evaluating Treatments for PTSD   150

                  Those Who Survived: Bobby Grey   156

Section VI   **Other Groups at Risk**   159

Chapter 26   Suicide on the Land: The Farmer's Dilemma   161

Chapter 27   Spirit Sickness and Soul Loss   166

Chapter 28   Suicide among Indigenous Peoples   171

Chapter 29   Children, the Elderly, and the Sleep-Deprived   176

Section VII   How Professionals Understand Suicide   181

Chapter 30   Two Views of Suicide from Evolutionary Psychology   183

Chapter 31   Suicide as a Public Health Issue   186

Chapter 32   The Archetypes of Suicide   191

Chapter 33   Why Mythology Is Personal   196

Chapter 34   The Psychophysiology of Suicide   202

Chapter 35   The Rational Emotive Approach to Suicidal Thoughts   206

Chapter 36   Beyond the Personal Self: Transpersonal Models   213

Chapter 37   Systems Approaches to Understanding Suicide   219

                 Those Who Survived: Marla   224

Section VIII **Prevention**   227

Chapter 38   Preventing Suicide   229

Chapter 39   REBT and Suicide Prevention   234

Chapter 40   Resilience Training and Suicide Prevention:
                 Did It Work?   240

Chapter 41   Skills for Self-Regulation   246

Chapter 42   Building a Better Teenage Brain   250

Chapter 43   Preventing Suicide behind Bars   258

Chapter 44   Spirituality as a Path away from Suicide   262

                 Those Who Survived: The Sister Who Lived   267

Section IX   Healing   269

Chapter 45   Achieving Self-Empowerment   271

Chapter 46   Deal with PTSD Nightmares First   275

Chapter 47   Nightmare Dream Revision and Lucid Dreaming   282

Chapter 48   Eye Movement Desensitization and Reprocessing   287

Chapter 49   Narrative Exposure Therapy   292

Chapter 50   Time Perspective Therapy   296

Chapter 51   How TPT Saved Jamie from PTSD   300

Chapter 52   Nature's Gift   305

Chapter 53   Psychedelics Old and New   310

Chapter 54   Vine of the Spirits   316

                  Those Who Survived: Saved by the Vine   322

Section X   Turning the Tide   323

Chapter 55   Turning the Tide   325

Index   335

Foreword

Suicide appears to be increasingly common in the United States, where suicide rates have hit their highest peak since World War II,[1] and the World Health Organization recognizes it as a global problem.[2] Within some historical and cultural contexts, suicide can be seen as a noble act—as in the traditional Japanese practice of *seppuku*, in which disgraced individuals disemboweled themselves as an act of restoring their lost honor—but these days it is rarely viewed favorably.

Yet, suicide has its allure within the contemporary West, which has been reflected in the title of this book. It raises many perplexing questions about life's meaning and how one should live. In fact, suicide could be seen as the primal human dilemma, as all of us face a world replete with unavoidable suffering as well as fleeting pleasure. As philosopher Albert Camus famously stated, "There is but one truly serious philosophical problem, and that is suicide."[3] To Camus, facing this question is necessary for confronting questions about meaning and purpose.

As a clinical psychologist, I occasionally encountered suicidal clients in outpatient settings and routine hospital consultations but later became fascinated by this area, so I consulted with a Crisis Stabilization Unit at a community mental health center, where most people being initially seen were actively suicidal, arriving with rope burns on their necks or bandaged wrists. Still later, I consulted with several prisons, where one of my main roles was to decide whether inmates placed on suicide watch were actually suicidal or just trying to game the system to get better housing.

For those who hold on to a heroic version of life, such as dedicating themselves to wars against cancer, social and environment injustices, and even war itself, the fundamental assumption is that life is precious and suicide an ungrateful squandering of its opportunities. It seems easier to excuse suicide in dire circumstances, such as intractable suffering during terminal illness.

However, I hazard that most Westerners see suicide as a failure rather than as a proclamation of one's freedom to live (or not to live) on one's own terms.

As the authors of this book have shown, there are many psychological theories and some solid research about what causes and what might prevent suicide. Even so, this ultimate act remains elusive, especially for those left behind. This can be especially painful when young and healthy people with a life apparently full of promise decide to end their existence.

This book is not an academic tome dryly examining scientific theories and data. In fact, the authors of this book are not "suicidologists"; they were curious about the epidemic of suicide in recent years. So it is a book about exploring a complicated topic, looking at a multiplicity of ideas from many perspectives, including the spiritual and transpersonal. Some chapters are practical, such as demonstrating how mental health practitioners use certain therapeutic approaches. Others are more abstract and scholarly. But all are thought-provoking and challenging. Rich case studies are given of people who have ended their own lives and of others who considered doing so, but who survived their "dark nights of the soul."

For anyone who is struggling with suicidal thoughts, or who knows someone who is, or who is dealing with the aftermath of a loved one's suicide, this book can be a source of insight and inspiration. Camus concluded, "In the end, one needs more courage to live than to kill himself." It is hoped that this book can help instill such courage for those during their own moments of truth.

Harris L. Friedman, PhD
Visiting Scholar, History of Science, Harvard University
Research Professor of Psychology, University of Florida
Clinical Psychologist in Private Practice

Notes

1. Centers for Disease Control and Prevention. (n.d.). Suicide rising across the US: More than a mental health concern. Accessed January 3, 2020. https://www.cdc.gov/vitalsigns/suicide/index.html.

2. World Health Organization. (n.d.). Suicide data. Accessed January 3, 2020. https://www.who.int/mental_health/prevention/suicide/suicideprevent/en.

3. Archon, S. (n.d.). 91 Albert Camus quotes on death, suicide, God, truth, philosophy, fear, rebellion, freedom, and more. Accessed January 3, 2020. https://theunboundedspirit.com/albert-camus-quotes.

Acknowledgments

The authors of this book would like to acknowledge the financial support of Drs. Robert and Zohara Hieronimus, Richard and Connie Adams, and the AUM Center in Maryland, offering educational opportunities pertaining to religious metaphysics, occult sciences, and the mystical arts since 1969. Rosemary Coffey and Steve Hart provided editorial support, and Alanna Bova, Pamela Hansen, and Steve Speer supplied valuable resource material.

To the Reader

There are so many factors in developing, treating, and recovering from the risk of suicide that we found we have written over fifty chapters! We gave each major topic its own section, with numerous chapters in each. It is not necessary to read the whole book at once. There are sections you may find most relevant at a particular time and others that can be read as time permits. If you are a health care professional, this book covers a wide range of at-risk populations, theories, and treatments, and perhaps some of them are approaches you may not have been familiar with before.

In trying to explain the reasons that people take their lives, we have listed many defeatist attitudes and emotions, challenging conditions, and life circumstances. Our intention has been to put things into realistic perspective and, by describing the many treatments now available, to provide hope and encouragement. We have included information about some indigenous and other non-Western societies, though there is room in this book for only a small sample of these, but perhaps it is enough to help our readers look beyond Western problems.

Telephone hotlines, rescue organizations, hospitalizations, and barriers being built at suicide "hot spots" are a few of the many resources now being used to prevent suicide. People in the public eye—entertainers, elected officials, and so on—are less afraid than in previous times to disclose their struggles and ultimate victories. Advances and innovations in health care—new treatments, social support, animal-assisted therapy, and more—have made the prospect of living with chronic illness less dreaded and feared.

We offer vignettes called "Those Who Survived" throughout the book to reassure and remind you that there is hope and that many people have survived their bleakest times and found renewed satisfaction in life. This element of the book—doses of encouragement—may remind you of some steps of prevention: Acknowledge the problem. Pay attention to mood. Challenge negative beliefs. Seek help and support. Take one more step, one more breath. Remember that others have made it through their darkest nights.

A Final Note

Our book is not intended to provide counseling or therapy but to give readers an overview of this important issue and some idea of the many causes and, more importantly, the many treatments and preventive strategies that have been devised.

Our book does not purport to cover the entire field of suicidology. What it represents is our personal quest to understand why some people want to kill themselves and why some of them do. We have paid special attention to three groups of people most vulnerable to suicide in the United States today—veterans and victims of assault and bullying—and we also highlight many other people who receive less public attention, such as children, teenagers, farmers, minorities, and people suffering from economic insecurity.

Please be aware that the presence of one factor or another does not necessarily mean that the person is suicidal. As we emphasize throughout the book, suicide is complicated, and no two cases are exactly alike. There are so many promising treatments being tested that we urge our readers to stay abreast of these encouraging advances.

When the Crisis Is Global: Coronavirus and PTSD

As we were completing this book, the world was struck by the coronavirus pandemic. This global upheaval triggered losses of life, livelihood, family, and treasure and induced prolonged stress, which can lead to post-traumatic stress disorder (PTSD). Health care workers are risking their lives to go to work. They are facing inexcusable shortages of equipment, caring for far more patients than normal, having to make wrenching decisions, and watching many patients die. They are the last face and voice many dying people will have known. Too many health care workers have sacrificed their lives. We salute them.

Health care workers face *moral injury* when forced to make life-and-death choices that violate their moral standards. They also face such questions as whether to stay home and protect their families or report to work, possibly carrying the infection from one place to the other.

People who had never before been regarded as heroes suddenly were seen in a new light: clerks and cashiers, trash collectors, letter carriers, and grocery store employees restocking shelves. With low pay and limited prospects, they are stressed and put at risk by crowds; some have died. We honor them as well and hope that, in the future, they receive the rewards they deserve.

Delayed, stumbling, and ill-informed responses from some public officials and others added to the uncertainty about this new plague. The capacity to *tolerate uncertainty in life* is an important marker of maturity. Even in ordinary life, people often make decisions without having all the information. They take risks without knowing the outcome, such as going on a first date with a stranger. An inability to tolerate uncertainty can lead some people to adopt dogmatic black-and-white thinking. As one of us (Riebel), says, "They'd rather be certain than right."

Those who have been spared and those who have recovered may experience *survivor's guilt*. Some spent days or weeks in a hospital, often seeing those around them die. The bereaved may be haunted by what-if questions: What if I hadn't insisted on going to that party? Why didn't I make peace with Mom before she fell ill? What if I hadn't believed the false reassurances that this was just "the flu" that would soon go away?

A new generation will have spent a significant portion of their childhood in extraordinary circumstances. Many children have been cooped up with anxious parents, only been allowed outside in strictly controlled conditions, been unable to meet friends in person or learn in a group setting, and were possibly exposed to adult desperation or domestic violence. These children have had to learn coping mechanisms with few role models to guide them. Their experiences could leave scars that only refugee children and those locked in internment camps know.

While it is too soon to know exactly what psychological consequences will linger, we offer some observations and suggestions. First, we want to reassure our readers that it is normal to have mental and emotional reactions to crises and that it is possible to manage them. The following coping mechanisms can help people through these troubled times and are especially valuable for those at risk for self-harm:

- Learn to tolerate uncertainty. (It is better than being certain but wrong.)
- Acknowledge your feelings and emotional reactions.
- Learn and use the many thinking and self-care skills we describe in this book.
- Share these coping skills with others.

Finally, try to remain open to facing the inevitable challenges of life, including the biggest trials of all: loss and death. Having faith in the larger picture is a humble recognition of our participation in something greater than ourselves, a stance of awe, humility, and wonder. The existential themes that run through this book are especially crucial for coping with the coronavirus pandemic and other emergencies that may arise in the future.

The Allure of Suicide

CHAPTER ONE

Who Is Attracted by the Allure of Suicide?

Carlton was very close to his mother, Cathy. Carlton, Cathy, and Gary, Carlton's father, lived in a beautiful home on Lake Michigan. Cathy had been an opioid addict ever since she was introduced to OxyContin during a minor operation. Carlton, seventeen, and Gary tried to get Cathy to stop using Oxy-Contin, but her supplier began to lace it with fentanyl, a powerful opioid that intensified her pleasure.

When Cathy died of an overdose, Carlton was bereft. He began to drink heavily. In a drunken state, he claimed to hear Cathy asking him to join her. Carlton's father urged him to seek professional help, but he refused. Instead, he walked into the lake, leaving a note that said he wanted to join his mother. To him, suicide was alluring.

Mildred lived in a suburb of San Francisco. Her friends knew that she was depressed, but they were not alarmed because she was on medication. Even her frequent walks across the Golden Gate Bridge seemed natural. After she jumped to her death, they felt guilty. "We should have known better. Those walks across the bridge gave us a clue." Like many others, succumbing to the mystique of the Golden Gate Bridge provided Mildred a dramatic way to end her life.

Why do some people kill themselves? What is the appeal that brings about this drastic act? Can the allure of suicide be prevented? In this book, we discuss the many triggers, at-risk groups, and means of prevention and healing that have been introduced to save lives. Carlton and Mildred were real people, known personally to one of us (Krippner), as are the others we have described in this chapter. However, their identities have been carefully disguised, and pseudonyms have replaced their real names.

In the late 1950s, one of us (Krippner) had a close friend and classmate, Finn, who delighted in telling him about his sexual exploits with good-looking men on the campus. However, these tales contained hints of self-hate. When Finn returned to school from summer vacation, he displayed photos of his fiancée and said that he was looking forward to being "a normal married man." Finn attended classes with confidence and stayed away from the bars and parks that had been the venues of his earlier sexual encounters. He was in good spirits when he left campus for the winter holidays.

Finn never returned. He drove his fancy red sports car into his garage, closed the doors and windows, and inhaled the noxious fumes coming through a tube he had inserted into his mouth. Apparently, Finn had been having a liaison with his fiancée's brother and had been caught in the act. Finn's suicide notes were filled with self-condemnation and apologies, telling his friends and family members that they should be glad he was out of their lives. But they were not. Friends and family members mourned Finn, saying, "If we had only known his feelings, we would have insisted that he receive help." Finn dreaded the thought that his straight arrow family and friends would hate him. After all, it was the 1950s, and even the brilliant gay computer inventor Alan Turing had killed himself. Finn thought death was the only escape from the terror of being found out and rejected.

Fred retired after serving as a highly regarded director of a celebrated museum. Now he finally had leisure time to enjoy his hobbies and his family. But his experiences from World War II came back to haunt him. Fred had joined the navy in 1942, lying about his age in order to enlist. He was sent to the Pacific, eager for action, which occurred all too soon. Japanese airplanes bombed and sank his small naval craft, and Fred was one of the few survivors. He could never forget the dead bodies and body parts floating in the water. He was so badly injured that it took him eight months to recover.

Fred spent his eighteenth birthday in a hospital bed. Every night, he took sedatives, but his sleep was interrupted by nightmares about the bombing and his dead buddies. He also felt terrible guilt. He asked himself, "Why did I survive? Others were worthier of living. They had families. They had careers. I'm just a teenager." Today, Fred's reactions would be called post-traumatic stress disorder (PTSD). Back then, it was written off as "battle fatigue," and precious little help was available.

Fred married and became a father and a workaholic. Family and work kept Fred from dwelling on his traumatic experiences. But once he retired, the nightmares returned with a vengeance. The pain was unbearable. Fred took his wartime service revolver and fired a bullet into his head. In a letter to his wife and children, Fred assured them that they were not at fault. He simply could not cope with the suffering, which had become a twenty-four-hour-a-day ordeal. For the people he left behind, the letter did not help. His family members asked each other why they had overlooked clues that would have prompted them to seek professional help for their beloved husband and father. Those who knew Fred believed "he had everything to live for." But they did not know what he was dying to escape.

For Carlton, Mildred, Finn, and Fred, the allure of suicide was greater than life itself.

Allure

We have used the term *allure* to describe those who find the idea of killing themselves compelling. Allure is tempting, enticing, even irresistible. For people in unbearable pain, suicide's allure can be all three.

We use the phrase *suicide-prone* to describe people who are suicidal or at risk for killing themselves. Unfortunately, there is no surefire way to make an accurate prediction. A 2019 survey covered seventy studies on suicidal thoughts and revealed that 60 percent of people who killed themselves had *not* expressed any thoughts about suicide when they were questioned beforehand. When interviewed by general practitioners, 80 percent of those who later tried to kill themselves did *not* express suicidal thoughts when asked. These studies were time-consuming because authors had to follow up with the interviewees to see how many eventually made suicide attempts. The authors concluded, "Our study suggests that suicidal ideation is not sensitive enough to be very helpful as a stand-alone screening test for suicide in psychiatric or non-psychiatric settings."[1] In other words, even asking people directly whether they are contemplating ending their lives is not a successful tactic.

In this book, we describe many people who are suicide-prone, especially three specific groups: people who have experienced war combat, sexual assault, or bullying. Many of the tragic stories we have known fall into one of these three groups. We have primarily focused on Western societies, especially the United States, which appears to be particularly susceptible to stressful and traumatic experiences.

War Combat

The term post-traumatic stress disorder (PTSD) first became well known following the U.S. defeat in Vietnam, which was often linked to the ensuing trauma and suicides of former soldiers. Surprisingly, psychiatric casualties occurred less often in Vietnam than in earlier U.S. wars. The rate of emotional breakdowns was twelve cases per one thousand soldiers, compared to thirty-seven per one thousand during the Korean conflict and at least twenty-eight per one thousand during World War II. An exact comparison is not possible because the studies used varying diagnostic criteria, but they still challenge the stereotype of the drug-addicted, suicidal, pathologically isolated Vietnam veteran that persists in many accounts of that tragic conflict.

Unlike Vietnam, where the draft provided a steady stream of soldiers, Operation Iraqi Freedom and Operation Enduring Freedom–Afghanistan have been fought by an all-volunteer army. Troops were deployed for tours of up to fifteen months at a time and were sometimes redeployed for longer periods. Imagine having to live with the daily stressors of roadside bombs, improvised explosive devices (IEDs), suicide bombers, handling human remains, killing civilians thought to be enemies, seeing fellow soldiers dead or injured, the sexual abuse of female soldiers (usually perpetrated by fellow servicemen), and the inability to end the violent situations resulting from ethnic and religious rivalries among the Iraqis and Afghans themselves.

Due to such combat stressors, these veterans were at a high risk for mental health disorders such as PTSD, depression, dissociation, and suicide-proneness. Since 2005, more soldiers and veterans have taken their own lives than those who were killed by enemy fire in those two intractable wars. In 2015, the suicide rate was 20.2 per 100,000 for active military members, 27.1 per 100,000 for the National Guard, and 24.7 per 100,000 for the reserves.[2]

Many veterans do not commit suicide until they return home from their tours of duty in Afghanistan or Iraq. Fred, the veteran of World War II whom we discussed earlier, is an example of this delayed reaction.

Sexual Assault

Sexual assault occurs when someone is exploited, violated, or abused in a manner directly related to sex. The gamut of sexual assault ranges from gang rape and torture to posting nude photos of someone on the internet without permission. The perpetrator of sexual assault can be a stranger, an acquaintance, or a family member. Dylan Farrow, in a highly publicized television interview, accused her father, Woody Allen, of sexual assault. When questioned about the vehemence of her accusation, she replied, "Why shouldn't I be angry? Why shouldn't I want to bring him down?"

The numerous cases of sexual assault by men of status and power have led to group protests, most notably the activist movement #MeToo, which was formed in 2006 by Tarana Burke, a survivor of sexual assault. The group's internet site erupted with millions of posts per month a dozen years later. Unfortunately, sexual assault is not new. Two decades earlier, the student of one of us (Krippner) had confided in him. When her family was invited to spend a weekend at the country estate of a well-known politician, Yolanda was delighted to have her own room with a large window through which she could see trees, wildflowers, and squirrels romping about. But in the middle of the night, her host entered the room, drew the curtain across the window, and forced himself on her.

He repeated the assault each night, warning her not to tell her parents or he would accuse her father of financial misconduct that would put him in jail. Yolanda tearfully recalled, "Who would believe me anyway? It would be the word of a twelve-year-old girl against a highly esteemed public figure. Also, I began to blame myself. Perhaps I had worn something that was provocative, a dress that was, in some way, seductive."

The incident was traumatic, and Yolanda entertained thoughts of suicide. She said, "I had lost my self-respect. Who would ever want me? I was lucky I did not get pregnant. If I had, I'm sure I would have killed myself." As a young adult, Yolanda entered psychotherapy, which helped her resolve the trauma.

Bullying

One of us (Krippner) went to church school with Phil, a farm boy like himself. Phil was not cut out for farming, and his father constantly ridiculed him for not "being a man" and helping with farm duties. He said, "Your sister is more of a man than you are." At school, Phil preferred to read science books and dreamed of discovering causes and cures of diseases. Phil did not attend sporting events and never dated, although he had several female friends, and he always volunteered to tutor younger children who were having trouble learning to read and write. Phil's male classmates bullied him, "accidentally" bumping into him on stairs or on the way to class, grabbing the cookies that his mother had put into his lunchbox, and throwing spitballs at him both in class and when he was heading home on the school bus. They called him a "sissy" and a "fag," though he had little idea what those terms meant.

Church school was a refuge for Phil. The pastor was very kind to Phil, who sought personal guidance from him and poured out his heart, saying, "I just can't take the bullying anymore." The pastor told Phil to pray and to ask God for strength. But it was too late. Shortly after a counseling session, Phil hanged himself. He was seventeen.

Bullying is aggressive behavior that involves a real or perceived power imbalance; the action is (or could be) repeated, producing anxiety on the part of the person being bullied. It may occur verbally or physically and in a variety of settings—the schoolyard, the classroom, in public places, and on the internet, where Facebook and other social networks often become the sites for hostile comments. Bullying also takes place in academic settings, such as primary and secondary schools and college. Bullying can occur in places of employment, where a person who has taken an unpopular stand may be shunned. In relationships, it may present as endless put-downs in public, contempt during private conversations, or domestic violence.

Many parents downplay reports that their sons and daughters have bullied classmates, saying, "They're just being kids." Parents of the students being bullied may tell their children, "Just ignore them," "You have to develop a thick skin," or "Why don't you fight back?" None of this well-meaning advice would have saved Phil. He was so sensitive that he could not ignore the taunts or fight back, much less develop a thick skin. What gifts might he have brought to the world if he had lived?

Misconceptions

Some readers of this book may assume that suicide springs from sadness. But sad people can be consoled, and sadness generally passes. By contrast, it is difficult for a family member or friend to console a person who is suicidal. The allure is too great. Other readers may assume that "positive thinking" will suffice. However, using a cliché such as "Look on the bright side of life" can backfire. The suicidal person may discover that there is no bright side and feel even worse for failing to benefit from the advice.

Other readers may assume that if someone is reporting for work, functioning well at social gatherings, and paying the bills, there will be no time or need for suicidal thoughts. After all, Fred (whom we discussed earlier) had a successful family and professional life. But every suicide is different. Anthony Bourdain, a celebrity chef and travel show host, was filming an episode in France when he hanged himself.

Bourdain's suicide undermines another assumption, that suicide follows a sudden trauma. Traumatizing experiences can predispose some people to suicide, but others may be temperamentally vulnerable to mood swings. Still others are motivated by an incurable illness, a desire for revenge, religious fanaticism, or a personal myth that dictates that they must end their lives.

Each suicide is unique. Bourdain's son attributed his father's death to a "broken heart." Bourdain's successes were no match for his troubled relationship with his paramour of many years. A close inspection of Bourdain's life yields earlier predisposing elements, including substance abuse. His coworkers recalled the dark moods that marked his final days. The romantic rebuff may have been the proverbial last straw.

Another puzzling celebrity suicide was reported in 2019. Alan Krueger, the chair of the White House Council of Economic Advisors, had completed his sixth book. The only forewarning was Krueger's abrupt halt to his tweets, which he had posted almost daily until two months before he took his life. So even the greatest successes in life do not guarantee that a person will overcome hidden despair.

We suspect that studying suicide's allure—and discovering what type of allure best describes the one appealing to a loved one at risk—may be more productive in identifying and securing the help needed. We invite the readers of this book to join us on this search.

Takeaway Points

At the end of each chapter, we will present a few takeaway points to assist readers in making maximum use of the material.

- "Suicide-prone" people are at risk for killing themselves.
- Suicidal people may be sad, but sadness alone rarely triggers suicide.
- The allure of suicide is especially powerful in at-risk groups of people: those who have experienced war combat, sexual assault, or bullying.

Notes

1. McHugh, C. M., Corderoy, A., Ryan, C. J., et al. (2019, March 4). Association between suicidal ideation and suicide: Meta-analysis of odds ratios, sensitivity, specificity and positive predictive value. *British Journal of Psychiatry, 5*(2), 1–12.

2. Center for Deployment Psychology. (n.d.). "Suicide in the Military." https://deploymentpsych.org/disorders/suicide-main.

CHAPTER TWO

Suicide Is Complicated

Around the world, some three thousand people take their lives each day—one death every forty seconds. Suicide is the tenth-leading cause of death in the United States. Since the beginning of the century, there has been a 50 percent rise in suicides among American females and a 21 percent increase among males. Although this book mostly focuses on three vulnerable groups (combat veterans, sexual assault victims, and the bullied), there are other groups at risk, including lonely senior citizens, people who are destitute and homeless, and people with chronic diseases. We will touch on these groups later.

Five Levels of Suicide

After surveying many books and articles on the topic, Canadian psychologist William Tillier concluded that "suicide is complicated."[1] Tillier rediscovered the work of Kazimierz Dabrowski, a Polish psychologist, who had uncanny insights into suicide. He was one of the experts who reported the link between suicide attempts and overexcitability (also called "emotional sensitivity"). This trait is difficult to measure, yet, according to Dabrowski, it is the overriding characteristic of those who tried to kill themselves or who brought the act to completion.

Dabrowski found several levels in the thinking and feeling patterns of suicidal people. At the lowest (first) level, suicide is a desperate attempt to escape from a difficult situation. Combat veterans with PTSD constantly find themselves in difficult situations, those in which guilt, shame, and fear often overwhelm them. Many survivors of sexual assault experience guilt, wondering whether they were somehow responsible for the assault or are now considered damaged. They may live in fear, afraid that they will be assaulted again by the same person or by someone else. Bullied persons have similar reactions, especially if the bullying is constant or comes from people they cannot avoid, such as schoolmates. They frequently live in a constant state of guilt, shame, fear, or all three.

At the second level of Dabrowski's spectrum, the emotions that suicidal people experience are chaotic, often propelling them into destructive behavior. Alcohol- and drug-related suicides are common at this level. Many of the combat veterans we interviewed tried to dull their anxiety and depression with alcohol. When that escape no longer worked, some of them could not resist suicide's allure.

Dabrowski's third level is existential and spiritual in nature. People considering suicide seem stuck in loneliness and despair, unable to contact their "higher selves." They may have a transcendent glimpse of humanity as a whole but only identify with its universal suffering, not its spirit of resilience. At the fourth level, they start to take an active role, imagining how to end their life. At the fifth level, hoping their pain will end with self-destruction, they make the *suicide attempt*.

Rarely, suicide at the fifth level may be an attempt to reach transcendental worlds. The Heaven's Gate adherents who killed themselves in the 1990s were convinced that aliens from outer space would carry them into another dimension. Some Muslim suicide bombers had been beguiled with promises of a paradise where they would be welcomed by lovely virgins.

Existence Matters

There are four modes of death: natural, accidental, suicide, and homicide. These categories may overlap. A person's suicidal impulses may contribute to a natural, accidental, or homicidal death through disregarding medical advice, living dangerously, carelessness, or unconscious suicidal behaviors, such as a drug overdose or traffic accident.

We will be using the word *existential* quite often in this book. An experience can be described as existential if it involves searching for meaning or purpose, asking fundamental questions about life, and taking responsibility for one's actions. Whether they know it or not, people constantly search for meaning.[2]

Existential psychotherapy tries to address the entire person, not just the person's behavior, feelings, and thoughts. It attends to subjective experience and attempts to find meaning in life. There are many research studies demonstrating that meaning in life tends to nurture people, improving longevity and relieving depression and PTSD.

People who manifest meaning feel that their lives make sense, that their existence matters to others, and that they have meaningful life goals. But suicide-prone people say that their life makes no sense, that nobody cares if they live or die, and that their only goal is to kill themselves. Existential psychotherapists attempt to evoke change at a deep level, not just relieve symptoms, and they are committed to helping clients find a sense of adventure and even awe in their daily existence.

Yolanda was fortunate to find a psychotherapist who focused on existential issues, identifying deep-seated ideas that had blocked her ability to integrate a traumatic experience and move past it. Having lost her self-respect, Yolanda was harboring such irrational beliefs as "Nobody will want me," "Maybe I was to blame," "I have no power." When each of these was brought to her awareness and discussed with her therapist, she began to see how unrealistic they were. What existential psychotherapists call the "willingness to live" finally returned.

The case of Ellen West is a well-known example of self-demise.[3] Ellen, a patient of Ludwig Binswanger, a pioneer in existential psychotherapy, was described by him as a "rebellious child" and a "passionate student," both examples of the emotional excitability so often linked with suicide. Ellen had an eating disorder; she loved food, but she feared getting fat, creating an intolerable situation (Level One). This conflict became the predominant focus of her life, as she continually tried to cope with a chaotic condition (Level Two). She also engaged in risky behaviors, such as dangerous horseback riding. Over the years, this condition morphed into an identification with the food she was eating (Level Three). Rather than destroy the food, she resolved to destroy herself, initiating several attempts at self-destruction (Level Four). Ellen West refused to eat, hoping to die from starvation. She stood outside naked and kissed children who had scarlet fever in an attempt to catch a fatal disease (Level Five). When these efforts failed, Ellen West took a lethal dose of poison (Level Six).

Binswanger admitted that he had been unable to dissuade his client from taking action on her obsession. It was an allure too great for even a skilled psychiatrist to counteract. Fortunately, most contemporary psychotherapists are less patriarchal than Binswanger. Ellen West's childhood behavior could have been an attempt to become assertive and establish her own identity; her adult rebelliousness and passion did not fit the stereotype of submissive female behavior expected in that time and place.

Misunderstandings

Many people view suicide attempts as initiatives to attract attention or manipulate others. This may be true in some instances. But even if a suicide attempt fails, there is usually an underlying desire to succumb to suicide's allure; attempters are not playacting, and dismissing the seriousness of signs of suicidality can be fatal. Ellen West's destructive behaviors, such as not following safety regulations while riding horseback, were not seen as suicidal by her husband or friends.

Another misunderstanding is that achievement and success dissuade people from suicide. We have already mentioned Anthony Bourdain, whose eminence as a writer, television star, and master chef did not deter him from taking his life. We also discussed Finn and Fred, one a successful teacher and the other a successful museum director. From the outside, they seemed to have "everything to live for," but people making those judgments did not have access to the inner worlds of tortured feelings and obsessive thoughts that led to their demise.

There are simplistic explanations of suicide that do not stand up under scrutiny. "Her work on Earth was done." "God called him home." "He was selfish and disregarded the welfare of his family." "She was possessed by an evil spirit." These convenient answers bypass suicide's complexity.

Another misunderstanding is that suicide is rare, so rare that many courses in mental health ignore it or treat it superficially. This is a gross error. In Canada, suicide is exceeded only by automobile accidents as a cause of death for people under the age of twenty-four. In the United States, more people die by suicide than from automobile accidents.

In addition, there is often a facile assumption that adolescents and children do not kill themselves. However, depression, loneliness, and sadness are increasingly common among young people, even in the days of Facebook and iPhones, which would seem to facilitate personal contact. But these technologies also facilitate bullying and sexual exploitation, which can contribute to the allure of death. The suicide rate for adolescents was much higher in the early part of the twenty-first century than it was in the latter part of the 1990s, especially for girls.

A final misunderstanding is the effectiveness of a single act of intervention. Some people take pride in aborting a suicide attempt by taking away a weapon found in a teenager's room, visiting a senior citizen who has complained of isolation and loneliness, or finding and destroying a lethal amount of medication in the cupboard of one's spouse. These are admirable actions, but they are not enough. As we will see, consistent, prolonged, and multifaceted help is required.

Trauma and Suicide

Survivors of PTSD usually move from predisposing conditions, to activating conditions, to maintaining conditions. Childhood trauma, such as bullying, may predispose a child to succumb to a later traumatizing event (such as combat stress) and the maintaining condition (PTSD). Even if the predisposing condition does not trigger thoughts of suicide, the activating and maintaining conditions may do so. We do not use the term *traumatic event* because no event (such as an earthquake) is traumatic to everyone who goes through it. Instead, we speak of *traumatizing events* and the resulting *traumatic experience.* We know of many people who have survived potentially trauma-tizing events, ranging from tsunamis to rape, without being traumatized. Other people are traumatized by what outsiders might see as minor events—belittling by a family member, receiving a low grade on a school examination, or being temporarily trapped in a malfunctioning elevator. Til-lier put it well: "It is the individual experiencing the trauma who defines its impact and, consequently, the intervention needed."

Childhood traumatic experiences may be linked with later suicidal attempts, suicides, and self-harming behavior, such as substance abuse, cut-ting, and other forms of self-injury. Self-harm is usually a dysfunctional attempt to regulate emotional excitability. When asked about his or her muti-lation, a cutter often responds, "Nothing else can relieve the tension."

Dabrowski observed that there is an interaction between one's age and the impact of the trauma. An adult might be surprised at how frightened a child is when watching a ghost story on television or hearing about the death of someone's pet. One of us (Krippner) had a personal experience of this nature:

> In 1942, my parents took me to see *Billy the Kid,* a Robert Taylor movie that romanticized the notorious outlaw's life and death. When Billy was shot and died, I broke into tears. My reaction was not traumatic, but, at the time, it seemed profound. My parents, of course, did not share my reac-tion, and consoled me. They said that Billy was only pretending to be dead. They were referring to Taylor's performance, and this consoled me. It was an important lesson in separating appearance from reality, a distinction that is a sign of maturity.

These parents had the wisdom to take the boy's terror seriously and to deal with it.

A specific event may be inconsequential to a person who is at Level One but a major trauma to a person at Level Three, or vice versa. There is consid-erable ambivalence at each of these levels; sometimes it is resolved early enough to keep someone from progressing to Level Five, the suicide attempt. Family and friends need to take every suicide attempt seriously. A poorly planned suicide attempt may be a genuine call for help, not merely an attention-getting ploy. At the earlier levels, a suicidal person wants to die but also wants to live. Family, friends, and therapists all need to provide hope and manifest caring to blunt suicide's allure.

In summary, suicide is complicated. There are no reliable markers for sui-cide and no dependable ways of predicting it. Overexcitability and emotional sensitivity are loose descriptions; even so, these traits may result from trauma, predispose one to trauma, or both. As we will later see, it may even protect against suicide. Norman Faberow, the cofounder of the Los Angeles Suicide Prevention Center, stated that each person becomes suicidal in his or her own framework.[4] Leo Tolstoy began his classic novel *Anna Karenina* with the phrase, "All happy families are alike; each unhappy family is unhappy in its own way." We might suggest that the latter statement also applies to suicide, recalling that, at the end of Tolstoy's novel, Anna threw herself in front of a train.

Takeaway Points

- People constantly search for the meaning or purpose of their existence.
- There is no dependable marker for suicide, but childhood trauma is one commonality.
- Suicides can be glimpsed through the lens of levels, but no two suicides are the same.

Notes

1. Tillier, W. (2018). *Personality development through positive disintegration: The work of Kazimierz Dabrowski*. Ana Maria, FL: Maurice Bassett.

2. Schneider, K., & Krug, O. (2017). *Existential-humanistic therapy*. Washington, DC: American Psychological Association.

3. Binswanger, L. (1958). The case of Ellen West. In R. May, E. Angel, & H. F. Ellenberger (Eds.), *Existence: A new dimension in psychiatry and psychology* (pp. 237–364). New York: Basic Books.

4. Faberow, N. L. (2005). The mental health professional as suicide survivor. *Clinical Neuropsychiatry, 2*, 13–20.

CHAPTER THREE

The Pioneer of Suicidology and What He Found

Émile Durkheim was born in France in 1858. His sociological text *Suicide* (1897)[1] was the first book to explore self-inflicted death in depth. Many of his insights are still relevant in the twenty-first century.

Durkheim argued that suicide was related not only to individual psychological factors but also to social factors such as financial, marital, and religious pressures. He emphasized *social integration*—the degree to which people feel that they belong to a group of other people, that life has meaning, and that they are a meaningful part of society. Durkheim proposed that those who feel connected to society are less likely to commit suicide.

Durkheim found that suicide rates were lower among women than men (at least in his study), that single people had a higher suicide rate than those in romantic partnerships, that parents had a lower rate of suicide than those without children, and that soldiers had a higher rate of suicide than civilians. He found four types of suicide that reflect an imbalance of two social forces: social integration and moral regulation:

1. *Anomic suicide:* Anomic suicide (from the word *anomie*, a lack of purpose, identity, or ethical values) reflects a feeling of not belonging, which is more likely to occur during the periods of intense stress and frustration that follow social, economic, or political turmoil, when changes in daily life can be rapid and extreme.

2. *Altruistic suicide:* Excessive social integration can influence some individuals to martyr themselves for the sake of a cause, group, or belief, such as the Japanese kamikaze pilots of World War II or suicide bombers in Iraq and Afghanistan.

3. *Egoistic suicide:* Like anomic suicide, egoistic suicide is the result of too little social integration and is often associated with a major personal life change, such as retirement, divorce, or a substantial loss. Elderly people who lose their personal emotional ties are the most susceptible to egoistic suicide.

4. *Fatalistic suicide:* Fatalistic suicide, like altruistic suicide, can occur under conditions of extreme social regulation or oppression, such as those suffered by slaves, jailed convicts, and prisoners of war.

The highly publicized death of Private Aaron Mitchell in 2019 serves as a tragic example of Durkheim's first type of suicide, anomic suicide. Private Mitchell was stationed in South Korea when he was informed that his husband, Rich Rosa, had killed himself in their Nebraska home. Mitchell returned for the funeral and shot himself the following day. The parents of the young couple requested donations for veterans' organizations and suicide prevention programs. Rosa's father told the *Army Times* newspaper, "We are without words to express how much we're grieving and how much grief we feel." Mitchell's commanding officer added, "His death affects every member of our formation."[2] While these mourning reactions reflect an encouraging acceptance of gay marriage, the loss of these two lives is tragic.

An infamous group altruistic suicide occurred in 1973. Jim Jones had established a "spiritual community" in South America. The People's Temple had enticed hundreds of mainly poor people from the United States to establish a community that would practice "apostolic socialism." When the venture went sour, Jim Jones called for an act of "revolutionary suicide." Some nine hundred people, one-third of them children, died.[3]

Not so well known is the suicide of Matome Ugaki in 1945. A Japanese fighter pilot, Ugaki was devastated when he heard about Japan's imminent surrender. He donned his uniform and climbed into his airplane, determined to be the last kamikaze pilot. American pilots gunned him down as soon as they calculated his trajectory, but he still died by suicide.[4]

The death of Fred, described in our first chapter, may have been an egoistic suicide. His retirement was a personal life change in which he lost his real social support group—the museum staff. In many ways, he was closer to them than he was to his family members, especially as his children became adults and moved away. Fred's home was so distant from the museum that he could not interact with his former staff often. The loss of these emotional ties and the aging process weakened his defenses against the emotional onslaught of traumatic wartime memories.

Egoistic suicide may also occur after a career reverses. The famed psychologist E. B. Boring wrote that "a theory which has built up the author's image of himself has become part of him. To abandon it would be suicidal or at least an act of self-mutilation." The *American Bar Association Journal* reported the suicide of a lawyer who had just lost a trial for the Bank of America, one of his major clients. At the same time, the North Carolina office that he had helped open was experiencing a decline. Both disappointments enhanced suicide's allure as his only option.[5]

Fatalistic suicide is the fourth of Durkheim's categories. We would apply this category to include those suffering from an incurable disease. Beloved award-winning actor Robin Williams took his life in 2014; family members attributed it to his depression over learning he had Lewy body dementia, an incurable degenerative brain disorder similar to Parkinson's disease. In 1961, Nobel Prize laureate Ernest Hemingway shot himself, a death attributed to deteriorating physical and mental health.

If the category were expanded to include despondency over drug addiction, we would include Jay. Raised in a show business family, Jay was a bright, good-looking young man who was the life of every party he attended. His ebullience hid his ongoing depression, and he refused the offer of treatment that his mother had presented numerous times. A single mother, she kept telling Jay how sorry she was that she often left him alone as a child due to her work. He was able to elevate his mood temporarily with heroin, which he obtained from a dealer in his neighborhood. Jay's bravado hid feelings of estrangement, and the drugs temporarily dulled the pain.

When Jay could not make payments, his dealer offered him a position as a pusher. Jay delivered drugs to local customers, some of them celebrities, while descending deeper and deeper into addiction. He confided in his sister, saying, "Don't be surprised if I kill myself someday. I am sick and tired of being a junkie." She did not take this prediction seriously, but one day she entered his room and found his inert body, which was riddled with needle marks. An autopsy detected traces of a half dozen illicit drugs in his system. Was this an unintended overdose or had he fulfilled his suicide prediction? We may never know.

The Fifth Category: Moral Injury

We propose an additional category. *Moral injury* occurs when people's experiences violate their deepest values. This is an existential crisis that threatens the meaning of one's very existence. It can occur in military service when an inept commander gives an order that would destroy civilians and their livelihood, when a newly appointed police officer discovers corruption in the department, or when an industrial worker learns that a company ignores safety standards to make more money. Moral injury often accompanies PTSD and can lead to suicide, as when a soldier who entered the military with high ideals encounters incompetent or corrupt leadership or who complied with an unjust order and suffers from subsequent guilt.[6]

Moral injury can even be found among pilots of unmanned aerial vehicles. They know their decisions cost lives. A few may imagine the infirm elderly victims and the helpless children whom they have sent to their deaths. Their risk may be as great as that of the ground soldiers who directly see, hear, and smell the results of their actions.[7]

Award-winning author, filmmaker, and social critic Michael Moore claims to have received thousands of letters from service members stationed in Afghanistan and Iraq.[8] Many of them are eloquent examples of moral injury, of shattered ideals and unmet expectations. One officer wrote, "I felt betrayed and used. As an officer, I am not supposed to show these feelings in front of the soldiers. We are supposed to put on a good face and ensure that the men and women we give orders to never lose sight of the mission and the risk at hand. The thing was, I didn't know what the mission was any more." A member of the U.S. Air Force wrote, "I'm ashamed of what I do. In past generations, serving in the military was always considered an honorable sacrifice. Many brave men and women have died for the idea of America. . . . What happened to this country? In a breath, we have come apart at the seams."

An infantryman serving in Southeast Baghdad wrote, "I am embarrassed to be a part of it. . . . It's just so ridiculous. . . . A Blackwater contractor makes $15,000 a month for doing the same job as my pals and me. I make about $4,000 a month over here. What's up with that?" A rifleman wrote from Iraq, "I have a choice to make and that choice becomes more clear every time a soldier dies to line the pockets of rich men who will never lose sleep over the blood they've spilled."

A veteran wrote Moore to thank him for making the movie *Fahrenheit 9/11* because it compelled him to become

> a more compassionate person and for showing me that everything is not as it seems. I have shared my views with a lot of fellow coworkers, and the response has ranged from very harsh to very accepting. . . . I was called into my platoon sergeant's office after the rest of the platoon provoked me into an argument about politics, and I was told that I was not allowed to give my views anymore because we have "young impressionable soldiers who can't hear those things because it lowers morale."

The U.S. Army has developed special units, such as Rangers and Special Forces, that have high standards for membership. They experience less than half the amount of PTSD than regular combat units, despite having more frequent and more intense engagements with enemy forces. These units have clearly defined goals and missions; their leaders are officers of high character who have been well trained. This combination of expertise and high standards provides some protection against postcombat stress.

In 2019, documents obtained through the Freedom of Information Act (FOIA) and other sources were published showing that presidents and leaders of the wars in Afghanistan and Iraq knew that these wars were failing, but they kept sending soldiers into combat and civilians to their deaths. In light of this appalling revelation, which resembles belated revelations about Vietnam, we fear that moral injury and disillusion with their leaders may make suicide more alluring than ever to soldiers who were manipulated with false promises. Vigilance is required![9]

Takeaway Points

- Human beings need to be part of a social group. They also need a moral code to guide their behavior. An imbalance in either is often associated with self-destructive acts.

- Moral injury, especially in times of war, can put people at risk for suicide.

- We must be vigilant on behalf of service members and veterans of recent wars.

Notes

1. Durkheim, E. (1951). *Suicide: A study in sociology.* Glencoe, IL: Free Press. (Original work published in French, 1897)

2. Myers, M. (2019, February 14). Following his husband's suicide, a soldier took his own life while waiting for the funeral. *Army Times* (online).

3. Fundakowski, L. (2013). *Jonestown stories.* Minneapolis: University of Minnesota Press.

4. Hoyt, E. (1993). *The last kamikaze: The story of Matome Ugaki.* Westport, CT: Praeger.

5. Weiss, D. C. (2009, May 11). Disappointments preceded suicide by lawyers at three major law firms. *American Bar Association Journal* (online).

6. Meagher, R., & Pyrer, D. A. (Eds.). (2018). *War and moral injury: A reader.* Eugene, OR: Cascade Books.

7. Matthews, M. D. (2014). Stress among UAV operators: Posttraumatic stress disorder, existential crisis, or moral injury? *Ethics and Armed Forces: Controversies in Military Ethics and Security Policy, 1,* 53–57.

8. Moore, M. (2004). *Will they ever trust us again? Letters from the war zone.* New York: Simon & Schuster.

9. Ellsberg, D. (2017). *The doomsday machine: Confessions of a nuclear war planner.* New York: Bloomsbury.

CHAPTER FOUR

Suicide among Minorities

Choosing death among ethnic groups and other minorities in the United States has not received adequate attention. In this chapter, we attempt to remedy that situation by focusing on suicide among African Americans, Native Americans, Hispanics, Asian Americans, and members of sexual minorities.

Historical Roots of Suicide among African Americans

Most African Americans are descendants of slaves who were brought to North America against their will and deprived of their personal freedom, their communities, their cultures, and their languages. In African civilizations, suicide was rare, but when it did happen, it was most frequently reported as a sign of resistance to Eurasian invasion and domination. The Yoruba culture of West Africa deemed suicide acceptable if done in defense of the community. Centuries later, during the Haitian revolution against France, an entire village jumped off a cliff rather than become enslaved.[1]

In contrast, enslaved Africans and their descendants were characterized by whites as having a cheerful demeanor and a low suicide rate. However, the stereotype was not accurate. On the Middle Passage, the horrific ocean voyage imposed on captured Africans for almost three centuries, some jumped overboard to their deaths. Depression was evident within black communities and could be glimpsed by outsiders in "blues" music. In the early 1900s, a black man, Ota Benga, was displayed at the St. Louis World's Fair and in the Bronx Zoo in the same cage as an orangutan. Harlem residents rescued Benga, and he went to live in Virginia with an African American family. But the damage had been done. Profoundly depressed, he took his own life in 1916.[2]

The stresses of acculturation had been present for centuries, but black communities and institutions such as churches acted as buffers. People of mixed ancestry often found themselves conflicted because of culture clashes. Even today, mixed-ancestry youth are more vulnerable than nonmulticultural African Americans to factors and behaviors that contribute to suicide. The rate of suicide among African Americans has rapidly increased since 1980, especially among black males between fifteen and nineteen years of age; the increase from 1960 to 2000 was 234 percent.[3]

Wright's Sociopolitical Model

Bobby Wright, a scholar and activist, argues that African Americans who take their own lives are victims of white supremacy. His social-political model targets structural factors in U.S. culture as bringing about massive depression and all-too-frequent suicidal behavior by African Americans. Wright's model acknowledges the presence of other factors, but he sees them as adding to the existing difficulty of black people's lives. He points out that suicidologists often discuss "own-life taking" as if it occurs in a vacuum. Wright's model posits "faulty, dysfunctional psychological adaptation"; factors of religiosity, African identity, socioeconomic status, stressful life events, and perceived "burdensomeness"; and thwarted "becomingness." Hence, the model holds that the structure of U.S. society is a key factor in the etiology of black suicides.[4]

To ignore the antiblack nature of the predominant U.S. society and its institutions is to deny reality. Wright's model argues for recognition that

- suicided and suicidal attempts by African Americans are qualitatively different from the same behavior by Euro-Americans;
- subsuming explanations of African American self-harm under Euro-American models is an example of the prevailing antiblack racism of U.S. institutions; and
- African American women are especially vulnerable to self-harm because of the additional burden of sexism in the dominant society and its institutions.

In 2009, the U.S. National Institute for Mental Health reported that "at some point before they reach 17 years of age, 4% of black teens, and more than 7% of black teen females, will attempt suicide."[5] One study found that among children under thirteen, the suicide rate was twice as high for black children than for white children.[6]

Daudi Ajani ya Azibo, an author and social critic, has listed structural realities that contribute to "own-life taking" behaviors of African Americans: a higher rate of deaths from "legal intervention" (such as police action), reduced longevity, a high rate of unemployment for males, and lower enrollment for health insurance, despite eligibility. This is why Wright claimed that "lynching by any other name is still lynching."[7]

Suicide among Native Americans

Native American lands were invaded and settled by Europeans. They, too, were deprived of their culture, and their communities were devastated by diseases and the new religions and laws that were forced upon them. In the twentieth century, Native Americans and Alaskan Natives had the highest rate of suicide of any U.S. ethnic group, and the rate has been rising since 2003. Approximately 36 percent of the deceased were between the ages of ten and twenty-four; in comparison, about 11 percent of Euro-Americans of that age killed themselves.[8]

A 2013 study found that, when compared to Euro-American suicides, Native Americans and Native Alaskan suicides were more likely to be associated with high alcohol intake, the death of a loved one by suicide, and a violent argument with an intimate partner. Depressed mood was significantly higher than among Euro-Americans, as was opioid use.[9]

Native Americans and Alaskan Natives are more likely to live in the countryside, where there is less access to mental health facilities. Furthermore, they are less likely to consider seeking out a social worker, psychologist, psychiatrist, or other clinician because seeking help from a mental health practitioner attracts considerable stigma among these groups.[10]

Before the European invasion, shamans and medicine people were available, but their number and influence have greatly declined. In addition, training in these roles can be laborious, sometimes lasting for a dozen years, a situation that may discourage new practitioners.[11] Tribal identity probably serves as a buffer in some cases, but can it also lead to "suicide contagion," as reflected in the frequent occurrence of suicides and suicide attempts by friends or family members following a completed suicide? There is no persuasive evidence to support the notion of "suicide contagion," but there are incidents of "copycat suicides," in which the suicide of a well-known person triggers a cluster of deaths, typically in the same manner as the original. In Goethe's celebrated novel *The Sorrows of Young Werther*, the central character shot himself after the woman he loved married someone else. Young men throughout Germany began to dress like Werther, and some shot themselves, leading to a ban of the book in several German cities.

Suicides among Hispanics

As a group, Hispanics (Latinos and Latinas) face many obstacles that can affect their health and well-being. They earn less than non-Hispanic whites and are more likely to lack health insurance coverage, hampering their access to mental health facilities. However, the practice of *colectivismo*—building a network of relationships through extended family members, friends, and fellow workers—helps to provide emotional safety nets. Church activities and social dancing are part of *colectivismo* as well.[12] According to the Centers for Disease Control and Prevention (CDC), about the same number of Hispanics attempt suicide as non-Hispanics, but a smaller percentage actually die.[13]

Hispanics have the highest rates of hopelessness and fatalism of all U.S. ethnic groups. Even though they may be depressed and socially withdrawn, their family and church ties serve as buffers.[14] Hispanic high school students report higher rates of self-harming behaviors than the general U.S. population of high school students. However, young people who are closely connected to their families or their teachers and who have moral objections to suicide are less likely to try to kill themselves.

Hispanics (U.S. governmental agencies' preferred term) are a multifaceted population from several countries, not a single monolithic group. Not all their family or community relationships are positive or healthy, but the longer an immigrant family stays in the United States, the more likely it is for a family member to harbor thoughts of suicide or to make an attempt. Hispanics born in the United States have higher rates of thoughts about suicide than Hispanic immigrants.[15] Apparently *colectivismo* weakens over the years if its ties are not reinforced.

Suicide among Asian Americans

Suicide is the eighth-leading cause of death for Asian Americans and the second-leading cause of death for those ages fifteen to thirty-four, similar to the same age range in the general U.S. population. Among all U.S. females between the ages of sixty-five and eighty-four, Asian Americans have the highest suicide rate of any ethnic group. Asian American college students are more likely than Euro-American college students to have suicidal thoughts and to have attempted to kill themselves. However, they are one-third as likely to seek help from a mental health practitoner.[16]

Suicides of Asian American students at prominent East Coast universities have attracted national attention, especially that of Luke Tang at Harvard University in 2015. After a failed attempt to take his life during his freshman year, Tang returned to the campus with the proviso that he receive mental health counseling. Tang's treatment was interrupted by a weeklong trip to China. He did not resume treatment on his return in August and killed himself in September. His grief-stricken parents established a foundation in his honor, and in 2018, his father filed a lawsuit against four Harvard officials for their "negligence and carelessness."

His death triggered a documentary and a Harvard-sponsored conference on Asian American mental health issues. George Qiao, the writer who helped organize the conference, disputed the racial stereotype:

> The story goes that Asian parents raise their children ignorant of the stress these expectations cause. Immigrant narratives overwhelm students with

the impossible demand of a return on interest. Asian kids are stretched so thin that only a lucky few don't suffer some kind of breakdown by the end of high school.[17]

Suicide among Sexual Minorities

Individuals who do not fit into the binary "straight male–straight female" categories have suffered terrible persecution, both personal and official, from Western societies that demand simple gender categories. The British designer Alexander McQueen took his own life, and some scholars believe that the great Russian composer Pyotr Tchaikovsky was coerced into doing the same. Besides their personal anguish, these deaths represent major losses to fashion and music.

Despite encouraging progress in recent decades toward tolerance for gender variants, prejudice and oppression continue in some places and for some people. Some religions, families, schools, and geographical regions remain forbidden or unwelcoming to them. Young people whose parents or social group reject them for their sexual orientation are often suicide-prone. The initialism LGBT (lesbian, gay, bisexual, transgender) often adds a "Q," for "questioning," because some young people do not know where they "fit." Those who find a support group, even one that is solely online, are less suicide-prone than those who feel completely isolated.[18]

Perhaps the most persecuted sexual minority comprises "trans" persons—those who fully identify with the gender *different* from the one they were assigned at birth. (We do not say "opposite" because we believe there is a continuum of sexual identities and behaviors, with no clear "opposite.") A depressing number of these people are murdered each year for their orientation, and others die by their own hands to escape the painful oppression. Young people who consider themselves "trans" are in desperate need of expert counseling; their nervous system is not fully mature, and they may latch onto the "trans" label to justify same-sex attraction and begin hormone treatment and irreversible surgery, when the solution may be more nuanced. One study discovered that postsurgery male-to-female transgendered people were twenty times more likely to kill themselves than others of the same background.[19] Some transgendered individuals have posted videos on You-Tube that warn young people not to rush into gender reassignment.

Conclusion

This brings us back to Wright's social-political model of ethnic suicide. History casts a long shadow. African Americans, Native Americans, Hispanics, and Asian Americans have all been targeted by the dominant Euro-American culture, each in its own way. Some progress has been made, but a residue lingers. Just as the children (and even grandchildren) of Holocaust survivors have exhibited aftereffects of the traumatizing experiences of their parents, the descendants of persecuted ethnic and racial minorities may continue to struggle. The social-political model calls for mental health programs that are not staffed exclusively by white people, who represent, even unconsciously, the values of the dominant and historically oppressive culture.

Takeaway Points

- Ethnic and sexual minorities often face structural and systematic oppression by the dominant culture.
- To be effective for minorities, suicide prevention and treatment need to question the values of the dominant culture, especially its oppressive features.

Notes

1. Jackson, J. (1990). Suicide trends of blacks and whites by sex and age. In D. Ruiz (Ed.), *Handbook of mental health and mental disorders* (pp. 95–110). Westport, CT: Greenwood.

2. Breggin, P., & Breggin, G. (1998). *The war against children of color: Psychiatry targets inner city youth.* Monroe, ME: Common Courage Press.

3. Roberts, R., Chen. Y., & Roberts, C. (1997). Ethnocultural differences in prevalence of adolescent suicide behaviors. *Suicide and Life-Threatening Behavior, 27*, 208–217.

4. Wright, B. (1981). Black suicide: (Lynching by any other name is still lynching), *Black Books Bulletin, 7*, 15–19.

5. National Institute for Mental Health. (2009). *Black teens, especially girls, at high risk for suicide attempts.* https://netdoc.com/black-teens-especially-girls-at -high-risk-for-suicide-attempts/.

6. Bridges, J. A., Horowitz, L. M., Fontanella, C. A., Sheftall, A. H., Greenhouse, J., Kelleher, K. J., & Campo, J. V. (2018). Age-related racial disparity in suicide rates among US youths from 2001 through 2015. *JAMA Pediatrics, 172*(7), 697–699.

7. Ajani ya Azibo, D. (2017). Suicide? (Re)introducing the Bobby Wright social-political model of African-U.S. own-life taking or African high-tech lynching. *Humanity & Society, 41*, 107–126.

8. Suicide Prevention Research Center. (2013). *Suicide among racial/ethnic populations in the U.S.: American Indians/Alaska Natives.* Waltham, MD: Education Development Center.

9. Cwik, M., Barlow, A., Tingey, I., et al. (2015). Exploring risk and protective factors with a community sample of American Indian adolescents who attempted suicide. *Archives of Suicide Research, 19*, 172–189.

10. Leavitt, R. A., Ertl, A., Sheats, K., et al. (2018, March 2). *Morbidity and Mortality Weekly Report.* https://www.cdc.gov/mmwr/volumes/67/wr/mm6708a1.htm?s_cid=mm6708a1_w.

11. Reichbart, R. (2018). *The paranormal surrounds us: Psychic phenomena in literature, culture and psychanalysis.* Jefferson, NC: McFarland.

12. Huff, C. (2018, October 15). As U.S. suicide rates rise, Hispanics show relative immunity. *Kaiser Health News.* https://khn.org/news/as-u-s-suicides-rates-rise-hispanics-show-relative-immunity.

13. Centers for Disease Control and Prevention. (2010). *Web-based inquiry statistics query and reporting system.* http.//www.cdc.gov/injury/wisqars/fatal.html.

14. Suicide Prevention Resource Center. (2010). *Risk and Protective Factors: Hispanic Populations.* https://www.sprc.org/resources-programs/risk-protective-factors-hispanic-populations.

15. Heron, M. (2011). Deaths: Leading causes for 2007. *National Vital Statistics Reports, 59,* 8.

16. Kuroki, Y., & Tilley, J. L. (2012). Recursive portioning analysis of long time suicidal beliefs in Asian Americans. *Asian American Journal of Psychology, 3,* 17–28.

17. Qiao, G. (2017, October 8). Why are Asian-American kids killing themselves? *Plan A Magazine.* https://planamag.com/why-are-asian-american-kids-killing-themselves.

18. McDermott, E., & Poen, K. (2016), *Queer youth, suicide and self-harm: Troubled subjects, troubling norms.* New York: Palgrave Macmillan.

19. Seelman, K. (2016). Transgender adults' access to college bathrooms, housing, and the relationship to suicidality. *Journal of Suicidality, 63,* 1373–1399.

CHAPTER FIVE

The Most Beautiful Alluring
Demon I Have Ever Known

According to a *Rolling Stone* magazine article, "All-American Despair" (2019), white men account for 70 percent of suicide cases, and the most rapid increases are in the forty-five to sixty-four age group. The states with the highest rates are Montana, Alaska, Wyoming, New Mexico, Idaho, and Utah, in that order. Brian Stauffer, the investigative reporter who wrote the article, relates how he drove through most of those states, "a place of endless mythology [where] the region has become a self-immolation center for middle-aged American men." Stauffer found "guns, lots of guns," observing that, in Utah, 85 percent of gun-related deaths are suicides.

Although high suicide rates in the rural West could be blamed on economic factors such as the Great Recession of 2007–2009, the rate was still climbing a decade later. A psychologist at the University of Utah told Stauffer that, during those years, there had been an increase in the "every-man-for-himself mentality" as opposed to "we're all in this together." A suicide prevention coordinator added, "There's still that cowboy-up mentality of 'I don't need any help. I'm not going to talk about my problems.' They see it as a weakness, especially when they have depression."

Stauffer interviewed a local reporter who had written a series of articles about suicide in the rural West. The reporter speculated that suicide might be the last obtainable option available after everything else had been exhausted. Admitting that he had considered suicide himself, he observed, "I used to shoot competitively in college. Now I won't own a gun. To me, suicide is the most beautiful, alluring demon I've ever known. She'll wear the gown and perfume, and procure the limo and the wine. She wants me, but I won't let her have me."[1]

This haunting conclusion tells how one man reframed his despair. As we will discover throughout this book, there are many ways to escape the allure of suicide.

Poverty and Suicide

These deaths of despair have been denied or ignored by many suicidologists. However, a 2015 study, the first of its type, clearly demonstrated such an association. Researchers analyzed data from sixteen states from 2005 to 2011, which included the major U.S. economic downturn from 2007 to 2008. A county-by-county analysis revealed the link between economic factors and suicide, even when unemployment and home foreclosures were ruled out. The link, which held for both genders, was especially strong during the recession years. As many became homeless, their dire situation pushed them over the edge. Others suffered from malnutrition, lacking the mental and physical stamina to think clearly about suicide's allure. Some people may have already been near the breaking point when the recession hit.

Unemployment usually plays a smaller role in suicides than poverty—except during this recession. In counties that had strong unemployment support systems, suicide rates were lower. The researchers identified the lack of resources at the county level as contributing to the deaths.[2]

A more positive note was provided by a 2019 working paper sponsored by the National Bureau of Economic Research. Higher minimum wages significantly reduced suicides that were not associated with drug overdoses. The same effect was noted for those with an earned income tax credit, especially among women. It was estimated that increasing both sources of income would prevent over one thousand suicides each year in the United States.

Lack of Attachment and Suicide

The "I don't need help" mentality mentioned above may suggest a lack of attachment, a frequently cited predisposing factor in suicide. The early bond of infants with their caregivers creates the foundation for future relationships. Different forms of attachment in infancy and early childhood have been linked to the individual's later emotional development and stability.[3] In healthy families, babies form secure attachments with their parents as naturally as they breathe, eat, smile, and cry.[4] Children from homes that consistently provide a safe, emotionally supportive, inclusive, and accepting social environment experience less distress in "strange" situations—such as when introduced to and briefly left alone with a stranger—and more easily form and maintain healthy relationships.

Children of parents who provide an inconsistent social environment or one of rejection, exclusion, or isolation tend to adopt more anxious or avoidant attachment styles, the former being so highly sensitive to rejection as to jeopardize the stability of relationships and the latter being so insensitive as to often lack the motivation necessary to form or maintain relationships. Unemotional parenting is especially harmful.

Good mothering begins before a child is born. An expectant mother who abuses drugs and alcohol or whose diet is faulty has already compromised the well-being of her child. If she is in a strife-filled relationship, quarrels and shouting raise her stress levels and those of the baby. Even genetic factors can be disturbed by poverty, financial instability, and family turmoil.

High Sensitivity and Suicide

About one in every five people can be termed *highly sensitive*.[5] This trait consists of heightened reactions to the five senses, acute awareness of even slight interpersonal difficulties, and a tendency to ruminate. This sensitivity includes a tendency not to consider consequences, whether positive or negative, when a stressful situation occurs. Highly sensitive people may feel hopeless, despondent, and worthless. Or they may think they are causing others so much trouble that those close to them would be better off without them.

On the other hand, highly sensitive people also engage in deep thinking and cognitive processing. They are more likely to wait to consider things again at a later time, when they will probably see their life from a different viewpoint. This uncertainty means they are less likely to make a suicide plan that they feel they must carry through. In addition, they tend to speak metaphorically, sometimes telling friends, "I feel so bad I want to kill myself." But this may just be a way to express how depressed they feel. Furthermore, highly sensitive people tend to have empathy; they are more aware of the drastic effects a suicide would have on the people around them.

So, in some ways, being highly sensitive protects against suicide. Some highly sensitive people become excellent psychotherapists and counselors. Others make their contributions in artistic, musical, and literary fields. Indeed, virtually any profession, including homemaking and parenting, is open to highly sensitive people who will bring a special dimension to their endeavors.

Ernest Hemingway was probably a highly sensitive person, but Stauffer observed, "What really killed Hemingway was one of the things killing American men today: a macho fantasy of a man who needs no one but himself." The celebrated writer's death in 1961 became one of the first suicides to be talked about openly in the United States. For most of his life, Hemingway endured mental illness, possibly bipolar disorder, and his family tree was wracked with suicides, including his sister, brother, granddaughter, and

father, who killed himself in 1928. Hemingway once commented, "I'll probably go the same way."

There have been conjectures that the suicide rate is unusually high among
gifted students because of their alleged emotional sensitivity. However, an
exhaustive study of the literature failed to support this claim.[6] Nonetheless,
special attention needs to be paid to this group's vulnerabilities, an issue
directly addressed by a 2018 study.[7]

Child Abuse and Suicide

When psychotherapists were questioned about their clients who had
killed themselves, they reported that more than half had experienced rejection or abandonment by their parents.[8] Obviously, this reflects poor attachment. But sometimes the parents exhibited violent behavior in the forms of
physical, psychological, or sexual abuse.

The term *abuse* is used by psychologists to describe interactions in which
one party behaves in a violent, demeaning, or invasive matter toward another
party, such as a child, a partner, or an animal. Sometimes the term *child maltreatment* is used to cover not only abuse but also neglect, exploitation (as in
forced labor), or trafficking (involuntary prostitution). Even though recorded
history contains numerous examples of child abuse and maltreatment, professional inquiry into the topic did not begin until the 1962 publication of
the paper "The Battered Child Syndrome" in the *Journal of the American Medical Association.*[9]

Intentional use of physical force against a child can take the form of hit-
ting, beating, kicking, sticking, belting, slapping, whipping, strangling,
burning, poisoning, or suffocating the child. Psychologist Alice Miller, the
author of several books on child abuse, would add spanking to the list,
which, according to Miller, can result in humiliation, guilt, shame, anger,
and other emotional consequences.[10]

Psychological abuse, which is often as harmful as physical or sexual abuse,
probably affects millions of American children each year. It can take the
forms of terrorizing, spurning, ignoring, isolating, ridiculing, degrading,
humiliating, or threatening a child. It can involve name-calling, harsh criticism, destroying a child's physical belongings, or killing the child's pet.

In *sexual abuse*, perpetrators involve a child in sexual acts for their own
stimulation or gratification. It may take the form of showing a child pornographic material or pressuring a child to engage in such sexual activities as
exposure, masturbation, oral sex, anal sex, or vaginal sex. The child can be
the active partner, the passive partner, or both. A study of several hundred
cases found similar rates of abuse across ethnic groups.[11]

In *sexual trafficking*, a child is manipulated or forced into performing sexual acts with adults or even other children for money, which is usually

pocketed by the perpetrator. In *exploitation*, a child engages in manual labor, pornographic films, or other activities for money, again, usually for the benefit of the perpetrator. Forcing children to become soldiers or to serve as sexual objects for soldiers often accompanies civil strife or terrorism.

Child neglect is the failure of a caregiver to provide needed food, shelter, clothing, medical care, or supervision to the point where the child's health, safety, or well-being is threatened. *Emotional neglect* is characterized by a lack of nurturance, encouragement, or support. *Educational neglect* is characterized by the caregiver's failure to provide or permit educational resources for a child. As we know, there is no list of traits or experiences that can infallibly predict suicide.[12] But there are also considerable data in which a path, perhaps one with many crossroads, can set someone on a suicidal journey.[13]

Caution should also be exercised with terms such as *child abuse*, which derive from the perspective of U.S. psychologists and psychiatrists. There are societies where children join the workforce at an early age, are harshly punished for their misdeeds, or are sexually initiated when young. We do not know whether such practices harm the children of those cultures. In our culture, there is evidence that many perpetrators of abuse were themselves abused as children. However, in the United States, abuse and other forms of maltreatment can result in suicidal behavior, attachment disorders, or other problems. Suicidologist Kristine Bertini refers to these factors as "the seeds of suicide."[14]

Takeaway Points

- Many factors appear to predispose people to take their own lives, but they differ from person to person.
- Suicide is rarely linear, and it is difficult to separate cause from effect.

Notes

1. Stauffer, B. (2019, June). All-American despair. *Rolling Stone*, pp. 70–79, 93–97.

2. Kerr, W. C., Kaplan, M. S., Huguet, N., et al. (2017). Economic recession, alcohol, and suicide rates: Comparative effects of poverty, foreclosure, and job loss. *Journal of Preventive Medicine, 52*, 469–475.

3. Bowlby, J. (1973). *Attachment and loss: Separation, anxiety, and anger* (2nd ed., Vol. 2). London: Penguin.

4. Hughes, D. A. (2018). *Building the bonds of attachment: Awakening love in deeply traumatized children.* Boulder, CO: Rowman & Littlefield.

5. Aron, E., Aron, A., & Jagiellowicz, J. (2012). Sensory processing sensitivity: A review in light of the evolution of biological responsibility. *Personality and Social Psychology Review, 16*, 262–282.

6. Gust-Brey, K., & Cross, T. (1999). An examination of the literature based on the suicidal behavior of gifted students. *Roeper Review, 22*, 28–35.

7. Cross, T. L., & Cross, J. R. (2018). *Suicide among gifted children and adolescents* (2nd ed.). Waco, TX: Prufrock Press.

8. Richards, B. M. (1999). Suicide and interfamilial relationships: A study from the perspective of therapists working with suicidal patients. *British Journal of Guidance and Counseling, 27*, 85–98.

9. Kempke, C. H., Silverman, P. N., Steele, B. F., et al. (1962). The battered child syndrome. *Journal of the American Medical Association, 181*, 17–24.

10. Miller, A. (2005). *The body never lies: The lingering effect of cruel parenting.* New York: W. W. Norton.

11. Roosa, M. W., Reinholtz, C., & Angelini, P. J. (1999). The relation of child sexual abuse and depression in young women: Comparison across four ethnic groups. *Journal of Abnormal Child Psychology, 27*, 65–76.

12. Goldstein, R. B., Black, D. W., Nasrahalla, M. A., et al. (1991). Sensitivity, specificity, and predictive value of a multivariate model applied to suicide among 1906 patients with affective disorders. *Archives of General Psychiatry, 48*, 413–422.

13. Brodsky, B. S., & Stanley, B. (2008). Adverse childhood experiences and suicidal behavior. *Psychiatric Clinics of North America, 31*, 223–235.

14. Bertini, K. (2009). *Understanding and preventing suicide: The development of self-destructive patterns and ways to alter them.* Westport, CT: Praeger.

THOSE WHO SURVIVED: WILLIAM STYRON

Not many book-length memoirs originate in psychiatric lectures. William Styron, the eminent author of *The Confessions of Nat Turner* and *Sophie's Choice*, was dismayed when a fellow author was publicly condemned for killing himself. Styron published an op-ed explaining the dangers of depression, which he understood all too well. In 1989, Styron discussed the topic and his experience at a psychiatric symposium that he later adapted into a magazine article. The following year, an expanded version came out in book form, which is still praised as an eloquent description of the disorder and credited for helping reduce its stigma.[1]

Styron took his title, *Darkness Visible*, from the seventeenth-century poet John Milton's description of Hell in his epic *Paradise Lost*:

> No light; but rather *darkness visible*
> Served only to discover sights of woe,
> Regions of sorrow, doleful shades, where peace
> And rest can never dwell, hope never comes
> That comes to all, but torture without end
> Still urges, and a fiery deluge, fed
> With ever-burning sulfur unconsumed.

Styron used his own depression, which was unrelenting, to put the experience into words:

> Mysteriously and in ways that are totally remote from normal experience, the grey drizzle of horror induced by depression takes on the quality of physical pain. But it is not an immediately identifiable pain, like that of a broken limb. It may be more accurate to say that despair, owing to some evil trick played upon the sick brain by the inhabiting psyche, comes to resemble the diabolical discomfort of being imprisoned in a fiercely overheated room. And because no breeze stirs this cauldron, because there is no escape from the smothering confinement, it is natural that the victim begins to think ceaselessly of oblivion.

Styron planned to kill himself but somehow summoned the energy to enter a hospital, where he made a full recovery.

> For those who have dwelt in depression's dark wood, and known its inexplicable agony, their return from the abyss is not unlike the ascent of the poet, trudging upward and upward out of hell's black depths and at last emerging into what he saw as "the shining world." There, whoever has been restored to health has almost always been restored to the capacity for serenity and joy, and this may be indemnity enough for having endured the despair beyond despair.

Styron lived for almost twenty years after his bout with suicidal depression, dying at age eighty-five, after receiving many literary honors.

Note

1. Styron, W. (1989). *Darkness visible: A memoir of madness.* New York: Penguin/Random House.

CHAPTER SIX

Dreams, Nightmares, and Suicide

No single behavior can predict which members of high-risk groups will commit suicide. In fact, many people who were never considered suicidal have killed themselves. However, an often overlooked factor is the predictive value of dreams and nightmares. People who kill themselves may have fantasies about suicide, just as if they were rehearsing the suicidal act. This rehearsal may take place in dreams and nightmares as well.

Dreams that precede or suggest suicide may contain childhood scenes of failure to make an emotional attachment to either parent, episodes of alienation, doomed relationships, unsuccessful business ventures, or disillusionment with the dreamer's church, government, or lifestyle. As the date for suicide approaches, the dreams may become unusually placid, as if welcoming the end. R. E. Litman, a psychiatrist who worked with many suicidal people, created a list of common dream themes:

- Death and dead people
- Destruction of oneself and others
- Being trapped and struggling to escape
- Taking leave (especially once suicide plans have matured)[1]

One of us (Krippner) became acquainted with a family that included a young woman we will call "Ming." Ming was seeing a counselor because of feelings of depression and inferiority that sometimes cascaded into thoughts of suicide. When the counselor met the entire family, she noticed how partial the family was to Ming's brother and how dismissive they were to Ming. Not surprisingly, Ming had nightmares in which she would try to kill her brother, and when that failed, she would try to kill herself. These dreams are examples of Litman's second category. Ming finally confided these nightmares to her therapist, who recognized that they served a problem-solving function. Killing her brother, a major cause of her stress, would not resolve the issue because a family is part of a system. Realizing this, Ming dreamed of suicide, Litman's fourth category. Dreams often exaggerate to make their point; once Ming got the message, these nightmares stopped.

Other researchers found similar results. In one study, dreams of suicidal clients were compared with those of depressed clients who were not suicidal. The dreams of both groups contained such themes as guilt, shame, and sadness. But the dreams of at-risk clients contained frequent themes of revenge, punishment, reunion with a loved one, self-disintegration, and confusion of the dreamer's body with that of another person.[2] Another study found that dreams reported by at-risk people contained images of being trapped, feeling helpless, and self-dissolution. Some dreams portrayed death as a liberator, with images of merging with a symbol that represents death, such as an ocean.[3]

The Adaptive Functions of Dreams

In recent decades, researchers have found that dreams perform several functions: reviewing waking life experiences, regulating emotions, reordering information in the brain, discarding obsolete memories, incorporating new experiences into the memory system, solving problems, and preparing for future events, especially those involving threatening situations.[4] Dreaming keeps the brain activated, serving as a type of "screen saver."

Many dream researchers believe that these functions were adaptive, that dreams played a role in human evolution and survival. Early humans who solved problems, regulated their emotions, stored important memories, discarded obsolete memories, and made plans while dreaming had an advantage over those who did not. Their genes entered the gene pool, passing on these advantages to future generations.

Ernest Hartmann, a former president of the International Association for the Study of Dreams (IASD), wrote that all dreaming is adaptive in one way or another. Dreams help people to adapt to stress, to recognize when a personal myth is no longer functional, to discover ways of responding to external threats, and to adapt to new social situations. According to Hartmann, dreams also illuminate unresolved emotional concerns, which are often triggered by a waking-life experience.[5] Carl Jung called this the most important function of dreaming.[6]

Nightmares and Suicide

Nightmares are dreams so disturbing that the dreamer awakens. They disrupt the ordinary dream's self-regulation of emotions during dreaming, resulting in negative moods upon awakening. This is especially true of nightmares that are associated with PTSD, which often replay the traumatic experience. Ordinary nightmares more commonly use symbols and metaphors to process negative experiences, something that PTSD nightmares seem incapable of doing. A PTSD nightmare might recall the dreamer's unwitting killing of a child because the dreamer mistook the child's toy for a weapon. By contrast, an ordinary nightmare might include a baby bird falling from its nest to its death because a human passerby bumped against the tree harboring the nest.

Night terrors are sudden arousals accompanied by panic, anxiety, and disorientation. As intense as nightmares, if not more so, night terrors involve irregular breathing, profuse perspiration, dilated pupils, and rapid heartbeats. They take place during deep, dreamless, non-REM sleep and are not uncommon among children, who may not remember them upon awakening. If they occur frequently during adulthood, they may be a symptom of PTSD or other disorders.[7]

In 2015, English investigators studied the nightmares of a large group of university students and then asked them about subsequent self-injury (such as cutting). The team reported that the content of nightmares predicted self-injury behavior better than any other single measure they had used. This suggests that there is continuity between dream life and waking life.[8] Mood upon awakening was an even better predictor of self-harm thoughts and behaviors than the content of nightmares.

In a 2019 study of several thousand Chinese teenagers, daytime sleepiness was correlated with suicidal thoughts (STs), suicidal plans (SPs), and suicide attempts (SAs). Besides falling asleep during the day, at-risk adolescents in this study reported insomnia, snoring, and inadequate nighttime sleep.[9]

Jesus at the Funeral

The following dream was reported to Scott Sparrow, a former president of the IASD, by a fifty-four-year-old woman:

> I was a confused and depressed individual, and the depression complicated the relationship and my life. I had been suicidal on and off since the age of fourteen, and I found myself feeling that way again. . . . One evening I became so low that I decided I was going to kill myself the next day. I had the plan worked out, and I was sure I would go through with it. Then I had the following dream:

> *I am standing at a lectern in a funeral parlor. I see about 50 people or more seated in front of me. I turn my head to the right, almost in slow motion, and see a casket. The lid is open. I am confused as to what I am doing here. I turn my head to the left, and I see Jesus standing in the back of the crowd. He is angry! He gently tilts his head forward and telepathically tells me to look inside the casket. I do so without question. I see my best friend Claire from 4th grade is dead. I am puzzled and surprised. I ask Jesus directly, "Why is SHE in there? It should be me!" He tilts his head forward again, gently but angrily, and again telepathically "orders" me to say the eulogy. . . .*
>
> *I felt I was inadequate and not the right person to do her justice. But Jesus gets VERY angry at this point, and this time he stares right at me with no head tilting and again telepathically "orders" me to do the eulogy. . . . I stare out into the crowd. The people are staring back at me. I see my best friend's father in the middle of the crowd. I look at him and begin speaking, I say, "She was my best friend. . . ." At this point I come to a complete stop. I feel the pain of every single person in that room all at one time, especially the pain of Claire's father. It is overwhelming and horrible. I turn to Jesus with tears of despair and regret, realizing how my suicide would affect others, I say, "I'm so sorry, I will never kill myself . . . never!"*

When I woke up from the dream, I sat up abruptly and continued repeating, "I won't kill myself. I promise I won't kill myself. . . . I'm so sorry." The dream stopped me from contemplating suicide. Even though I still have suicidal feelings, on and off, even to this day, the dream always reminds me of the consequences. I know I will NEVER act on these feelings because of this dream.[10]

The Varieties of Nightmare Experience

Fariba Bogzaran and Daniel Deslauriers have identified several types of nightmares that could be associated with thoughts of suicide. The *anxiety* nightmare centers around a fear for one's safety or that of a loved one, usually including a failed attempt to save oneself or another person. The dreamer can be paralyzed, unable to either flee or fight. Or the dreamer might be active, running from danger or fighting a terrifying attacker. The attempt is futile, and the dreamer, upon awakening, is relieved that it was "just a dream." However, the dreamer should not miss the opportunity to learn from the nightmare's metaphors. The anxiety in the dream and the relief upon awakening may mirror the thought that suicide would be a longed-for awakening from the nightmare of daily life.

The agonizing *distress* nightmare is marked by depression, grief, discouragement, guilt, shame, confusion, anger, or a combination of these. These nightmares often pose an existential issue: "I need to kill myself in penance for my horrible sins"; "I am so ashamed of what happened that I can never face the world again"; or "I am so depressed that nothing seems worthwhile, not even life itself." Sometimes these dreams end in death, either self-inflicted or brought about by a circumstance or a dream character.

Bogzaran and Deslauriers describe the *alienation* dream as one in which the dreamer is separated from family, community, or life itself. The dreamer is portrayed in the dream as an outsider, one who is making so little impact on the world that he or she might as well not exist. No thought is given to the advantages of living apart from the mainstream, only to the pain and agony felt from being rejected or simply not "fitting in." The rejection might be romantic, sexual, political, economic, social, or a combination.[11]

These and other varieties of the nightmare experience have in common a sense of hopelessness, helplessness, and a lack of meaning—precisely the feelings that people at risk for suicide often express in their letters, texts, and conversations. Perhaps these nightmares are calls for help, and a friend, family member, or loved one should take them seriously.

In 2019, Kathleen Jacob, an investigative reporter, interviewed Allen Chapman, a veteran who had served in Afghanistan. Chapman was taking ten pills a day to treat PTSD and depression. He told Jacob, "I didn't want to go to sleep. . . . I was killing people and cutting up body parts and chopping up their body, and it was always with a knife." One of the drugs prescribed by the VA doctor was prazosin, a medication used for blood pressure. But the nightmares got worse, and Chapman stopped taking the medication, fearing its side effects. A study conducted at Augusta University confirmed Chapman's suspicions; reports of this nature were not uncommon. Furthermore, study participants taking a placebo showed a greater improvement than those taking prazosin. As a result, the U.S. Food and Drug Administration (FDA) has not listed prazosin as a drug useful in treating PTSD.[12]

Like many PTSD nightmares, Chapman's repeats the traumatic experience, killing civilians while in combat. Rather than helping Chapman face the existential issues expressed in the dream, the VA practitioner prescribed medication, unfortunately choosing a drug that often leads to suicide rather than preventing it.

Takeaway Points

- Dreams and nightmares can be useful predictors of suicide attempts, and there is evidence that they are more accurate than an at-risk person's waking thoughts and behaviors.
- These dreams and nightmares may suggest methods for suicide prevention, if used with insight and creativity.

Notes

1. Litman, R. E. (1995). The dream in the suicidal situation. In J. Natterson (Ed.), *The dream in clinical practice* (pp. 283–299). Northvale, NJ: Jason Aaronson.

2. Maltsberger, J. T. (1993). Dreams and suicide. *Journal of Suicide and Life-Threatening Behavior, 23*, 56–62.

3. Soubrier, J. P., & Vedrinne, J. (Eds.). (1983). *Depression and suicide.* New York: Pergamon.

4. Krippner, S. (2017). Foreword. In R. J. Hoss & Robert J. Gongloff (Eds.), *Dreams that change our lives* (pp. 5–6). Asheville, NC: Chiron.

5. Hartmann, E. (2011). *The nature and functions of dreaming.* New York: Oxford University Press.

6. Jung, C. G. (1971). *The portable Jung* (J. Campbell, Ed.). New York: Viking.

7. Nielsen, T. A., & Levin, R. (2007). Nightmares: A new neurocognitive model. *Sleep Medicine Reviews, 11*, 295–310.

8. Hochard, K., Heym, N., & Townsend, E. (2015). The unidirectional relationship of nightmares in self-hurtful thoughts and behaviors. *Dreaming, 25*, 44–58.

9. Liu, X., Liu, Z., Wang, Z., et al. (2019, February). Daytime sleepiness predicts future suicidal behavior: A longitudinal study of adolescents. *Sleep, 42*(2), 1–10.

10. Sparrow, S. (2017). Embracing spirit. In R. J. Hoss & Robert J. Gongloff (Eds.), *Dreams that change our lives* (pp. 235–242). Asheville, NC: Chiron.

11. Bogzaran, F., & Deslauriers, D. (2012). *Integral dreaming.* Albany: State University of New York Press.

12. Jacob, K. (February 18, 2019). *Fox News* (online).

CHAPTER SEVEN

Mental Illness and Suicide

Most suicidologists we have studied assert that the majority of suiciders do not meet the criteria for mental illness. Thomas Joiner and his colleagues disagree, stating that suicide is "an exemplar of psychopathology" and that all suiciders are mentally ill.[1] To support this position, they cite the danger of *suicide contagion*, the accidental deaths of innocent bystanders, and the hardship imposed on friends and relatives, any one of which is indicative of psychopathology. Suicide is in so great an opposition to the "biological imperative" that Joiner and his associates refer to this "derangement" as far more serious than psychosis or mania.

But other suicidologists take a more moderate perspective, listing the types of mental illness most closely linked with suicide, such as panic disorder (intense fear and anxiety without a reasonable cause), borderline personality disorder (extreme and inappropriate emotional responses), and the schizophrenias, all of which are marked by a departure from ordinary reality. What do all three have in common? Impulsivity—an onlooker never knows what will trigger a suicide attempt, and it is unlikely that the suicider does. Alcohol and substance abuse are also linked with suicide, as are extreme mood swings and poor judgment; none of these, by themselves, qualify as mental illness.[2]

A 2010 issue of *European Psychiatry* explored the frequently cited findings that no factor or combination of factors could reliably predict a suicide attempt and that suicidal behavior was not associated with any specific type of psychiatric disorder. However, poor decision-making appeared to be related to the inability to cope with stressful life situations and high sensitivity to negative social stimuli, such as angry faces. Disadvantageous decision-making was underlined by genetic factors, including the brain's serotonin production.[3] Twins have a higher rate of mental illness but a lower risk of suicide than the general population.[4]

French philosopher Albert Camus once stated that there is only one serious philosophical question: whether or not to commit suicide. This idea would sound bizarre to most people, who go through life with a sense of meaning and purpose, believing that they carry out their tasks for positive and even profound reasons. However, not everyone is so fortunate. Someone may decide that his daily activities are done through force of habit. Another person may see herself as nothing more than a mechanical drone. From this point of view, behaviors and desires may seem absurd, a feeling that may make one's belief system (or personal mythology) inadequate to survive the storms of life. Camus was a leading existential writer; his philosophical query about suicide strikes at the heart of the human search for meaning.

Fawn Journeyhawk's Spiritual Emergency

For most of her life, Fawn Journeyhawk had experienced unusual phenomena, such as jolts of energy running through her body, dreams that seemed to predict future events, visions that felt as real as her everyday perceptions, and voices that had no identifiable source. She consulted a physician, who promptly put her on medication and told her that she was suffering from a "psychotic break" and might have to be institutionalized. The medication did not stop her visions and voices, and Fawn considered suicide preferable to incarceration in a mental hospital.

One of Fawn's Native American friends suggested that she see one of us (Krippner), and for the first time, Fawn received a completely different diagnosis. Fawn was informed that her experiences resembled those of men and women who were being called to become shamans and that her best option would be to visit a Native American healer. Fawn had never heard the term *shaman*, but she investigated the concept and located Dead Grass, an Anishinaabe traditional pipe carrier, who took her on as a student.

This was the beginning of Fawn's remarkable career as a shaman and ritualist, renowned for successfully treating extremely difficult cases of mental and physical illness. A doctoral dissertation was written about her journey; she established several "medicine camps" in various Western states and soon had students of her own. Serendipity, or perhaps her guiding spirits, had saved her from an ignominious ending and kept her talents from being wasted.

Fawn's story is an example of what psychiatrist Stanislav Grof and his associates have called *psychospiritual crises*.[5] If correctly understood and treated, they can result in psychological and physiological healing, even personal transformation. These episodes can be found in the life stories of shamans, mystics, and spiritual leaders. Grof used the term *spiritual emergencies* to describe some of these conditions and listed eleven of them, acknowledging that several overlap. These could lead to suicide if improperly managed.

1. Shamanic crises (such as experienced by Fawn)
2. Kundalini experiences (jolts of bodily energy, typically in the spine)
3. Unitive consciousness (feelings of "oneness" with others or the cosmos)
4. Psychological renewal (feelings of death and rebirth)
5. Psychic openings (information from nonordinary sources)
6. Communication with "spirit guides" (such as hearing "voices")
7. Past-life experiences (memories from earlier incarnations)
8. Near-death experiences (recalled by those who had been declared deceased)
9. Encounters from outer space (visits from "aliens")
10. Possession experiences (shift of identities)
11. Alcoholism and drug dependence (misuse of substances)

Grof and his associates have presented treatment regimens for each of these spiritual emergencies, hoping to turn them into life-changing spiritual "emergences." It requires a well-trained and skillful therapist to distinguish a potentially transformative experience from mental illness because there are usually alternative explanations, such as vivid hypnagogic, presleep experiences, or misinterpretation of sensory and auditory phenomena.[6] Some observers feel that pathological experiences have sometimes been romanticized and idealized by Grof and his associates. Even so, the unusual material in these reports may be of value in Jungian, Gestalt, psychosynthesis, bodywork, expressive arts, and other transpersonal therapies.

Grof's work and the contributions of others had an impact on the American Psychiatric Association's *Diagnostic and Statistical Manual for the Classification of Mental Disorders*, which added a category for "spiritual and religious problems" in its fifth edition.[7] These issues were described as nonpathological crises in which the process of growth and change has become overwhelming and chaotic. Membership in a cult, so-called mystical experiences, and the questioning of one's faith, especially during a terminal illness, were included.

Discernment and training are needed to distinguish those cases that meet the criteria for spiritual and religious problems from those that are symptoms of schizophrenia or other psychosis. This process, which is used when a clinician is not yet sure which of several similar illnesses a person has, is called *differential diagnosis*.

Harry: Borderline Personality Disorder

One of the authors of this book was personally acquainted with a family whose son we will call "Harry." Harry's parents had never wanted children, but once his mother became pregnant with him, they decided against having an abortion, simply vowing not to have another child after this unwanted one was born. Following a rough childhood and a series of disruptive incidents in high school, Harry's parents took him to a psychiatrist, at the school's insistence.

Harry was diagnosed as having borderline personality disorder, a condition characterized by mood instability, poor social relationships, and self-destructive behavior that includes suicidal tendencies. Psychotherapy was recommended, but Harry's parents delayed it. His politically ambitious father was running for office and feared that his son's diagnosis would cost him votes. His socially ambitious mother had similar fears regarding her social standing. They told themselves that if their son was just "borderline," he was not extremely disturbed.

This is a tragic case of one word making a big difference. The term *borderline* was chosen long ago to refer to disturbances that were more serious than *neurotic* but less serious than *psychotic*. As the years passed and more was understood, borderline personality disorder was found to be serious indeed; in fact, it is a significant risk factor for suicide. But the name has unfortunately remained.

Harry left home and moved to another city, where he rented an inexpensive room and found a job as a waiter. One of Harry's coworkers, Cleo, told Harry that she was making extra money as a prostitute and suggested that Harry consider entering the same profession. His good looks and athletic build would ensure him a bevy of customers, both male and female. Harry eagerly accepted her offer and was soon making enough money to rent an apartment. He told Cleo that if he were ever arrested, his parents would be mortified—much to his delight.

Harry began to buy illegal opiates, but these substances had an adverse effect on both his jobs. He reported late for work and forgot appointments with his "dates." His lack of social skills alienated him from his coworkers at the restaurant, and he was soon fired. Cleo told him that he was also at risk of losing his other job because he was getting a negative reputation among his clients for his unpredictable behavior. He also got into political arguments with his dates, even though they usually had no interest in discussing politics.

After two years, Harry moved back home, where his parents welcomed him, albeit with mixed feelings. Having no siblings and no educational or vocational ambitions, Harry was lonely much of the time. His father was now mayor of their town, but he had loftier goals in mind. His mother was rarely at home; her husband's official duties had given her a wider social arena, and she was enjoying every minute of it. If Harry manifested signs of suicidal ideation, they did not notice them.

Harry found a local drug dealer to supply him with opiates. He had no close friends and was not skillful enough to find sexual partners. Instead, he developed a fetish—masturbating while talking with the pet panda doll he slept with as a kid. The panda began to talk back to Harry, cajoling him to consider suicide; such a deed would shock the community and embarrass his parents. Harry relished both outcomes.

One morning Harry did not show up for breakfast. His mother discovered his lifeless body hanging from a rafter in his room. He had announced his plan on social networks and quickly received the prominence he had never achieved while he was alive. Contrary to Harry's expectations, his father capitalized on his son's death. He became a spokesperson for mental health and was elected to the state legislature. Harry's mother, deluged with condolences, founded a working group to fight opioid addiction that resulted in considerable positive media exposure. They blamed their son's demise on his opioid dealer and quickly burned his panda.

We do not know about Harry's neurobiology, but we do know that he was diagnosed with borderline personality disorder. His upbringing might not meet the strict definition of child neglect, but Harry seems to have considered it in those terms. It would be too easy to say that Harry's suicide was *caused* by failed attachment, his borderline personality disorder, or his use of opioids. Like others we will meet in this book, there may have been many causes.

What if Harry had received the psychotherapy that was recommended? We know that borderline personality disorder has a high risk of suicidality, especially when accompanied by depression or substance abuse. One of the best approaches shown to prevent suicide is dialectical behavior therapy, which combines cognitive behavioral techniques, such as learning interpersonal skills, mindfulness, and how to regulate emotions and tolerate distress. The therapeutic alliance is a powerful factor,[8] as trust and a sense of safety are necessary for growth to occur. One research participant said, "I was able to stop the suicidal behavior when the caring team stayed by my side and believed in me."[9]

Takeaway Points

- Some writers state that all suiciders are not mentally ill, but most others take a less extreme position.
- An unsatisfactory resolution of existential questions regarding life's meaning and purpose underlie a number of suicides and suicide attempts.

Notes

1. Joiner, T. E, Hom, C. R., & Silva, C. (2016). Suicide as the derangement of the self-sacrificial aspects of eusociality. *Psychological Review, 123*, 235–254.

2. Range, L. M., MacIntyre, D. R., Rutherford, D., et al. (1997). Suicide in special populations and circumstances. *Aggression and Violent Behavior, 2*, 57–63.

3. Courtet, P., Guillaume, S., Malafosse, A., & Jolliant, F. (2010). Genes, suicide, and decisions. *European Psychiatry, 25,* 294–296.

4. Tomassin, C., Juel, K., Hol, N. V., et al. (2003). Risk of suicide in twins: 57-year follow-up study. *British Medical Journal, 307,* 373–394.

5. Grof, S. (2010). *Healing our deepest wounds: The holotropic paradigm shift.* Santa Cruz, CA: Multidisciplinary Association for Psychedelic Studies.

6. Cardena, E., Lynn, S. J., & Krippner, S. (2014). *Varieties of anomalous experience* (2nd ed.). Washington, DC: American Psychological Association.

7. American Psychiatric Association. (2013). *Diagnostic and Statistical Manual* (5th ed.). Washington, DC: American Psychiatric Association.

8. Bedics, J. D., Atkins, D. C., Harned, M. S., & Linehan, M. M. (2015). The therapeutic alliance as a predictor of outcome in dialectical behavior therapy versus nonbehavioral psychotherapy by experts for borderline personality disorder. *Psychotherapy, 52*(1), 67–77.

9. Holm, A. L., & Severinsson, E. (2011). Struggling to recover by changing suicidal behaviour: Narratives from women with borderline personality disorder. *International Journal of Mental Health Nursing, 20,* 165–173.

CHAPTER EIGHT

Teenage Suicides

Teenage deaths by suicide were relatively stable until 2010, but then they started to rise. Suicidologists have long pondered what they call the "gender paradox." For decades, girls reported thinking about suicide more often than boys and made more suicide attempts. However, more boys died from suicide. Previously, girls tended to use less deadly means, such as poison, while boys more often used lethal means, such as firearms. But girls have begun to use more deadly means, such as drowning and suffocation.[1] Some girls try to kill themselves by taking massive doses of their parents' prescription drugs or their own medication for attention deficit disorder, hyperactivity, or depression. Within the past decade, rates have more than doubled each year, the rate of suicide among girls eventually outpacing the suicide rate among boys. What is so wrong that our young people are killing themselves?

Is It the Technology?

In 2019, there were media reports about an alleged spike in young people's suicides following the 2017 release of *13 Reasons Why*, a popular Netflix series about a girl who ends her life. In the nine months following the series' release, there were nearly two hundred more youth suicides than expected, given historical and seasonal trends. A coauthor of the study, from the U.S. Institutes of Mental Health, which helped sponsor the study, called teenage suicides "a major public health crisis." Netflix included warnings with some of the episodes and created a website that provided information about crisis hotlines and other resources. Netflix also cited a study carried out at the University of Pennsylvania that found *fewer* suicidal thoughts among young people who watched the entire season when compared to nonviewers.[2]

Christopher Ferguson, a psychologist, added that if *13 Reasons Why* did spark suicide contagion, suicides would be especially disproportionate among girls and young adults who watched the series and continue to increase as the show was streamed. None of this took place. Suicides were actually increasing before the series was released, and no increase was noted in the month following its release. Ferguson reported data from at-risk viewers who watched the entire series. For them, the suicide rate decreased, and their willingness to help others increased. However, there was an increase in negative outcomes for those at-risk viewers who stopped watching the show.[3]

Having studied the effects of all suicide-related fictional media, Ferguson found no evidence for "suicide contagion." He recalled the attribution of rising crime rates to media violence in the 1970s, a claim that failed to be supported by research. Ferguson concluded that reactions to shows like *13 Reasons Why* are highly individual, helping some, not helping others, and having no discernible effect on most.[4] Ferguson and another psychologist, Patrick Markey, also studied the effects of video games on violent behavior and found no overall negative impact. Instead, certain video games appear to have positive effects on users' cognitive skills and overall mood.[5]

Experts disagree regarding the link between smartphone use and teenagers' well-being. One study linked iPhones, Android phones, and similar devices to disrupted sleep patterns and increased thoughts about suicide.[6] Ferguson and Markey found no such link, stating that part of the problem is an ongoing one for psychological science, namely, the tendency for scholars, the media, and professional guilds such as the American Academy of Pediatrics (AAP) to hype weak results that link social media and television to unhealthy behaviors by an unsuspecting public. We find some of these efforts, such as the AAP recommending that parents limit their kids' screen time, to be misdirected. We also worry about the potential for undisclosed conflicts of interest (such as offering consulting services or paid talks to tech companies) among scholars on both sides of the debate. Professional groups particularly need to be more responsible about not marketing faulty science to policy makers and the public.[7]

Religious and Spiritual Beliefs

Previous research has examined several risk factors for child and adolescent suicide, but little attention has been paid to religious and spiritual beliefs. A 2018 study conducted by researchers from Columbia University and the New York Psychiatric Research Institute found that children whose parents had religious affiliations, either Protestant or Catholic, were less likely to think about or to commit suicide, whether their parents were active churchgoers or not. For children of parents who were said to take their religion seriously, there was a 40 percent decrease in the risk of suicidal behavior. However, church attendance was not associated with this decrease. The sample size was only 214, so this question must be studied with larger groups.[8]

Sexual-minority adolescents (LGBTQ: lesbian, gay, bisexual, transgender, or questioning) are more likely than their heterosexual peers to plan or attempt suicide, with 25 percent having reported suicide attempts and 40 percent having reported seriously considering suicide. Sexual-minority boys reported four times more suicide attempts than their heterosexual peers. However, teen girls were more likely than teen boys to report attempting, planning, or considering suicide.[9]

School Violence and Suicide

School violence has taken many lives and triggered additional tragedies. More than a quarter of mass-shooting survivors develop PTSD, according to the National Center for PTSD. Sandy Richman, who lost his first-grade daughter in the 1999 massacre at Sandy Hook Elementary School, killed himself in March 2018, just a few days after two student survivors of the Marjory Stone Douglas High School shooting in Parkland, Florida, took their own lives. Two members of the Columbine community, a star student athlete and the mother of a student who was paralyzed in the school attack, also killed themselves after that 1999 shooting.

The assailants in most school shootings are young men with mental health issues, which raises questions about male teenagers and their frustrated search for identity. To be a man today, says filmmaker Jennifer Siebel Newsom, is to fight for success and sex, to reject empathy, and to never cry. This stereotype persists despite decades of feminist critique and the prevalence of news stories about men showing their feelings. The result is often depression, anxiety, and violence. Siebel Newsom's film, *The Mask You Live In*, includes interviews with youth program leaders, psychologists, sociologists, and candid middle school students. Boys are four times as likely to be expelled from school, and suicide is their third most common form of death. The term *toxic masculinity* is sometimes used when these harmful stereotypes are discussed.[10]

Harry Revisited

Let's take another look at Harry, the young man we met in chapter 7. We know that he was diagnosed with borderline personality disorder, and he apparently lacked attachment to his parents. He was lonely and took opioids.

But let's remember the theme we repeatedly emphasize in this book: suicide is complicated. Each person may have numerous reasons for wanting to die. It would be too easy to say that Harry's suicide was *caused* by failed attachment, his borderline personality disorder, or the effect of opioids on a brain that was not yet mature. Life does not take a linear path; cause and effect interact over the course of a person's life. Major research studies are underway, both in the United States and Europe, that are following the development of teenagers' brains, which are vulnerable to any number of stresses, ranging from contact sports to alcohol and drug use. Impulsive behavior, such as a suicide attempt, often characterizes an immature brain. Later, we will find that there are ways to strengthen the thinking of young people whose brains are still developing.

Takeaway Points

- There is no convincing evidence that the use of smartphones and social media is directly related to suicide among adolescents.
- The teenage brain is still developing; alcohol and drug use can have an adverse effect upon this development.

Notes

1. Spiller, H. A., Ackerman, J. N., Spiller, N. E., & Casavent, M. J. (2019). Sex- and age-specific increases in suicide attempts by self-poisoning in the United States among youth and young adults between 2000 and 2018. *Journal of Pediatrics, 210,* 201–208.

2. Tanner, L. (2019). Study: Kids' suicides spiked after Netflix's "13 Reasons." https://news.yahoo.com/study-kids-suicides-spiked-netflixs-13-reasons-212216175.html.

3. Ferguson, C. (2019). Results don't back TV show's link to suicide: Commentary. *Orlando Sentinel* (online).

4. Ferguson, C. (2015). Does movie or video game violence predict societal violence? It depends on what you look for and when. *Journal of Communication, 65,* 192–212.

5. Markey, P., & Ferguson, C. (2017). *Moral combat: Why the war on violence and videogames is wrong.* Dallas, TX: Holly Hill Books.

6. Carbone, J. T., Holzer, K. J., & Vaughn, M. G. (2019). Child and adolescent suicidal ideation and suicide attempts in the Healthcare Cost and Utilization Project. *Journal of Pediatrics, 206,* 225–231.

7. Ferguson, C., & Markey, P. (2019, March 27). Blaming social media for youth suicide trends is misguided and dangerous. *The Inquirer* (online).

8. Kelly, L. (2018, August 13). Religiosity linked to lower teen suicide rates. *Washington Times,* p. 13.

9. Winerman, L. (2018, March). LGBTQ teens face higher suicide risk. *Monitor on Psychology,* p. 76.

10. Matos, K., O'Neill, O., & Lei, Xue. (2018). Toxic leadership and the masculinity contest culture: How "win or die" cultures breed abusive leadership. *Journal of Social Issues, 74*(3), 500–528.

CHAPTER NINE

Physician-Assisted Suicide

Suicide is often unpredictable and poorly planned. One exception is physician-assisted suicide. Western medicine has prolonged human life, but its practitioners often fail to face the end of life frankly with their patients, even those who are clearly close to the end. However, some physicians attempt to assist terminally ill or severely disabled patients in ending their lives.

Historical Perspectives

The Hippocratic oath, devised by Greek physicians from the third century BCE, states, "To please no one will I prescribe a deadly drug or give advice that may induce death." This oath became part of a modern physician's moral code. Admirable as it may sound, it has hampered attempts to legalize physician-assisted suicide to relieve terminal individuals of unbearable suffering.

Outside the sphere of Western medicine, several indigenous tribes practiced euthanasia before their lands were colonized. The Caribs practiced euthanasia on the grounds that the terminally ill were possessed by evil spirits; the longer they clung to life, the more powerful the malevolent spirits would become, endangering the community. Euthanasia has been practiced both as population control during times of famine and as an act of mercy. The Kalinago inhabitants of the island of Grenada sent the aged and the terminally ill into the afterlife with the aid of herbal poisons, convinced that they were sparing the infirm both inconveniences and pain.[1]

Contemporary Developments

Both physician-assisted suicide and other forms of euthanasia are opposed by mainstream Western medicine, as expressed by the World Medical Association, and by religious institutions, such as the Lutheran Church's Missouri

Synod and the Roman Catholic Church. Islam is slightly more moderate, holding that the life of gravely ill people should be ended "only when absolutely necessary."

However, change has been coming for decades. In the Netherlands, physician-assisted suicide has not been punishable since the 1970s, provided it has been carried out by a specially trained physician. Canada gives its terminally ill citizens the right to refuse medication, intravenous feeding, or "heroic" interventions that would prolong their lives. The Belgian Parliament legalized euthanasia in 2002 for competent adults and emancipated minors. Furthermore, with the support of the Association for the Right to Die with Dignity, a Belgian pharmaceutical company announced the development of "home euthanasia kits" in 2005. In Switzerland, euthanasia cannot be prosecuted, assuming the physician has no selfish motive.

In the United States, philanthropist George Soros initiated the Death in America Project to support the legalization of euthanasia and physician-assisted suicide.[2] The Compassion and Choices organization in the United States, formerly known as the Hemlock Society, supports the right to control the time and manner of one's death. This society supported Oregon's 1997 law, upheld by the U.S. Supreme Court, to allow physicians to prescribe lethal drugs to terminally ill patients who want to end their lives.

As populations age worldwide, many governments and public opinion leaders have addressed this issue in a responsible manner, facing ethical dilemmas for which there is no clear-cut consensus. For instance, there is no definitive reason to distinguish severe psychological stress from physical pain; one can be just as excruciating as the other.

Some advocates support *passive euthanasia* (withholding a surgical procedure or vital medication) but reject *active euthanasia* (administering a toxic substance or other fatal procedure). Finally, it is worth pondering why many advocates of euthanasia to spare pain and suffering in animals do not extend the practice to humans whose dire medical situations are equally agonizing.

Data from Psychical Research

Survival of some part of the human psyche following bodily death has been assumed by organized religion for centuries. However, serious study of this possibility only dates back to the founding of the British Society for Psychical Research in 1882 and the American Society for Psychical Research in 1885. Members of these societies use disciplined inquiry to explore this possibility. Topics they investigated are now a part of mainstream psychology, including near-death experiences, out-of-body experiences, hypnosis, and dissociative identity disorders (formerly referred to as multiple personalities).

Near-death experiences (NDEs) are reported by people who were pronounced dead by medical personnel but then revived; they have provided accounts, some of them quite detailed, about their time on the "other side." Near-death experiences have also occurred outside the presence of medical personnel. Bruce Greyson, a psychiatrist, has looked at common elements in the reports from people who had NDEs following suicide attempts. Of course, not every person experienced every insight listed here.

- They experienced a sense of "cosmic unity" that they were part of something greater than themselves.
- The problems that drove them to suicide seemed less important when viewed from the perspective of this "cosmic unity."
- The NDE enhanced their life, giving it more value and meaning and making life more precious.
- The NDE made their life more "real" than it had been before.
- The NDE enhanced their sense of self-worth.
- The NDE gave them a sense of "bonding" with other people.
- The NDE convinced them that suicide was not the way that their life was meant to end.
- The "life review" they experienced in their NDE helped them evaluate their life in a more constructive way.
- Their personal situation was enhanced as a result of the NDE.
- They became convinced that their suicide attempt had been ethically incorrect.
- They experienced the death of the negative part of themselves so that the positive part could go on.
- The NDE made them reluctant to make another attempt to end their life.[3]

Greyson observed that half of these elements were transcendental in nature, whereas suicide prevention and counseling focus on practical matters, such as reality-oriented problem-solving. However, some people choosing death may contemplate transcendental issues. Our readers may notice the similarities between the reports of Greyson's group and those from survivors of Golden Gate Bridge suicide attempts. In both cases, they went through transitions that changed their lives in remarkable ways.

From the beginning, the work of the psychical research societies was subjected to hostile criticism or ridicule. Nonetheless, the investigators persisted, obtaining data from several sources, including alleged communications with the dead by "mediums" who claimed to "channel" messages from deceased persons and "after-death communications," in which ordinary people reported messages from loved ones in dreams, in daytime imagery, or electronically (as in instrumental voice communication).

Some of the data scrutinized by the psychical researchers were fraudulent or attributable to such ordinary processes as coincidence, wishful thinking, or projecting meaning onto ambiguous phenomena. However, the most interesting finding for many people is that NDE descriptions of the afterlife differ from conventional religious teachings. For example, there are very few mentions of a hell-like realm or a Supreme Being who doles out justice. This was especially notable in the case of "messages" received from people who had committed suicide.

In 2006, two psychologists, Pamela Rae Heath and Jon Klimo, published the results of their extensive research on after-death communications (ADCs) from people who had killed themselves. They combed the psychical research literature; Jewish, Christian, Kardec Spiritist, and Islamic publications; and interviews with mediums and other investigators. The reports, which exceeded fifteen hundred in number, exhibited many similarities. These, of course, do not prove the validity of the reports, as ordinary explanations could have applied to most, if not all, of them. With that caveat in mind, here are the main themes uncovered by Heath and Klimo:

- When people are suffering and near the end of their life span, physician-assisted suicide and other forms of euthanasia are likely to be acceptable, but if they kill themselves before their "life purpose" has been manifested, they will remain in anguish until the time at which their life purpose would have been attained.

- The grief of loved ones left behind is not helpful to the deceased, who carry this burden with them, hampering them from "moving on." It is better that survivors release their grief, anger, and guilt.

- From the perspective of the "spirit world," intent and motivation are all-important. In euthanasia, the intent is to end suffering. In altruistic suicide, the motive is to save others.

- Even though there is a hypothetical life purpose for everyone, the choice is personal. Self-destruction is rarely a solution. People need to take responsibility for their actions, both in this life and afterward.

Heath and Klimo include existential perspectives about choice and meaning in their discussion. Existentialists differ from each other regarding an afterlife, but they offer the challenge that life is worth living even if physical life is all there is. Heath and Klimo point out that William James was haunted by depression throughout his life, but he never wavered in his conviction that life is worth living.[4]

Is there one specific life purpose for each person? We do not know. But people come into the world with a genetic inheritance and circumstances that manifest or stunt their potentials. One's ability to make choices may not be as straightforward as one might hope. But one can certainly adopt attitudes, rational beliefs, and personal myths that assist optimal functioning in those circumstances, whatever they may be, and provide a person with meaning and purpose in life.

Because of the taboo surrounding this topic, many people are unaware of options to die a peaceful death without the help of a physician. If people simply stop eating and drinking, they will die in a few weeks. One could consult a mental health professional, one with whom the suicidal person could engage in a life review and discuss the rationale for taking one's life. Sometimes such a professional can propose means of alleviating pain that neither suicidal people nor their physicians had considered. A mental health professional can also discuss the effect that one's demise would have on family members, a consideration often ignored.[5] However, physician-assisted suicide and other forms of euthanasia may well be justified for some of those in unbearable pain, and this is why we respectfully consider them in this book.

Takeaway Points

- The practice of physician-assisted suicide, which has a long history, can be found in many cultures. A case can be made for using it or other forms of euthanasia in cases of intractable pain.
- People whose lives have been changed by near-death experiences report transformations similar to those of some survivors of suicide attempts.

Notes

1. Krippner, S. (1989). Mythological aspects of death and dying. In A. Berger, P. Badham, A. H. Kutscher, et al. (Eds.), *Perspectives on death and dying* (pp. 3–13). Philadelphia, PA: Charles Press.

2. Krippner, S., & Kasian, S. J. (2009). Cross-cultural perspectives on euthanasia and physician-assisted suicide. In M. C. Bronson & T. R. Fields (Eds.), *So what? Now what? The anthropology of consciousness responds to a world in crisis* (pp. 136–163). Newcastle upon Tyne, UK: Cambridge Scholars Publishing.

3. Greyson, B. (1992). Wish for death, wish for life: The NDE and suicide attempts. In E.-S. Mercier (Ed.), *Death transformed: Research into real-life experiences of the approach of death* (pp. 135–145). Paris: L'Age du Verseau (in French).

4. Heath, P. R., & Klimo, J. (2006). *Suicide. What really happens in the afterlife?* Berkeley, CA: North Atlantic Books.

5. Werth, J. L. (2013). Assisted suicide. In D. Lester & J. L. Rogers (Eds.), *Suicide: A global issue, Vol. 2, Prevention* (pp. 209–218). Santa Barbara, CA: Praeger.

THOSE WHO SURVIVED: COLIN WILSON

Colin Wilson, a writer and existential philosopher, decided to kill himself when he was sixteen. His father had thwarted Wilson's desire to attend college and become a scientist, so he went to work in a wool-processing factory to help support his family. Even though he was exhausted at the end of each day, Wilson became a voracious reader. He read a play by George Bernard Shaw in which a character described his search for meaning. Wilson had never given the topic much thought, but, upon reflection, he realized that he had no sense of purpose. This insight reinforced Wilson's thoughts about suicide.

When visiting his old school to borrow some books, Wilson encountered his former headmaster, who arranged for him to become a laboratory assistant at a nearby college. Wilson was pleased to escape the factory, but he soon realized that he had lost his desire to become a scientist. Still, working in the chemistry laboratory enabled him to take classes and continue his daily reading. One day in the laboratory, Wilson noticed a bottle of hydrochloric acid. He knew that a swig would kill him in a few seconds. He removed the stopper and inhaled the distinctly almond smell.

At that moment, a strange event took place. Wilson wrote, "I became two people. I was suddenly conscious of this teenage idiot called Colin Wilson, with his misery and frustration, and he seemed such a limited fool that I could not have cared less whether he killed himself or not. But if he killed himself, he would kill me, too. For a moment I felt that I was standing beside him and telling him that if he didn't get rid of this habit of self-pity he would never amount to anything."

Wilson continued, "It was also as if this 'real me' had said to the teenager, 'Listen, you idiot, *think how much you'd be losing,*' and in that moment I glimpsed the marvelous, immense richness of reality, extending to distant horizons." Wilson put the stopper back on the bottle and went back to work, feeling "relaxed, light-hearted, and totally in control." Wilson now had a life purpose: to become a writer.

Wilson went on to develop a philosophy of existentialism that was fundamentally optimistic. In *The Outsider*, he discussed creative writers of the nineteenth century who were outsiders in one way or another. Many of them killed themselves or ended up in hospitals for the insane, unable to maintain their creative visions. But Wilson held that one need not wait for "peak experiences" to occur; one could discipline one's imagination to induce them, especially during times of boredom or despair. This "act of will," Wilson maintained, is the existentialist's answer to feelings of negativity. Learning how to generate it became the aim of his life. He was never allured by suicide again.[1]

Note

1. Wilson, C. (2004). *Dreaming to some purpose: An autobiography.* London: Random House.

SECTION II

Suicide in the Military

CHAPTER TEN

Daryl Paulson's Story

All the personal accounts in this book are authentic cases. Some will appear under the authors' names; others will use pseudonyms. This one is told by one of the authors of this book, Daryl Paulson.

Returning from Combat

Let me tell you about my experience returning from combat in South Vietnam. For those of us who survived the "'Nam," our day to leave the country finally came. We were going back to the "world"—a name we gave the United States—back home to round-eyed, friendly, warm, and affectionate women. Home to a world where the streets were paved and there were flush toilets, hot and cold running water, food other than C-rations, and plenty of cold beer.

When we boarded the commercial 707 jet and took off, we were singing, "We've got to get out of this place, if it's the last thing we ever do," by the rock group the Animals. We were so excited that tears were streaming from our eyes.

We flew directly to Okinawa. Even in our extremely dirty and smelly combat utilities (clothes worn in combat), we were relaxed and comfortable, for there were no more night ambushes, no more firefights, no more rockets and mortars attacks. I remember waking up startled, but remembering I was out of Vietnam, I relaxed—I even slept. We were ordered to turn in our combat clothes and to shave and get haircuts. We were able to keep our jungle boots—the ones we had worn for the thirteen months we were in Vietnam.

In Okinawa, I took steam baths to wash away all that I had experienced in Vietnam. It took three or four days to get everything ready for our flight to the United States. Then we boarded another 707 jet and headed home. I don't think there was anyone on the plane who was not incredibly happy. Alas, unknown to us, the biggest battles forced on us were the battles we were to face at home.

When our 707 landed in Southern California, I was secretly preparing for a hero's welcome. I think all of us reasoned that we would get a doubly strong welcome because we had fought, even without explicit government plans to win the war. For example, Congress or the president would decide to bomb North Vietnam one week but stop bombing the next. This on-again, off-again strategy had terrible effects on our morale. We wondered, "Why the hell are we here if our leaders cannot make up their minds whether to fight the war or bail out?" Given the unusually hard conditions, we now thought we would be rewarded.

As we walked out of the plane to our homecoming reception, I saw only *three* people waiting for us. That was it! They were Marine wives who had volunteered to serve cookies and Kool-Aid to us. Where was everyone else? Where were the women to welcome us home?

We were escorted to waiting military buses and driven to Camp Pendleton Marine Corps Base for discharge or reassignment. During the drive, some college-age people screamed obscenities at us and flipped us the bird. I can still remember them yelling something about us being "warmongers."

At Camp Pendleton, we were swiftly processed and bused to Los Angeles International Airport to schedule flights home. I went to a bar to have a couple of drinks while waiting for my flight. This was an especially big event for me. It was my first legal drink in the United States and in a bar, for now I was twenty-one. I felt like being friendly, so I tried to start a conversation with two women sitting next to me; they ignored me. Then I tried to talk to a couple of guys, but they, too, ignored me. I felt like a misfit. This is when I realized that no one cared that I had served in the Vietnam War.

The lack of concern for what I had been through was even apparent with my friends. Things were different now. I noticed that they not only did not care about the war but also that I was now different from these guys. They were caught up in being "cool" and contriving to attract women. I just did not care. I had seen too many people killed from my own unit as well as hundreds of North Vietnamese soldiers I had tried to kill in retribution. I had faced thirteen months of not knowing whether I would die that day. Now, to worry about my hair or a woman seemed petty and meaningless. To protect myself from the meaninglessness of this life, I found a friend that night—one who would keep me calm and mellow for the next two years. That friend was Budweiser beer.

The first several weeks back in the United States and adjusting to civilian life were hard on me, particularly when I had to describe the Vietnam experience to my friends. I thought to myself, "How could I describe that *hell* in words?" I felt anger, frustration, fear, and hate all welling up inside of me. I felt like beating the table in utter frustration, but instead I calmly took another drink of beer. I said, "It was really bad," and left it at that. But I knew—not only consciously but in the center of my being—that something was terribly and painfully wounded within me. My friend did not really care. He was more interested in collecting information to support his anti-war beliefs. For me, however, it was different. He had opened a huge wound inside me. I recalled the men from my unit who were killed: John O., John B., José, Peter, Jocko, Fraize, Rocko, Lieutenant Smith, Pork Chops, and Glen. What had they died for? They died for nothing. I took another drink of beer . . . and another . . . and another.

Other combat veterans had similar experiences. Joey, for example, went back to college and his fraternity when he returned. He found, however, that he was no longer wanted. The fraternity brothers no longer wished to associate with him. He was "flawed." He was a Vietnam veteran. He could not deal with that, so he ended it by shooting himself in the head.

Art, a fellow Marine Corps combat veteran and the person I went to boot camp with, went to college. He suppressed the entire Vietnam experience and never spoke a word about it to his nonmilitary friends. He found that he was harboring tremendous amounts of guilt. To compensate, he tried to be all things to all people—the best, most caring friend to both the women and the men he knew. In the process, however, he denied his own needs. He put on a good show, but his inner conflict was betrayed by his ever-present need for a drink: R&R—rest and recreation—on the rocks.

As Art continued to avoid himself and his inner needs, his guilt and inner conflict became worse. He compensated by being even nicer to the people he knew. Finally, under this self-imposed pressure, school became too much of a burden for him. He dropped out, left the country, and went to live in Cozumel, Mexico. There, Art began to question his involvement in Vietnam. Had he screwed up? What if he had not gone to defend the country? What if he had been wrong? He assuaged those questions with even more alcohol.

Art was not alone in this introspection. I think all of us combat veterans shared a sense of condemnation. We felt a kind of deep guilt, which sent terror to the very core of our being. If we had been wrong about the war, were we not like Nazi criminals? Was there really a reason to keep on living? How could we live with ourselves, having seen and experienced all the brutalities of war and survived, only to realize that our involvement served no positive purpose?

I sensed the overt damage within myself. I realized something was very wrong with me. I remembered fantasizing about how warm and caring I would be when I got back from Vietnam. I would find that special woman and devote my life to our relationship. The entire time I was in Vietnam, I thought to myself how nice it would be to be held by a warm, loving woman, to watch her laugh and smile. I fantasized over and over about what it would be like.

Instead, I found that I did not really like to be with women; they made me nervous. To be held by a woman made me feel very vulnerable. Instead of feeling good, I felt terribly sad and afraid in her arms. It was almost like being a little boy again, in need of a mother to hug away my pain. But I was twenty-one years old, too old to need a mother figure. Since these vulnerable feelings, I thought, were a sign of my weak character, I began avoiding any emotional closeness with women.

I did find that I could get physically close to a woman when I drank alcohol. Drinking made relationships with women much easier; I did not feel vulnerable and could use them for sexual gratification. After all, what was a woman for except to have sex with? Many other veterans with whom I talked shared this experience. In fact, our new motto became, "Find them, feel them, f*** them, forget them." We had to distance ourselves from any meaningful emotional encounter with women because we felt that we could not share with them what we had experienced. How could you tell your girlfriend what it was like for you to shoot another human being? How could you tell her how vulnerable and scared you had felt, never knowing, the whole time you were in Vietnam, whether you would live another hour? How could you tell her what it was like to kick dead NVA soldiers because you were so angry at them for killing your friends? I was afraid to tell any woman what it was like.

How could I tell her about the horror I felt watching a dump truck taking the corpses of seventeen of my friends to be embalmed? How could I tell her what I felt when I watched their blood drip and flow from the tailgate onto the ground? How could I tell her how deeply I hurt, of the agony I was in, how gnawing my suffering was? How could I tell her that the pain and guilt followed me like a beast tracking its prey? How could I tell her that the pain hounded me at night, during the day, and even while making love? What would she think of me if I told her? I feared that if any woman knew this about me, she would freak out, go into convulsions, vomit, and totally reject me for being such a disgusting human being. What was I to do? I did what seemed best: I kept it to myself, and I drank and drank and drank.

So did most of the other veterans I knew, and because we drank so much and so often—while pretending it was partying—it was hard for others to recognize it as a way of masking our own pain. But, God, it was.

I was getting worse and worse. Then, one day, it happened. I had an anxiety attack. I was sitting in an accounting class when I suddenly felt as though I were dying. My heart began to pound; I was becoming dizzy, and my eyes would not focus. I began gasping for breath and sweating profusely. I began to freak out. I walked out of class, pretending everything was okay, and went immediately to the student health service. The doctor who examined me could find nothing wrong. To me, this meant that something very serious was wrong. I began to relive feelings of being near death, as I had in Vietnam. This totally confused me. It was the beginning of my post-traumatic stress disorder (PTSD).

I suffered five more panic attacks before the doctor sent me to a psychiatrist. I did not relish the idea of having mental problems, but I needed to be spared this new form of suffering. The psychiatrist disinterestedly asked me what my symptoms were. I told him, and he prescribed two kinds of tranquilizers as well as an antidepressant and told me to take it easy. That was the last thing I could think of doing, I was so distraught with my life. I tried, though. I tried to enjoy target shooting with my .22 rifle, but I began to physically shake so badly while aiming that I could not shoot. Shooting had been my favorite pastime, and now it was gone.

I tried to go on relaxing picnics with my friends, but I became too uneasy, even with the tranquilizers, to enjoy the picnic. I kept feeling that someone—the enemy—was hidden in the trees, stalking me, just as I had felt in Vietnam. At times, I became so tense and anxious on the picnics that I had to drink a couple of belts of whiskey just to get through the ordeal.

No fear was worse than the fear I felt during thunderstorms. Even though I knew thunder was caused by lightning, the sound of thunder and the bright flash of lightning sent me right back to Vietnam. It felt as if I were undergoing a rocket or mortar attack. I would drop to the ground to protect myself from the incoming rounds.

Other veterans I have talked to reported similar experiences. They have had panic attacks when a fire alarm is set off, when a helicopter flies over them, or when hearing firecrackers on the Fourth of July. This period is pure hell for combat veterans. Initially, upon our return, we expected to have gained some positive feelings from our Vietnam experiences. We found instead that the quality of our lives was slipping fast, especially as we began to experience panic with benign events.

For the returning Vietnam combat veteran, there was nothing of value that he could share. There was only pain, remorse, and anguish. Instead of being treated as the hero, he was shunned by his friends for being a veteran; he was shunned by the World War II and Korean veterans for losing the war, by the hippies for being a warmonger, and by himself for allowing himself to be duped by his country. Vietnam was not a war to save the enslaved Vietnamese people; it was not fought to protect America. It was a cruel joke and a cruel turn of fate for the veterans who fought it. It seemed just one more thing that they had screwed up in their lives.

Faced with the realization that there was no positive meaning to be found in my participation in Vietnam, I was thrown into an existential crisis. My entire world was collapsing. I could only suffer and drink, and suffer and drink, and suffer and drink. My world continued to fall apart, as I realized and felt to my core that my involvement in the war had been for no positive purpose. Over and over in my mind, I lamented how I had trusted the government, and it had betrayed me. Over and over, I asked myself, how could the politicians have done this to us?

Plagued with guilt, I tried to find a place where I could go for forgiveness, to get away from this hell. I felt too guilty to go to God and church, for I had killed, I had injured, and I had tortured my fellow human beings with intense delight. No, I could not go to God or church, for I had too much blood on my hands. I reasoned that no one wanted me now, not even God, for I had killed His children. Faced with the fact that other guys had been killed and not me, I felt extremely guilty. I saw no reason why I should be alive when they had died.

I felt completely alone and totally isolated. I lived in an alien world with which I could not communicate. I did not fit in with the other college students, because I was a Vietnam veteran, but I did not fit in with the military either. I spent a little of my time studying, but mostly I drank to assuage the pain of life's all-too-obvious meaninglessness. The recurring visions and dreams of the killing I had seen and the killing I had done began to intensify. I could not stop visualizing and reliving the emotional scenes of my comrades' deaths. Even the alcohol was not taking the edge off. I could not sleep, and I could not bear the pain of being awake. I could only suffer and hurt and despair over the meaninglessness and aloneness I endured, but even these were not as painful as the guilt.

One night, I looked at my loaded .38-caliber revolver with perverse pleasure, thinking that I could end it all. My suffering would be over in a flash, and I would have the last laugh. One 158-grain hollow-point in my brain, and it would all be over. But, as I looked at my gun, I thought about the biblical Job's suffering and how it had been for a purpose. Then I thought about my comrades who had been killed and the despair they would feel if there was no one to tell their story. I started to cry, deciding then to stay drunk until I found a therapist who could help me. For the next year and a half, I remained mostly drunk. Incredibly, though, I finished college and went to work for my father. Even more incredibly, I got married. However, the marriage made me feel guilty because I did not fully love the woman. I had no feelings left inside; I was a hollow hole of a human being.

I finally found the therapist I needed, one who not only knew psychotherapy but who cared about me as a person. This match is essential to save lives of suicide-prone veterans. It saved mine.

Takeaway Points

- In recent U.S. wars, more veterans have died of suicide than in combat, especially the wars that followed Vietnam.
- With the right therapist, psychotherapy can save lives of suicide-prone veterans.

CHAPTER ELEVEN

Hard-Earned Insights from Combat Experience

In chapter 10, Daryl Paulson describes his own experience in Vietnam and how the PTSD that resulted brought him close to suicide. In this chapter, he presents what he learned from that ordeal. In retrospect, he would like to share these insights with our readers.

Paulson's Schema

Now I believe that I understand how suicide ideation in Vietnam War combat veterans can occur. I have developed a schema (explanatory theory):

1. Immaturity,
2. The overwhelming of the psyche through combat experiences,
3. The lack of close ties to assist healing,
4. The worsening of the sense of guilt, and
5. The feeling that there is no way out.

Immaturity

In the Vietnam War, the basic service member was between eighteen and twenty years of age, at which point the brain is not fully mature. In addition, many service members had not developed their social skills fully because they had stressors at home. Perhaps they did not have enough love, were immature in handling their relationships, were trying to get attention by fitting in, or needed to escape a difficult economic situation. They did not have an authentic, well-integrated sense of self; that is, they did not know who they were, what direction to take in life, what their values were, or where they were going. Nevertheless, their hormones were raging. They needed a sense of purpose—and perhaps a sense of adventure—so they enlisted in the military.

Overwhelming Psychological Experience of Combat

When young people are thrown into combat, they find out how temporary life is. They witness other people, including friends, being killed and wounded. They may kill some enemy soldiers themselves. They are shot at and have mortars and rockets explode nearby. Many of their activities are reduced to the level of survival. In Vietnam, they had to serve in combat for at least twelve to thirteen months, depending on which branch of the service they were in. Later, soldiers served for a period of six to eight months, returned home for a few weeks, and then went back into combat for another six months.

Lack of Closeness

As children, we usually have a close attachment with our parents. Without their support, a part of us dies, physically or emotionally. When we are teenagers, we start to separate from our parents to form a close, even intimate, relationship with another person, usually of the opposite sex. We build friendships. We intend to remain in those relationships our whole life, or at least for long periods of time. But combat soldiers have had such feelings of emotional closeness drummed out of them in boot camp. When they went into combat and witnessed good friends being killed, they narrowed their concern to survive. They developed a new type of emotional closeness with their buddies, one focused on doing their duty while staying alive.

When they return, they find it very difficult to get close to another person, especially someone who has little idea of the ordeal they went through. As a result, they usually find it difficult to relate to fellow workers and students. Veterans have difficulty in shifting from combat experience to everyday civilian life. Typically, they do not discuss their combat experience with nonmilitary peers. Combat veterans often feel isolated and separate, lacking social support. Many have some form of PTSD and have trouble securing a stable job and housing.

Sense of Guilt

Veterans who survived the war feel lucky that they did so, but sometimes they have "survivor's guilt," which is extremely taxing. In combat, the entire fire team or squad or company often felt incredibly close to death, which spurred the term "band of brothers." Each soldier depended on the others to get him or her through this ordeal. When they survive and others do not, they often feel guilty, perhaps thinking, "The other soldiers gave their lives for me." This gets increasingly worse as time goes by. For example, when they get married, they may feel guilty because their best buddy is dead and cannot get married. The guilt often becomes so overpowering that they drink and take drugs to ease the pain.

No Way Out

The combination of immaturity, psychic trauma, lack of closeness in civilian life, and a sense of guilt may eventually overwhelm many combat veterans. It may feel as if there is no way out of their hopeless situation, so suicide becomes the only viable option.

Background

In his article "More Veterans Commit Suicide Than Were Killed in Vietnam," John Ketwig suggests that the biggest battles faced by these young men were the battles they faced at home.[1] This article is one of several that drew people's attention to the Vietnam veterans' plight.

The PBS TV series *The Vietnam War* forced us to recall those times. The names of 58,315 combat veterans are etched into the Vietnam Veterans Memorial Wall in Washington, DC. Not appearing among those names are the larger number of veterans who have committed suicide since returning from Vietnam.

Combat veterans' suicides have become more common and prevalent since the Vietnam War, rising at an alarming rate since the wars in Iraq and Afghanistan began. The Centers for Disease Control and Prevention (CDC) found that the risk of suicidal thoughts increases dramatically between the ages of thirty-five and sixty-four. It appears that the average suicide rate is 13.7–17.6 per 100,000 people. In veterans, these figures are significantly higher.[2]

Since 2001, about two million soldiers have been deployed to Afghanistan and Iraq. Upon returning to the United States, most do not look for outside assistance for their PTSD. When the Vietnam veterans were shunned by American society, too many of them felt rejected and cast aside. In my opinion, the Veterans Administration (VA) failed miserably by not helping most of these individuals. I feel that the VA has been unresponsive to the rise in suicide rates in the aftermath of the wars in Iraq and Afghanistan and ignored the alarming connection between PTSD and suicide. People who experience PTSD are 5.7 times more likely than others to take their lives.

In 2013, the VA released a study that covered suicides from 1999 to 2010. It showed that about twenty-two veterans committed suicide every day, or one every sixty-five minutes. More recently, the VA found the suicide rate among veterans to be about thirty per one hundred thousand veterans per year, compared with the yearly civilian rate of about fourteen per one hundred thousand.[3]

Despite these sobering figures, the National Institutes of Health has only spent about $70 million on suicide research in recent years. It spends ten times that amount on cancer research, even though cancer kills fewer people than suicide. In the meantime, suicide and suicide attempts cost the U.S. economy about $100 billion per year, most of it in lost productivity. There are also massive psychological costs. For example, there is so much stigma associated with suicide that families will often cover up the fact and invent another cause of death. The American Association for Suicidology and other professional organizations are attempting to reduce this stigma, but it remains entrenched, notably in the military.[4]

Causes

The U.S. Department of Veterans Affairs discovered that veterans are more likely to develop symptoms of PTSD for reasons that include the following:

- Spending a longer amount of time in combat
- Having a lower level of education
- Undergoing more severe combat conditions
- Knowing other soldiers around them who were killed
- Having a brain or head trauma
- Being female

For many service members, being away from home for long periods of time can cause problems at home or work, which adds to the stress. This may be even more so for National Guard and Reserve troops who had not expected to be deployed for a long duration. Almost half of those who have served in the current wars have been in the National Guard or Reserves.[5]

Other Contributing Factors

Many combat veterans have difficulty transitioning back to civilian life. Many use their G.I. Bill or other education benefits, which often facilitate their return. However, the pursuit of education among veterans can aid in the transition to civilian life or, by contrast, aggravate postservice conditions linked to a higher likelihood of suicide. Veterans pursuing education, utilizing the post-9/11 G.I. Bill, are more likely to have protective factors related to socialization and reintegration than those who are not. They are characterized by the following:

- Difficulty relating to fellow students
- Difficulty in coping with their military experiences in an academic environment
- Lack of support or understanding of service-connected disabilities
- Negative stigmas related to military service
- Feelings of isolation
- Feelings of separation
- Lack of social support
- Difficulty establishing a stable or reliable income

Although higher education can pose many difficulties for returning veterans, research studies indicate that veterans often benefit from transitioning from the military into higher education. College often requires student veterans to work and interact with classmates. Most academic institutions have student veteran organizations and resource centers specifically designed to aid military veterans. Military education benefits, primarily the post-9/11 G.I. Bill, pay for tuition and provide a housing stipend to student veterans. Education benefits often give them an income, a goal to reach, and socialization opportunities with the general population.

So that is my story and my overview of the information that has been collected by government agencies relevant to the allure of suicide and the difficulty resisting that allure.

Takeaway Points

- Daryl Paulson used his combat experience in Vietnam to develop an explanatory schema to account for veterans' suicides.
- Veterans often have difficulty returning to civilian life; too many of them think that suicide is the only way out.
- Funding for research is hard to obtain, despite the seriousness of the problem.

Notes

1. Ketwig, J. (2019, February 21). More veterans commit suicide than were killed in Vietnam. *Roanoke Times.* https://www.roanoke.com/opinion/ commentary /ketwig-more-veterans-commit-suicide-than-were-killed-in-vietnam/article _2d841f24-c167-50bd-9e0b-02e42feb98d1.html.

2. Jakupcak, M., Cook, J., Imel, Z., et al. (2009). Posttraumatic stress disorder as a risk factor for suicidal ideation in Iraq and Afghanistan War veterans. *Journal of Traumatic Stress, 22,* 303–306.

3. Pilkington, E. (2014, May 23). US military struggling to stop suicide epidemic among war veterans. *The Guardian*.

4. Carney, J. (2014, April 13). Why are so many older veterans committing suicide? *National Journal*.

5. Nicks, D. (2014, January 10). Report: Suicide rate soars among young vets. *Time*.

CHAPTER TWELVE

The Parking Lot Suicides

Daryl Paulson is not alone. Military veterans returning from combat zones often face problems that are unjust compensation for their service: physical injuries, difficulty finding jobs and housing, and, worst of all, traumatic memories, stress, and learned responses that can lead to PTSD.

Over a century ago, the first expert on suicide, Émile Durkheim, recognized one psychological aspect of this risk.

> Émile Durkheim, the great sociologist, theorised as to why suicide is so common among military personnel—not simply because of the devastating effects of war, or because of their easy access to weapons, but because of the depersonalising effect of army training: "Military esprit can only be strong if the individual is self-detached, and such detachment necessarily throws the door open to suicide."[1]

The term *self-detached* sounds like a prerequisite for making it possible to commit acts of war—and to suffer ill effects afterward.

In 2019, a veteran killed himself outside the Veteran Affairs medical center in Cleveland, the fourth veteran suicide at a VA facility that month. The Cleveland death happened outside the facility's emergency room, one of several that have taken place in a VA parking lot, likely as a protest against lack of treatment or inadequate treatment by the VA.[2] These veterans were probably in pain, feeling that the VA was their last source of help. When they were put on a long waiting list or treated in a perfunctory manner, they may have turned to suicide as a form of protest.

A Parking Lot Suicide in Minnesota

Justin Miller was a thirty-three-year-old Marine Corps veteran who checked himself into the Minneapolis Department of Veterans Affairs hospital early in 2018. After spending four days in the mental health unit, he walked to his truck in the VA parking lot and shot himself. Shortly after his death, Miller's parents received a package from the VA; it included bottles of antidepressants and sleep aids prescribed to Miller to treat his PTSD.[3]

Miller's death was one of several that had occurred within a year in the parking lot of campuses, hospitals, or other VA facilities. A Marine colonel, Jim Turner, wearing his uniform and medals, sat on top of his VA records and killed himself outside a Florida VA office. He left a note commenting about the 22 military suicides reported per day, Turner's relatives claimed that he was unable to get the appointment he wanted with a mental health specialist. Even so, the VA claimed that it had prevented 233 suicide attempts within that same span of time.[4]

Nine million people, amounting to 62 percent of veterans and their families, depend on the VA for medical care. Obtaining that care can be frustrating because veterans are often asked to demonstrate that their injuries were connected to their service duties. An independent assessment of VA services by the RAND Corporation concluded that VA mental health care can be as good as or better than private health care plans, but there is a great variation across facilities. The Minnesota VA where Miller shot himself did not properly check out his access to firearms or schedule follow-up appointments.

Six Medications and Ten Prescriptions

Some specialists have proposed that these suicides were a way of protesting a system that had failed veterans. John Toombs, an Afghanistan War veteran, hanged himself on the grounds of a VA medical center in Tennessee. He had enrolled in a program to treat his PTSD, depression, and substance abuse, but he was asked to leave because he did not follow instructions, such as the timely pickup of his medications. Shortly before he took his life, he wrote on his Facebook page that he was "feeling empty." He added, "I dared to dream again. Then you showed me the door faster than last night's garbage." Toombs took a video just before he hanged himself, saying, "I came for help, and they threw me out like a stray dog in the rain." A nurse at the facility believed that Toombs's death could have been prevented.[5]

Toombs had served as the man riding on the back of a convoy in Afghanistan, watching for anyone who posed a threat to his team. When he returned home, his father said the change was so drastic that he found it difficult to recognize his son. "He just wasn't the same person. He said, for him, the main thing was being helpless and hopeless. If he was in a position that felt helpless and hopeless, that's when it kicked in the worst." Toombs's father added that getting released by the drug rehabilitation program was one of those "helpless and hopeless times." At the time of his death, Toombs had six medications in his system that listed suicidal thoughts as a side effect.

When questioned about this, the VA defended their procedures. However, Sergeant Allen Chapman, who served with Toombs and who lives with PTSD himself, told a reporter that this had not been his experience. "I can go to the VA and request a certain medication and there's no questions asked." Chapman claimed that his ten current prescriptions are refilled without any discussion regarding how they make him feel.

An article in the *Washington Post* about the "parking lot suicides" stated that veterans are 1.5 times as likely as civilians to die by suicide, after adjusting for age and gender. The veteran suicide rate was 26.1 per 100,000 compared with 17.4 per 100,000 of civilian deaths. Every year since 2008, there have been over 6,000 reported veteran suicides.[6]

A Parking Lot Suicide in Massachusetts

Not all parking lot suicides are forms of protest again an institution. Sometimes a parking lot is simply a convenient site for the last private act of someone's life. That was the case when a teenager in Massachusetts decided to commit suicide in a Kmart parking lot.[7]

Michelle Carter and Conrad Roy III were teenagers with mental health problems; both had attended therapy. Conrad had been on his high school's honor roll and was an all-around athlete. They kept in touch by phone calls, e-mails, and texts. Although early messages showed that Michelle had encouraged Conrad to return to therapy and not think about killing himself, her later texts advocated suicide, describing how he should do it. For example, she wrote, "It's probably the best time now because everyone's sleeping. Just go somewhere in your truck. And no one's really out right now because it's an awkward time. If you don't do it now, you're never gonna do it."

At the time of his death, he had been taking Celexa, which carries a warning that it may increase suicidal thoughts and behaviors for young people. In 2014, Conrad died in a Kmart parking lot after inhaling carbon monoxide produced by a water pump in his truck. Michelle was in constant contact with him in the hours leading up to his death, talking him out of his doubts, point by point. The final step was when Conrad got out of his truck and called her. She told him to get back in. In her indictment, the grand jury charged her with "wantonly and recklessly" assisting Conrad's suicide.

A psychiatrist testified that Michelle's behavior was a result of "involuntary intoxication" from antidepressants first prescribed when she was fourteen. Nevertheless, she was convicted of involuntary manslaughter and served a fifteen-month prison sentence.

The last therapist Conrad saw practiced cognitive behavioral therapy, which has a solid record of success. However, the time Conrad spent with this therapist was minimal in comparison with Michelle's onslaught of phone calls, texts, and e-mails. In his younger years, Conrad had endured physical and emotional abuse from his father and grandfather. He had made an unsuccessful suicide attempt when his parents divorced. Conrad's stellar high school record gained him admission to the college of his choice, but he had decided not to attend. Michelle entered the picture, showering Conrad with affection and attention. Conrad's vulnerability, perhaps abetted by prescription drugs, made him an easy target for Michelle's taunts. Shortly after Conrad's death, Kmart closed its parking lot.

Takeaway Points

- The suicide site often provides clues to the suicider's motive. At other times, it is simply the most convenient location.
- Many suicide-prone people take dangerous prescription drugs, despite the fact that their packages state that suicidal thoughts may be a side effect.
- There are limits to a bully's right to free speech when a vulnerable target's life is at stake.

Notes

1. Francis, G. (2019, November 22). What I have learned from my suicidal patients. *The Guardian* (online).

2. Slack, D. (2019, April 30). Veteran dies by suicide outside Cleveland VA hospital Monday, lawmakers demand action. *USA Today.*

3. Britton, P. C., Bohnert, K. M., Ilgen, M. A., et al. (2017). Suicide mortality among male veterans discharged from Veterans Health Administration acute psychiatric units from 2006 to 2010. *Social Psychiatry and Psychiatric Epidemiology, 52,* 1081–1087.

4. Ibid.

5. Jacob, K. (2019, February 18). Study shows drug commonly prescribed to veterans could be making suicidal thoughts worse. *Fox News* (online).

6. Wax-Thibodaux, E. (2019, February 7). The parking lot suicides. *Washington Post* (online).

7. *CBS News.* (2017, August 3). Texting suicide case: Michelle Carter sentenced to serve at least 15 months. (online).

CHAPTER THIRTEEN

An Integrative Treatment of PTSD

Bart Billings, a licensed clinical psychologist, presented a unique and compelling perspective in February 2010, when he testified before the U.S. Congressional Veterans Affairs Committee. His topic? How the use—rather, the misuse—of psychiatric medications for treating post-traumatic combat stress plays a major role in military suicides.[1]

Billings had been working in the field of mental health for half a century. He had spent over three decades in the U.S. Army as both an enlistee and a commanding officer, reaching the rank of colonel. After retiring from the army, Billings founded the Annual International Military and Civilian Stress Conference, bringing together experts and survivors to discuss important issues such as suicide. Holding that post-traumatic stress was a normal reaction to an abnormal experience, he rephrased Viktor Frankl's statement that an abnormal response to an abnormal situation is normal behavior.[2] Billings draws upon his own personal experience to explain how the resulting post-traumatic *stress* can usher in PTSD.

In addition to his military service and years of counseling veterans, Billings did considerable research on PTSD. He discovered that some widely used medications did no better than placebos in reducing the symptoms of PTSD and related disorders and that effective psychotherapy was more successful. "Talk therapy," he maintained, establishes involvement, caring, and trust, which the client can apply to social situations. Billings designed an integrative wellness program combining individual and group talk therapy, career counseling, nutrition, exercise, sports, and yoga—but no medication.

Reviewing the research on military and veteran suicides, Billings discovered that prescription drugs were involved in one-third of the cases. And contrary to the opinion that soldier suicide results from the stress of war, 85 percent of military suicides had never seen combat, and 51 percent had not even been deployed. When Billings contacted a historian who had been studying prisoners of war in Vietnam, he was told that of the eight hundred survivors he had studied, seventy-two died in captivity, but none from suicide. Billings attributed this statistic to the fact that the prisoners of war were not administered brain-altering medications while in captivity.[3]

Billings was pleasantly surprised in 2015 when the House Committee on Veterans Affairs Subcommittee on Oversight and Investigations held a hearing on prescription mismanagement and veteran suicide. This group was reacting to the skyrocketing opiate prescriptions, finding thirty-three unexpected deaths at just one facility for veterans. Billings was frustrated by the responses offered by representatives of the VA. They seemed concerned but were not providing answers, giving only short, concise statements. They also refused requests for information made by members of Congress until they were reminded that Congress has every right to that information. These representatives appeared to employ what the military calls SERE: survival, evasion, restraint, and escape tactics taught to service members to prepare them in case they are captured. The subcommittee members were not in enemy hands, but they behaved as if they were.

The Military "Family"

Billings believes that the military needs to bring more of a family structure into its ranks. In the basic military organization, each squad consists of about a dozen soldiers. The squad leader could serve in a role analogous to an older sibling. The first sergeant resembles a mother, and the platoon leader is analogous to a father. The company commanders and battalion commanders take on grandparent-like roles. When a soldier wants to discuss her feelings about a brother lost in warfare, she might go to a physician "uncle." She may be treated warmly, or she may be told that her uncle is busy but will give her some medicine. For a while, this relieves the pain, but she eventually needs a more potent dose. Her siblings note that she is acting "stoned" or like a "zombie." So she sees another uncle, one who listens patiently to her story and helps her cope with the loss. She begins to feel better and is assisted by her siblings, who also mourn the loss of their brother.

Billings states, "This is how the military should be set up. Each member of the squad is aware of the other members of the squad." If the squad is close-knit, every member should be aware of every other member. This would even assist soldiers following deployment; if members of the "family" were deployed together, they could help each other make the transition to civilian life.

General James Mattis asked that families and neighbors of returning soldiers treat the veterans with respect and gratitude. Rather than viewing them as "damaged," the community should look for ways that the military service equipped these men and women with unique potentials. They learned a great deal through their potentially traumatizing circumstances and can make valuable contributions in civilian life.[4] There are several first-person accounts of harrowing military service that eventually ended in transformations.[5]

Changing Rates

Suicide rates in the military were lower than those in the general population until 2005, but they surpassed the civilian rate in 2008, according to the Army Suicide Prevention Task Force. The task force discussed the role of substance abuse in many of these suicides, reporting that 29 percent of active duty suicides between 2005 and 2009 involved alcohol or drugs. In 2009, almost one-third involved prescription drugs, higher than in the general population. The abuse of prescription drugs is involved in one out of three army suicides. This statistic came as no surprise to Billings, as the use of brain-altering medication in the military increased almost 700 percent from 2005 to 2011.[6] If one looks at the list of possible dangers accompanying these drugs, one will note that the first warning is "suicidality." This may be an example of truth in advertising.

Soldiers having suicidal thoughts tend to be younger than thirty and have legal problems, failed romantic relationships, or medical issues. A U.S. medical school studied soldiers on their first tour of duty. Those most at risk were early in their career, were younger, had a previous mental health problem, and were female.[7]

In recent wars, severely injured soldiers are more likely to survive than in previous wars, albeit with injuries, especially to the brain. A traumatic brain injury (TBI) can be detected by a brain scan when there is noticeable tissue damage and noticeable impairment in behavior, such as motor difficulties or problems maintaining balance or coordination. Soldiers with TBI are four times as likely to commit suicide as those without this diagnosis. In wars in the Middle East, deaths and injuries due to improvised explosive devices (IEDs) are unusually high. These survivors are often referred for psychiatric help because of such symptoms as depression, forgetfulness, and frustration. Billings notes that psychiatrists, who are not necessarily experts in brain injuries, are likely to prescribe medication. Brain-altering medications, according to Billings, should not be the immediate intervention in most cases of TBI or automatically prescribed for post-traumatic stress.

Billings advocates greater use of physiatrists, who are practitioners of physical medicine and rehabilitation. They specialize in the treatment of brain and spinal cord injury, muscular diseases, injuries due to diabetes and strokes, and aftereffects of gunshot wounds and burns. They collaborate with rehabilitation therapists, speech therapists, occupational therapists, and nurses knowledgeable about prosthetics. They often make referrals to specialists in such mind-body treatments as biofeedback, neurofeedback, relaxation training, and hypnosis—none of which require brain-altering medicines.

These practitioners have studied the autonomic nervous system (ANS), a division of the peripheral nervous system that influences the function of the internal bodily organs. The ANS regulates specific body functions, including heart rate, digestion, respiratory rate, pupillary response, urination, and sexual arousal. It is the primary mechanism in charge of the flight-or-fight response. To introduce brain-altering medication into this delicately balanced system, according to Billings, is to risk doing more harm than good.

Billings is among those who have identified the dangers of a drug cocktail that combines the antidepressant Paxil, the antipsychotic Seroquel, and the benzodiazepine Klonopin (used to treat anxiety). This cocktail is regularly prescribed by VA psychiatrists, even though several veterans who returned from Iraq with PTSD died in their sleep after taking it.[8]

Integrative Treatment for PTSD

What would Billings advocate instead of overreliance on psychiatric medication? He and his associates have developed a wellness program that includes the following:

1. A complete physical examination;
2. A plan for psychological, social, and vocational counseling;
3. An individually tailored wellness program that includes exercise, biofeedback, yoga, relaxation exercises, breathing exercises, guided imagery, nutrition, vocational planning, and spiritual counseling;
4. Regular meetings with specialists; and
5. Evaluation to determine whether medication is needed and, if so, what type.

Billings found hypnosis to be very effective in treating PTSD. With hypnosis, clients can be taught how to relax, concentrate, and block out distractions. Clients can even be taught self-hypnosis to reinforce suggestions. Progressive relaxation and deep abdominal breathing can help decrease physical and mental tensions.

Meditation is the self-regulation of one's attention. Tai Chi and Qigong are moving meditations; the person does not have to sit still for long periods but instead moves slowly in sequences of postures. In guided imagery, a partner or healing professional acts as a gentle director of attention using visual images. Veterans can learn how to place their trauma in a mental "compartment" separate from their everyday experiences.[9]

An American Sniper

Medicine alone cannot help at-risk soldiers and veterans.[10] Although they have not focused on PTSD, as Billings has, Peter Breggin,[11] a psychiatrist; Gary Greenberg,[12] a clinical psychologist; and Henry Bauer,[13] a biochemist, have pointed out the dangers of overprescribing what Billings calls "brain-altering medication," what Greenberg calls "mind-altering medication," and what Breggin refers to as "mood-altering medication" created by "Big Pharma," the pharmaceutical companies that manufacture them.

Critics of Big Pharma claim that these drugs do not always have the effects claimed for them. Moreover, among the potential side effects listed on the packaging are suicide, violence, and criminal activity. Breggin criticizes the misuse of some psychiatrists' favorite drugs: Prozac, Paxil, Zoloft, Adderall, Ritalin, Concerta, Xanax, and Zyprexa. As we have noted before, nondrug interventions such as hypnosis can attain similar results without the potential side effects. Bauer observes that, if there is a "wonder drug," it is the placebo, the positive effect of patients' expectations and suggestions when given a substance by a practitioner they trust.[14] A reasonable critic would not ban all mind-altering medications but would caution against their indiscriminate use.

Billings's perspective is provocative and worth considering, especially when applied to specific cases. Chris Kyle was a Navy SEAL and war hero; the book and movie *American Sniper* were based on his life. After saving many American lives and killing numerous adversaries in Iraq, Kyle returned home to help veterans at the local VA hospital. He often took them to the local firing range, thinking that this form of active involvement would help them process some of their emotional issues.

One veteran, Eddie Ray Routh, diagnosed with PTSD, was among those whom Kyle and a friend took to a firing range. Without warning, Routh shot and killed them both. A week before the tragedy, Billings had been interviewed on the radio and asked whether veterans with a PTSD diagnosis should be allowed to purchase firearms. Billings replied absolutely not, especially if they were taking brain-altering medication. During Routh's trial, it was revealed that traces of both legal and illegal drugs had been found in his system. Perhaps the illegal drugs were partly to blame. But Billings does not think the risk of overusing prescription medication is worth it, and neither do we.

Restrictions on gun sales, such as background checks, could allow time for self-reflection and reconsideration. Jesse Bering, a communications scientist, observed that there is no better predictor of suicide than simply having access to a firearm. During a one-year study of California firearms sales, suicide was the leading cause of death, accounting for 25 percent of that group's fatalities. When women buy handguns, they are more likely than men to turn them on themselves. Of the deceased females in the California study, over half were suicide victims.[15]

Americans who live in states with high rates of household gun ownership are almost four times more likely to die by gun suicide than those in states where fewer households own guns. This relationship remains strong even when controlling for poverty, unemployment, serious mental illness, and substance abuse. Over a dozen studies on the topic indicate that having access to a firearm triples one's risk of death by suicide. This elevated risk applies not only to the gun owner but to everyone in the household.[16]

Takeaway Points

- The misuse of pharmaceutical medication can have negative side effects, including suicidal thoughts and suicide itself.
- At times, pharmaceutical medication can be part of an integrative program for treating soldiers and veterans with a PTSD diagnosis.

Notes

1. Billings, B. (2017). *Invisible scars: How to treat combat stress and PTSD without medication* (2nd ed.). New York: Paradies/Inspire, LLC.

2. Frankl, V. (2006). *Man's search for meaning.* Boston: Beacon Press.

3. The documentary *The Hidden Enemy: Inside Psychiatry's Covert Agenda* exposes the covert operation behind military suicides. http//www.cchr.org/documentaries/the-hidden-enemy.html.org.

4. Mattis, J. N. (2015, April 15). The meaning of their service. *Wall Street Journal.*

5. Seymour, A. (2016). *Psychedelic Marine.* Rochester, VT: Park Street Press.

6. Friedman, R. (2013, April 7). War on drugs. *New York Times,* Opinion (online).

7. Mozes, A. (2015, July 9). Newly enlisted army soldiers at risk of attempted suicide: Study. https://consumer.healthday.com/general-health-information-16/military-health-news-763/newly-enlisted-army-soldiers-at-risk-of-attempted-suicide-study-701176.html.

8. Tighman, A. (2010, May 26). Psychiatric drugs killing U.S. military vets in their sleep. *Marine Corps Times.*

9. Boscarino, J. A., & Figley, C. (2009). The impact of repression, hostility, and post-traumatic stress disorder on all-cause mortality: A prospective 16-year follow-up study. *Journal of Nervous & Mental Disease, 197*(6), 461–466.

10. Gordon, C. (2013, December 4). Why medicine alone can't help our veterans. *HuffPost.* https://www.huffingtonpost.com/chrisanna-gordon/why-medicine-alone-cant-help-our-veterans_b_4386587.html.

11. Breggin, P. B. (2008). *Medication madness: A psychiatrist exposes mood-altering medications*. New York: St. Martin's Press.

12. Greenberg, G. A. (2013). *The book of woe: The DSM and the unmaking of psychiatry*. New York: Blue Rider/Penguin.

13. Bauer, H. H. (2011). Medicine to make you mad. *Journal of Scientific Exploration, 25*, 351–363.

14. Shapiro, A., & Shapiro, E. (1997). *The powerful placebo: From ancient priest to modern physician*. Baltimore, MD: Johns Hopkins University Press.

15. Bering, J. (2019). *Suicidal: Why we kill ourselves*. Chicago: University of Illinois Press.

16. Everytown for Gun Safety. (2018, September 10). Firearm suicide in the United States. https://everytownresearch.org/firearm-suicide.

THOSE WHO SURVIVED: JIMMY STEWART

Academy Award–winning actor James "Jimmy" Stewart is beloved for his performance as George Bailey in *It's a Wonderful Life*. But did you know he served honorably, even heroically, in World War II? The Princeton graduate was already an experienced pilot, but he was rejected for being too old (thirty-two) and too thin to enlist. Nonetheless, Stewart persisted and joined the U.S. Army Air Forces. He was assigned safe stateside jobs: starring in recruiting films, training younger pilots, and attending rallies. In 1944, frustrated with this behind-the-scenes work, he asked to be transferred to war zones in Europe.

By now a captain (he ultimately retired as a brigadier general), Stewart flew dangerous combat missions over Germany, where so many fellow airmen were lost in battle that he was eventually grounded for being "flak happy," as they then called combat stress. After the war, he was depressed, could hardly focus or sleep, had nightmares, and refused to talk about his experiences in the war. Does this sound familiar? Today we call it post-traumatic stress disorder (PTSD).

Despite his condition and doubts, Stewart plunged back into his acting career. He drew upon his PTSD to enhance his darker roles in such films as *Rope, Rear Window,* and *Vertigo* as well as late scenes of *It's a Wonderful Life*.

Stewart was happily married for forty-five years and lived to the age of eighty-nine. He received honors for his military deeds, his acting skills, and his philanthropy.

SECTION III

Sexual Assault and Suicide

CHAPTER FOURTEEN

Two Cases of Sexual Assault

Sexual assault is an atrocious act that harms the victim in numerous ways, some of which are long-lasting. Sexual assault by a person in power can be especially devastating because the abused person often thinks that no one will believe him or her. Until recently, the victims were often right. Yolanda, whom we discussed in chapter 1 of this book, did not report her abuse by a well-known politician for this reason. We will open this section on sexual assault by telling our readers two poignant stories illustrating the dilemma faced by Yolanda.

The first account was written by Gail Hayssen, who allowed us to use her name. Gail was first sexually assaulted when she was fourteen. The aftereffects were still evident when she wrote this account in late 2018, several decades later.

Gail's Story: Trauma Hidden in My Body

I've spent the past four days in a fetal position. I'm just gradually coming out of it. I'm typing this with one finger. As painful as it is—as raw and vulnerable as I feel—I am still driven to write this.

I had never understood what post-traumatic stress disorder (PSTD) is. I think of my veteran friend Ed, who won't go out on the lake in my pontoon boat because of his combat experiences in Vietnam. They occurred fifty years ago. I have asked him so many times, "Come on, let's go out and cruise the lake—beauty, nature, wildlife. We'll have a great time." He always replies, "I'm busy."

But now I see a pattern. Something similar happens to me each time I have intense dental work. I realize how I've been protected from terrible pain by keeping it hidden in my body.

In my fifties, I was sedated for a wisdom-tooth extraction. As I came out of the dreamy state, I found no one in the room with me, and I was crying hysterically. I felt no pain in my mouth—but the pain in my entire body was debilitating. I was so weakened by intense emotions that it was hard to walk. My friend Kim and the secretary were the only ones in the waiting room. My sobbing had cleared the place. I didn't know what happened or why I was crying so much as Kim helped me to the car. As we drove home and the drugs started wearing off, my body became flooded with images of my first time in a dental chair for a root canal. And I remembered Leonard, the nice Bayside dentist who molested me.

I was fourteen and still a virgin, raised in a family by a dad who did not believe in medical or dental care. So I asked friends for help when my tooth had become so infected it abscessed. A nurse I met said her friend was a dentist, and he owed her a favor. I don't remember what Leonard used to sedate me. He was pulling my pants down around my firm young legs and shoving his hand up me, telling me it was important for him to check me out. After he sedated me, I don't know what happened.

A few years ago, I was preparing for work on the same tooth. I thought I might have a reaction again, so I met the dentist, described the problem, and explained that I needed gentle care when she redid the root canal. I was comforted to know that this was an office staffed by women. I thought they would be sensitive to my issue.

Instead, on the day of surgery, with my mouth propped open as she worked inside me, her focus was on dictating a text message to her assistant. I was in a room of people lined up like cattle, drooling with their mouths open. The dentist never asked how I was doing. There was no concern for the dental trauma I had experienced decades earlier.

My body held all the memory, the pain, the vision of the man who molested me. When I got out of the chair, I just ran out of that office and crumbled in the stairwell, crying my heart out. My husband came chasing after me. Again, I felt humiliated, unheard and unseen by these women, even after I had told them about my sexual-abuse dental history. I wrote a letter to their office explaining everything but never received any return calls or message—only a bill for a thousand dollars.

Last month, in my sixties, I needed a tooth extracted. I found myself in the kindest, most caring dental office ever, where my tooth was pulled out. I was only numbed, not sedated. It was as positive and pain-free an experience as you could ever want—and the valium to relax me beforehand certainly helped. I was laughing and joking as my husband assisted me to the car.

I figure, great. This is an amazingly positive experience. It's Tuesday at noon, and I'll go home, take meds, and go to sleep, hoping I will not have any excruciating tooth pain. Instead, I wake up paralyzed in pain. And just like before, it's not in my mouth. It's in my entire being—every muscle in my body screaming in pain. My heart hurts so much I just hold my hands over it, as if I could somehow give it the tender love and care it has not received. I am so overcome by the rage, anger, and deep guttural sobbing coming out of this four-foot, eleven-inch body that is Gail.

I'm lost in images and details of every #MeToo story my body holds. Molestations from a Hindu monk at the age of seven, him rubbing against my body and holding me so I cannot escape. Beatings from my father for eating ice cream. A mother who locks me in a dark dirty basement. A relationship with an abusive alcoholic. Images of men and women who have physically and mentally abused me throughout my life.

From Tuesday until Friday, I'm in a fetal position—my body crying out, sobbing, having no control when it surges up and overtakes me. Then I am so full of anger that I must break stuff and throw things until I snap inside, to let this old deep crap release itself where it hides deep in the cells of my inner body, despite years of psychotherapy, body therapy, meditations, retreats, and self-help. I don't want anyone to see me in this raw, vulnerable state. I get into a bathtub, knowing this can help calm me down.

As I lie in the tub feeling the warmth of the water, I'm enveloped in feelings of worthlessness. Visions of being raped with a gun to my head by someone I barely knew. Having my family say and do hurtful things, like keeping secret who my real mother was, having a sister raised as my cousin, the family denying this fact, and her refusing to accept me as her sister. Being betrayed by my family, being treated with no respect for my feelings, or even just ever including me with my brothers and sisters.

I have never heard the words *I am sorry for what happened to you. I should have protected you.* In this black hole, dark thoughts arise. I'm so hopeless, helpless, and alone; I can't grasp any reason for my life to go on. As a teenager, I was lost in that black hole. I was confused by all the lies, abandonment, and betrayal. I took aspirin and other pills, hoping to end my misery. Instead, I was terribly sick with stomach pain.

Ending my bath, I sit on my little stool, realizing these harmful thoughts are trying to take over my being. This old tape from my youth was back in my head. How dare these thoughts return, as if I were in this state of mind in my adult life.

For a year I've read constantly about famous people and their horror stories of men in places of power—their #MeToo stories. Let me tell you, this week's tooth removal taught me the power and the length of time represented by these violations to my body, these pains of family rejections, which are still rearing their ugly heads, no matter how much time, how much work, how much therapy, how much unconditional love I have received.

I never heard an apology from any of these men and women who hurt me as a child and adult. My father and mother told me those things were all my fault. My mother's miserable migraine headaches were my fault. The fact that men molested and raped me, my Dad says, was my fault. The fact that at fourteen I had to find a dentist to get out of pain was my fault—for eating candy.

This is what my body holds inside that I do not see. Instead, I make family Thanksgiving dinners for thirty years. I love and care for my father until he dies, waiting or hoping he will say, "I'm sorry." But he says nothing. I keep trying for years to connect to this sister-cousin and other family that I know of, but nothing positive or loving comes of it.

I let go of it all years ago. I'm no victim. It's made me stronger and more compassionate. I always forgive. And I still feel love for this father, this mother, this family. I have a wonderful, joyous, exciting life. I'm surrounded by loving family and friends in a beautiful, peaceful setting. But when the past comes up after a dental experience, the days that follow are like living in a hell fighting demons. I never want my three children to know even a minute of such painful mental and physical abuse.

When Ed comes by today, I am going to tell him I will never tease him or push him to go to the lake again. The lake, my happy place that brings me peace and serenity, could bring on the dental experience for him. It can turn from Lake Sonoma to the Mekong Delta.

Now I understand the true meaning of PTSD and how I could not function for four days even after a positive dental experience. These women who come forth are not exaggerating how these traumas affect their lives. From what I have experienced, it remains in the cells of the body.

Ruth's Story: Coming Out of the Closet of Shame

Ruth Moore, who also has given us permission to use her name, wrote the following account of sexual assault. A navy officer assaulted her when she was eighteen.

I was seventeen when I joined the navy. I was eighteen when I was raped by an officer.

I'd just been deployed to the Azores in Portugal. I was in a club. He came over to me and said, "Could you come outside for a minute? I need to talk to you." I didn't think it was unreasonable. He was my supervisor, and it was loud in the club. I didn't think it was wrong, but I was naïve. I was so young.

When we were outside, he put a knife to my mouth and said if I made a sound, if I screamed, he'd kill me. He raped me outside the club, in the bushes. Nobody saw anything. The day after, when I reported it to the chaplain, he advised me to forget it and move on. But how could I move on? My life had been destroyed by an act that lasted no more than ten minutes.

I was raped a second time by the same officer for having dared to talk. I tried to commit suicide by taking an overdose and was thrown into jail for attempting to destroy government property. My body was the government property! I was then transferred against my will to a psychiatric unit in Maryland, where I was interned for four months, including four weeks when I was strapped down on my bed.

I was scared. I was confused. I was angry. They tried to portray me as crazy, and I wasn't. I had no support. No medical help. My records had been destroyed, so there was no proof of the rape. And since they diagnosed me as crazy, they said I had made it up. This was just the start of a long process of exclusion and denial.

The navy forced me to waive my rights to the Department of Veterans Affairs, stating that I had medical care through my former spouse, a service-man, which was not wholly accurate. Following an injury after he came back from assignment, he started to do drugs, got hooked, and became violent. One day he beat me, so I packed my bags and left. I had nowhere to go. No money. I slept in my van for two weeks. We got divorced after twelve years together.

From 1991 to 2003, I was denied all types of benefits from the Department of Veterans Affairs. I was prevented from getting the psychological or medical help to which a veteran is usually entitled. The irony is they acknowl-edged that I had PTSD but claimed it was not service connected. So, I had no eligibility for health benefits. In 2003, I contacted a counselor outside the VA system who was the first to tell me, "There's nothing wrong with you. You're not crazy. You must have PTSD." It was the first time I had heard of it, and he was the first person since I was raped in 1987 to say, "I believe you."

In 2004, I obtained a military allowance for depression. I then went back to school to get a teacher's certificate and most of my benefits, not only for my disability rating but for life. A military counselor who specializes in helping rape victims went through all my files. When she saw that some evidence had never been taken into account, she had the strength to ask the military to live up to its responsibilities. Not only did they end up taking on the treat-ment of my PTSD, but in 2010, I received a document stating, "We find that more likely than not you were assaulted in the military." The best part was that they gave me a very rare clause, which is called "total and permanent," meaning that my case can never be reopened or challenged.

But the happy ending was still to come. On May 28, 2014, twenty-seven years after the fact, I had a phone call while I was working at my farm in Maine, where I was living with my daughter and my second husband. I had boots on at the time because I was digging a ditch. Butch came out and told me a VA representative was on the phone. I had no idea what she wanted.

When she told me they wanted to apologize for what had happened, and they were sorry that "it has taken this long," I started shaking. Butch was with me. We put the phone on loudspeaker. We couldn't move. And when she said, "We're very sorry, we made a clear and undeniable error" in not dealing with my first complaint filed in 1993, I was shaking even more.

Then she told me I was going to receive $405,000 in compensation, and I almost passed out. I literally collapsed on the floor. My husband and I were both holding each other, not knowing what to do. That was just WOW. The military was giving me apologies!

Although the money helped out, it was nothing compared with the apology I had given up hoping for. I hope, above all, that my case will help other victims seeking compensation.

My aggressor was never investigated, prosecuted, or disciplined. I don't know where he is now, but, as my husband says, he's probably living a quiet life somewhere, enjoying his retirement on a tidy pension. He gave me a sexually transmitted disease, which undoubtedly caused the nine miscarriages I suffered later on. It was not hard to prove. I was married, my husband didn't have it, and the person who attacked me was later treated for it.

How many other abused women soldiers still suffer in the shadows, rejected by the military they were prepared to die for, while their rapists continue unpunished and even promoted? Many, far too many.

Takeaway Points

- Sexual assault by those in power can be devastating to people of any age, especially to the young.
- The aftereffects of sexual assault, in both mind and body, are often associated with suicide attempts.

CHAPTER FIFTEEN

Sexual Assault Can Lead to Suicide

As psychologists dealing with the connection between assault and suicide, we will not discuss the medical issues of physical injury and sexually transmitted diseases. Instead, we look at the ways sexual assault is also an attack on the mind and soul and sometimes on relationships.

How does sexual assault contribute to the risk of suicide? Look at the aftereffects: powerful emotions of fear, rage, and shame; reasonable fears of renewed attack by the same person or by others; loss of trust in one's body and the ability to defend oneself; loss of the sense of security in certain places or in all unfamiliar places; and sometimes a sense of guilt and self-blame, usually misplaced.

The Grim Statistics

Sexual assault includes rape, molestation, unwanted touching, harassing, threats, and stalking. Every ninety-two seconds, an American is sexually assaulted or raped; 91 percent of the victims are women, mostly between the ages of twelve and thirty-four. Every nine minutes, a child is assaulted. According to the National Sexual Violence Resource Center (nsvrc.org), more than one in five women and nearly one in seventy-one men experience rape at some point in their lives. Over half of female victims were raped by an intimate partner, another 40 percent by an acquaintance. From other sources, we learn that 20 percent of gender-nonconforming college students have been sexually assaulted, compared to 18 percent of college females and 4 percent of college males. Fifty-five percent of assaults occur in or near the victim's home, 12 percent at or near a relative's home, and 8 percent while the victim is at work. These statistics are regularly compiled by the Rape, Abuse and Incest National Network (RAINN), using reliable sources, many of them from the U.S. Departments of Justice and Health and Human Services.

You may be surprised to know that men, too, have been sexually assaulted. These crimes occur as hazing rituals in fraternities, attacks from fellow soldiers or prison inmates, or kidnapping, rape, and murder by serial killers. Add to that the possibility that the crime is often discounted, and the investigation is just further insult.

On September 30, 2019, *Time* magazine described a confrontation two women had with U.S. Senator Jeff Flake, who had announced he intended to vote with the Senate Republican majority to confirm Brett Kavanaugh as an associate justice of the U.S. Supreme Court, despite credible testimony of past sexual molestation by Kavanaugh. One of the two women, Maria Gallagher, spoke of her rage and pain:

> I was sexually assaulted, and nobody believed me. I didn't tell anyone, and you're telling all women that they don't matter, that they should just stay quiet because if they tell you what happened to me, you are going to ignore them. Don't look away from me.

The second woman, Ana Maria Archila, chimed in with her own story of sexual assault.

Flake nodded and remained silent.[1] But he later rethought his position and demanded that the FBI investigate.

The two women may have made an impact on this one man, but the "investigation" was paltry; Kavanaugh was confirmed. Sadly, this was not a surprising outcome. There is a long history of sexual assault in the United States that typically affects those who have been barred from political power or are underrepresented.

Even teenagers can be rapists. In a 2013 report funded by the U.S. Department of Health and Human Services, Joann Schladale described a long list of violence among adolescents: bullying, harassment, hazing, verbal abuse, emotional abuse, physical assault, sexual assault, destruction of property, arson, murder, self-harm, and suicide. Negative effects can not only occur to the victim of violence but also to the witnesses.[2]

In 2017, after the histories of sexual assault by film producer Harvey Weinstein and other powerful men came to light, hundreds more women came forward with additional accusations. When asked what took them so long to speak up, they said they *had* spoken up—only to be denied, dismissed, discounted, and "dragged through the mud." It is a national disgrace that thousands of rape evidence kits have never been tested to be used in criminal trials. Only five out of one thousand rapists ever spends time in prison. For many victims, for whom #MeToo came too late, the assaults ended with their suicide.

Some Progress in Prevention and Treatment

Fortunately, RAINN's statistics are not all grim. Between 1993 and 2019, the number of reported sexual assaults fell by more than 50 percent. This may be due, at least in part, to increased public awareness fueled by women's movements and activists. In October 2017, actress Alyssa Milano asked her Twitter followers to reply "me too" if they had been sexually harassed or assaulted, a reference to a Me Too campaign initiated by Tarana Burke in 2006. For countless women, and some men, it was the first time they had been invited to discuss their experiences, some of which had resulted in suicide attempts.

Genuine progress requires more than just providing protection. True solutions get to root causes. A United Nations commission (www.unwomen .org) is devoted to women's issues that are global in nature. In a discussion of "rape culture," the organization made several proposals that could be implemented at community levels. We paraphrase some of them below:

- Replace the *rape culture* with a *culture of consent*. Rather than listening for a "no," men must make sure there is an enthusiastic "yes" from all involved.

- Dismantle the root causes. Rape culture means men believe they are entitled to sex whenever they want it and bear no responsibility for the consequences of their actions. Rape culture is allowed to continue as long as men are required to be strong and dominant, while women and girls are less valued and their protests are ignored.

- Do not accept such excuses as, "She was asking for it," "I knew she wanted it," and "She was dressed like a slut." What a woman was wearing during an assault is irrelevant. What the man *thinks* she thinks is irrelevant.

- Enforce zero tolerance. Leaders of schools, colleges, universities, businesses, law-enforcement departments, and governments must make clear that they are committed to zero tolerance, and it must be practiced every day, with no exceptions.

- Realize that rape culture takes many forms in different societies, going beyond the narrow notion of a man assaulting a woman as she walks home alone at night. It encompasses child marriage, female genital mutilation, incest, and rape as a weapon of war.

- Donate to organizations that empower women, amplify their voices, support survivors, and promote companies started and staffed by women.

- Listen to the survivors. Each rape victim has a story to tell, but too often there are few listeners. Hearing their stories can be therapeutic for them and educational for you.

Three Women Advocates for Mental Health

Pop music and movie icon Lady Gaga was repeatedly raped by an acquaintance at the age of nineteen, but she did not know how to process the assault and developed PTSD. Gaga first revealed her assault in 2014 and made her PTSD diagnosis public in 2016 to address the common misconception that PTSD only affects war veterans, stating, "Many associate PTSD as a condition faced by brave men and women who serve countries all over the world. While this is true, I seek to raise awareness that this mental illness affects all kinds of people, including our youth." She told Oprah Winfrey that she advocated mental health classes in schools and was working to implement this:

> I take an oath as a commitment today to work with you. It's 2020, and for the next decade and maybe longer, I'm going to get the smartest scientists, doctors, psychiatrists, mathematicians, brain surgeons, and professors in the same room together; and we're going to go through each problem one by one; and we're going to solve this mental health crisis.[3]

Ariana Grande is another singer who has become a mental health advocate. In 2017, she survived a suicide bomber's attack during her concert in Manchester Arena, England, which killed two dozen people and left her with PTSD. In 2019, she recalled the anxiety and dizziness she felt, realizing later that these were signs of post-traumatic stress. She stated, "It's hard to talk about this because so many people have suffered such severe, tremendous loss. But, yeah, PTSD is a real thing. I know those families and my fans, and everyone there experienced a lot of it as well. I don't think I'll ever know how to talk about it and not cry."[4]

The October 21, 2019, issue of *Time* magazine cited one hundred "new generation leaders" who, in the magazine's opinion, are changing the world. One of them was Oluwaseun Ayodrji Osowobi from Nigeria, whose organization Stand to End Rape has reached thousands of people. Its services include training for health workers and counseling for survivors. Given the risk that some rapes lead to suicide, it has probably saved countless lives as well.

Takeaway Points

- Sexual assault is disturbingly common in the United States and around the world, and it can leave great harm in its wake.
- *Rape culture* dismisses or trivializes sexual misbehavior and must be tackled at its root causes.

Notes

1. Lenz, L. (2019, September 19). Shouting into the void. *Time*.

2. Schladale, J. (2013). *A trauma-informed approach for adolescent sexual health*. Freeport, ME: Resources for Resolving Violence.

3. Burke, P. (2019, October 21–28). Survivors are also voters. *Time*, pp. 33–34.

4. Gillespie, C. (2020, January 6). Lady Gaga tells Oprah she was "repeatedly" raped at 19 and developed PTSD. *Healthy Living* (online).

CHAPTER SIXTEEN

Sexual Assault in Churches and Faith Groups

Sexual assault by so-called spiritual leaders is unfortunately not unusual. Since the first highly publicized revelations in 2002, there have been dozens of reports of men, women, and children who have been sexually abused by Roman Catholic priests.[1]

One of us (Krippner) interviewed two young men who had been abused by priests and heard two very different stories. Alwyn (not his real name) was sixteen when Father Joseph told him that he was under such tension that sex was the only way he could find relief. Alwyn agreed to have sex with the priest, if Father Joseph would not have sex with any other boy. Alwyn made this condition because he wanted to protect other boys. Father Joseph agreed, and the two of them had consensual sex until Alwyn left for college. During the interview, Alwyn said, "I felt pleased that I could help him out because he was doing a pretty good job as a priest."

The other young man's story was not so positive. Marco (not his real name) was fifteen when Father Julius told him, "Having sex with me is like having sex with Jesus. You are very special to me, and I will offer prayers for you and your family every night." Marco believed him and enjoyed the gifts he received after each sexual encounter. Then Marco discovered that Father Julius had told the same story to several other boys. Feeling betrayed, Marco made a suicide attempt, swallowing a bottle of his mother's sleeping medication. He survived, but he stopped going to church.

Later, Marco testified in a lawsuit that cost the church millions of dollars in damages. He lamented, "I received my share of the money, but it can never buy back my faith." When asked why he did not become an Episcopalian, a Buddhist, or a member of some other group, Marco replied, "You simply don't understand. Once a Catholic, you are always a Catholic. I have stopped going to Mass but still think of myself as a Catholic. Anything else would be a betrayal on my part. And I have had enough experience with betrayal."

Alwyn, on the other hand, still goes to Mass. He mused, "I am what you might call a 'cafeteria Catholic.' I don't agree with the church on birth control, but I do support its concern for the poor."

In 2009, an investigative reporter revealed that nearly four hundred Southern Baptist church leaders and volunteers had faced credible accusations of sexual misconduct in cases involving over seven hundred victims. Over half of the accused were convicted or made plea bargains. The Southern Baptist Convention, according to the reporter, treated the accusations as isolated cases. Debbie Vasquez told reporters that she was fourteen when the pastor of a rural Texas church first molested her. The abuse continued for years, and she became pregnant at nineteen. When the pastor said the sex was consensual, his church took no action. While the governing body of the Southern Baptist Convention also took no major action, its current president has called for taking the issue "more seriously than ever before."[2]

One American denomination, the Mormons, practiced and defended "plural marriage" (polygamy) until political considerations in the late nineteenth century made it expedient to abandon it. One splinter group, however, practices it to this day (the Fundamentalist Church of Jesus Christ of Latter-Day Saints, or FLDS). When the supply of women runs short, the men claim younger and younger females. Eventually, teenage boys are summarily expelled from the community, leaving the field to the men. Girls as young as fourteen are forced into marriage, vulnerable to sexual exploitation that is condoned and encouraged by their community.[3]

Abuse in South America

Sexual abuse by "spiritual" leaders appears to be widespread. Ayahuasca, a mind-altering tea made from plants in the Amazon, is used as a sacrament in certain South American religious groups. In 2016, a young woman claimed that she witnessed the leader of one of these groups engage in sexually inappropriate behavior toward most of the women in a group he was leading. Because the women had drunk the tea, they were especially vulnerable. As a result of her testimony, the leader was reported to the police and severely punished.

The previous year, João Teixeira de Faria, a prominent Brazilian "spiritual" leader known as "John of God," was charged with abusing hundreds of women who had come to him requesting healing. Some of them were suicidal following these experiences. He was best known for performing "spiritual surgeries," during which he would cut into the abdominal wall with a scalpel, insert a scalpel up the nose, or scrape the cornea of the eye with a knife. Many people claimed to have been healed, and about two thousand visited Abadiânia each week. One of us (Krippner) participated in an analysis of tissue samples taken from ten of Teixeira's clients following the "spiritual surgeries." Only one of the ten samples showed signs of pathology; yet, two-thirds of the clients reported some improvement in their conditions.[4]

In 2018, Zahira Lieneke Mous described how she had come to see Teixeira, hoping he could heal her long-lasting effects of past sexual assault. After she told him about her condition, the staff left the room.

> I was alone with him. As I told him I wanted to heal my sexual trauma, he nodded and stood up and asked me to stand in front of him with my back toward him. He touched my body. He smelled me. I had been in awe of this man and believed in a miracle. Simultaneously something crept up in me, feeling he's a dirty man, but I kept believing in his healing powers. He took me into his bathroom adjacent to his office. He put me in front of his mirror. . . . He stood behind me, grabbed my hand, and put it on his dick. I froze. . . . As I'm writing this, my palms are sweating, and my heart is pounding in my chest.

As reports of this nature kept being posted, Teixeira's daughter Dalva asserted that her father had abused and raped her between the ages of ten and fourteen.[5]

On the Other Hand . . . How a Church Can Help

For some, religion offers social support and a purpose in life. For example, a 2018 study indicated that children whose parents are religious are less likely to harbor suicidal thoughts or to take their own lives. Compared with children whose parents were not especially religious, this group showed a 40 percent lower risk of suicide. The effect was stronger for girls than for boys, though frequency of attending religious services did not affect the suicide rate one way or another.[6] But these reports of abuse threaten the role that religion has played in suicide prevention.

Psychologist Karen Mason published a suicide prevention handbook for members of the clergy that provides practical and evidence-based advice. She suggests that suicidal people do the following:

- Keep a list of reasons to live, one that can be augmented as time goes on.
- Create a number of "coping cards" that can be referred to when one is in a crisis.

- Build a "hope kit" that contains memos from happy times in life: a shell from a beach, a flower from a prom, or photos of beloved friends and family members.

Mason provides procedures for pastoral care, noting that pastors are usually equipped to provide "first aid" not "surgery." She advises that having a pet animal nearby or soothing music playing during a session may set the stage for a productive conversation. Listening and acceptance are required if a clergy member is contacted by a suicidal person.[7]

Mason's advice may help fill a tragic void. A 2017 survey by Lifeway Research revealed that most of the one thousand Protestant pastors interviewed believe that their church is equipped to intervene with people at risk. However, very few people who kill themselves have sought help from their church, and only 4 percent of those who have lost loved ones reported that their church was aware of the problem. You may recall the story of Phil, who was undergoing pastoral counseling when he suicided. Perhaps his life could have been saved had the pastor been better trained, but we will never know.

The Lifeway Research study was supported in part by the Southern Baptist Convention, so the possibility of antireligion bias is unlikely. In addition to the pastors interviewed, one thousand churchgoers were surveyed. One out of three revealed that a close friend or family member had suicided, and one out of three of the deceased had attended church during the months before dying. Half of the survivors noted that their church had reached out to them in some way, offering counseling, visitations, a referral to a psychotherapist, or access to logistical and financial help.

The majority of churches endorse some form of counseling for either the suicider or the survivors. About 40 percent of the pastors reported receiving formal training in dealing with suicide-prone parishioners, and about half have posted the National Suicide Hotline phone number (800-273-8255) in their church publications. But churchgoers also reported that community members were more likely to gossip about the suicide than to offer help to the survivors. Another disconnect is the report that about half the pastors claimed to address mental health issues in their sermons, but only 12 percent of parishioners agreed with that statement. Half the pastors had a list of local mental health practitioners on file, but only 16 percent of church members knew this.

These data represent Protestant congregations and may not be applicable to other denominations. However, organized religion can clearly play an important role in suicide prevention, treatment, and follow-up. This is the irony. Clergy members of several major denominations, both Christian and non-Christian, have engaged in sexual abuse, sometimes of young children. The amygdala, hippocampus, and related parts of the brain play important roles in religious experience, but they are also involved in feelings of fear, sexuality, and rage.[8] The biblical verse, "The Lord giveth, and the Lord taketh away," could well apply to religion itself and how it can bring out both the best and the worst of human behaviors.

Is It Everywhere?

Christianity is not the only tradition in which sexual misconduct occurs. Krishnamurti and Kalu Rinpoche are among many spiritual leaders whose sexual deceptions were eventually revealed. Jack Kornfield, psychologist and meditation teacher, studied many erring teachers and found that power, money, substances, and sex were the main problem areas (just as they are for many other people).[9] But faith leaders have extra tools to justify themselves, charisma, or excuses such as "It was a spiritual teaching" or "I'm helping so many people that I need some comfort." Moreover, their followers may be motivated to protect their image of the pastor or rabbi or swami as holy, ignoring or denying evidence of misconduct. Their idealization of the leader and need for guidance open the door to betrayal.

Takeaway Points

- Sexual assault by members of the clergy is widespread and has led to suicidal behaviors among some victims.
- However, religion can also be a bulwark against suicide. Many religious groups have created helpful suicide prevention and treatment programs.

Notes

1. Martel, F. (2019). *In the closet of the Vatican: Power, homosexuality, hypocrisy.* London: Bloomsbury.

2. Hopkins, A. (2019, February 11). Hundreds of Southern Baptist leaders, volunteers accused of sexual misconduct in bombshell investigation. *Fox News* (online).

3. Brower, S. (2011). *Prophet's prey: My seven-year investigation into Warren Jeffs and the Fundamentalist Church of Latter-Day Saints.* New York: Bloomsbury.

4. Moreira-Almeida, A., Moreira de Almeida, T., Gollner, A. M., & Krippner, S. (2009). A study of the mediumistic surgery of John of God. *Journal of Shamanic Practice, 2,* 21–31.

5. Nogueira, F. (2019, July/August). The not so divine acts of medium "John of God." *Skeptical Inquirer,* pp. 11–13.

6. Smietana, B. (2017, September 28). New research: How can churches help prevent suicide? *Facts and Trends* (online).

7. Mason, K. (2014). *Preventing suicide: A handbook for pastors, chaplains and pastoral counselors.* Downers Grove, IL: IVP Books.

8. Joseph, R. (2002). Sex, violence and religious experience. In *Neurotheology: Brain, science, spirituality, religious experience* (pp. 469–524). San Jose: University Press California.

9. Kornfield, J. (2000). *After the ecstasy, the laundry: How the heart grows wise on the spiritual path.* New York: Bantam.

CHAPTER SEVENTEEN

Sexual Assault in the Military

Perpetrators of sexual assault fall into four general categories. The *opportunistic rapist* takes advantage when the victim is most vulnerable, such as during sleep. The *angry rapist* encounters the victim while in a state of rage, sometimes because the victim denied a request for sex or perhaps because an earlier incident resulted in suppressed anger that was focused on an unfortunate victim. The *bullying rapist* wants to demonstrate his (or her) power. And the *sadistic rapist* enjoys making victims suffer in ways that are frequently bizarre. Investigators have found all four types of rapists in military settings.

Sexual Assault and Sexual Trauma

The U.S. Department of Defense (DOD) defines *sexual assault* as intentional sexual conduct characterized by the use of force, threats, intimidation, resort to authority, or activities when the victim does not or cannot consent. Sexual assault includes rape, forcible sodomy, and other unwanted sexual conduct. According to the DOD, only one out of ten people registers an assault. This low rate is due to fear of retaliation, embarrassment, or the suspicion (all too well-founded) that no action will be taken.[1] Most researchers believe that sexual assault on males (perpetrated by any variety of assailant, including groups of women) is severely underreported, even more so than sexual assaults of women. One survey of the literature placed the estimate at between 5 percent and 8 percent and noted the absence of effective coping strategies regarding the shame, distress, or depression following the assault.[2]

Self-loathing and guilt, common aftereffects of sexual assault, stem from understandable but maladaptive beliefs that need to be confronted directly by counselors and psychotherapists. Young soldiers are trained to be aggressive and are called upon to perform risky and complex activities, despite having social skills and neurological systems that are immature. It should be no surprise that sexual assault on one's fellow soldiers is an unfortunate consequence of their situation, especially when raging hormones or combat status are added to the mix. Sexual assault also interferes with the bonding that is essential to optimal functioning of military units.

The Veterans Health Administration has found that both men and women who experienced sexual assault are at increased risk for suicide, even after adjusting for age and mental health status. About 1 percent of male veterans and 21 percent of female veterans reported military sexual trauma; suicide rates were significantly higher for them.[3] The American Psychological Association defines *sexual trauma* as a disturbing experience associated with sexual activity, such as rape, and notes that it is a common cause of PTSD.[4]

When the U.S. Army investigates a reported sexual assault, the chain of custody of evidence must be controlled, and the statements and data must be preserved. To this end, the interrogator's line of questioning before, during, and after the interview must be objective, precise, and thorough. The interrogator needs to have a strong understanding of both male and female genital anatomy to be able to include both internal and external characteristics and both normal and abnormal variations of these anatomies. This knowledge will aid in the accurate detection of genital injuries, the preparation of documentation for legal purposes, and the accurate diagnosis and treatment of injuries, sexually transmitted diseases, and pregnancies. In 2005, the DOD changed its regulations to allow service personnel to *report* sexual assaults without *prosecuting* the offender.[5] This action was taken to allow for a more complete assessment of the case, as many victims felt they had legitimate reasons for not wanting to initiate prosecution.

Sexual assault is so feared and leaves such violent injuries that it has been one of the primary weapons of war on foreign soil. It is now designated "a crime against humanity" by the Geneva Conventions. However, rape regularly occurs in modern-day conflicts, such as those in Somalia, Kashmir, Bosnia, Afghanistan, and Iraq.

The Consequences

A physical examination following sexual assault has two primary purposes: to provide health care and to collect evidence. Physical injuries need to be treated so that they can heal without subsequent complications. The pattern of injury also has legal significance. However, the location of the genital injury provides only a partial description of the trauma.

One study of injuries from sexual assault revealed that the most commonly damaged areas for both genders were the soft tissues of the anus and those between the thighs. There were almost as many lacerations to other parts of the body due to the victim's resistance or to the sadistic propensities of the perpetrator. For women, the most commonly reported injuries occur in the vagina or vaginal areas. For both men and women, injuries result from penetration with a penis, fingers, or foreign objects such as pens, pencils, and other things that require surgical removal. For both genders, the consequences can include abrasions, burns, cuts, fractures, scrapes, strains, tears, and even traumatic brain injury. An ill-informed physician or nurse may attribute rectal or vaginal bleeding to hemorrhoids or state that the victim probably engaged in consensual sex. In either case, the refusal to be taken seriously can initiate a reaction that leads to suicide.

There are psychological consequences as well. Nondisclosing survivors may resort to wearing long-sleeved clothing, bracelets, or makeup to disguise the consequences of their assault. In these instances, suicide might result when disguise has not worked and the evidence of the assault is apparent. Marilyn Sawyer Sommers has called for a multidimensional definition of *genital injury* to allow for a more holistic approach to health care and the science of criminal justice.[6]

Ryan Leigh Dostie's Story

Ryan Leigh Dostie enlisted in the army at the age of twenty. Although raised in a conservative Christian home, she had a rebellious streak and looked forward to working in military intelligence. Fluent in Japanese, she was determined to learn Farsi during her stint in Iraq. Shortly after being posted at Fort Polk, Louisiana, Dostie went out drinking, came back drunk, shut the door, and went to bed. Her unlocked door was opened by a fellow soldier, who climbed into her bed and raped her.

To add insult to injury, Dostie was ridiculed by the rapist and his friends when she was dismissed from two platoons, standing at attention in a formation of one. When appealing her cases at the Judge Advocate General's office, she was asked, "Do you really want to ruin this guy's life?" Told to move on, she was sent to Iraq. She learned Farsi but found little use for it, as the people around her were military personnel who spoke English. PTSD hit her very hard. She went into a coma, and when she recovered, Dostie seriously considered killing herself.

Dostie described her service in the book *Formation*, published in 2019.[7] She described herself as being "so in love with the Army," even though she found it unprepared for women like her whose activities challenged standard operating procedures. After her discharge, she experienced a wide gamut of PTSD symptoms and entered cognitive behavioral therapy. It did not help her, but antidepressant medication did—for a while. Admitting that her story has no completely happy ending, she commented, "You never actually get over rape or war. You just have to carry it always, and it sits inside you, filling in the places where other things are lost and gone."

However, Dostie was encouraged by a 2018 DOD report. There were almost seven thousand accounts of sexual misconduct involving service members in 2017, a nearly 10 percent increase over those reported in 2016. Her efforts may have made a difference in victims' willingness to report, along with an apparent decrease in sexual assaults, reported or not. Dostie went to college, married a former Marine, had a daughter, and became a writer. Her book was widely praised as gritty, deep, and honest.

Takeaway Points

- Sexual assault in the U.S. Armed Forces can lead to suicide, but it is underreported, especially by male survivors.
- The physical and psychological consequences of sexual assault are often long-lasting, requiring both medical and psychotherapeutic intervention.

Notes

1. Gilberd, K. (2017). *Challenging military sexual violence: A guide to sexual assault and sexual harassment. Policies in the U.S. Armed Forces for servicemembers, MSV survivors and their advocates.* San Jose, CA: Military Law Task Force.

2. Tewksbury, D. (2007). Effects of sexual assault on men: Physical, mental, and sexual consequences. *International Journal of Men's Health, 6,* 22–25.

3. Kimerling, R., Makin-Byrd, K., Lauzon, S., et al. (2016). Military sexual trauma and suicide mortality. *American Journal of Preventive Medicine, 50*(6), 684–691.

4. VandenBos, G. R. (Ed.). (2007). *APA dictionary of psychology* (p. 847). Washington, DC: American Psychological Association.

5. Sexual Assault Prevention and Response Office. (2006). *Department of Defense F407 sexual assault in the military.* Washington, DC: U.S. Department of Defense.

6. Sommers, M. S. (2007). Defining patterns of genital injury from sexual assault: A review. *Trauma, Violence, and Abuse, 8,* 270–290.

7. Dostie, R. L. (2019). *Formation: A woman's memoir of stepping out of line.* New York: Grand Central Publishing.

SECTION IV

Bullying

CHAPTER EIGHTEEN

How Bruno Was Bullied to Death

To open this section on bullying, we will tell you about another tragic suicide. Names and locations have been disguised, but the facts are authentic. A friend of Bruno's wrote this account for us.

"Mom! Can we please go to McDonald's and get Bruno some hamburgers?"

My daughter Shenandoah explained that Bruno had not eaten all day because his mom had been out with her new boyfriend. Bruno's parents were separated and getting a divorce. Bruno's dad was aggressive and hot-tempered. I had had a long day, yet I agreed with her request. When we arrived at his home, Bruno came out to the car to greet us. He seemed polite and assertive, strong but broken. I had to remind myself that he was still a kid, just a seventh-grader.

Bruno and Shenandoah had attended middle school together. Bruno confided in her and felt safe, and Shenandoah nourished her soul in giving him guidance and love. Things at Bruno's home were harsh. His dad hit and bullied him and made derogatory comments. Bruno's mom was manipulative; she used Bruno as a foil in her perpetual duels with her husband. Bruno was lost. He got into trouble in school and started smoking weed. Sometimes he needed to rebel and let his heart roar, to scream and let out the pain.

Instead, Bruno transmuted his anger by protecting other kids who were being bullied. Psychologists call this *sublimation*—turning one's pain into something useful. He would get in the way of the bully and prevent him from harming the kids. As Bruno grew taller and stronger, he got into more and more trouble, often as a result of protecting kids who were bullied. His behavior was misunderstood and punished. No one at school realized that he so empathized with these kids because he was being bullied by his father. He could not protect himself from his dad, but he could control the way he protected others. Bruno made sure the little guys and the nerds were respected and safe. But his actions were not seen that way by the teachers and his parents. In their eyes, Bruno was an uncontrollable troublemaker.

One October morning, Bruno was on his way to school. The path trailed around a beautiful setting that consisted of ancient oaks, bays, and native plants. It was cold and foggy when Bruno found his best friend, Iver, hanging dead from the limb of a tree. Imagine his shock, horror, and sadness. A suicide note was later found. Apparently, Iver missed his mom so much that, one year after her death, he chose to take his life on the same day of the week, at the same hour, and the same minute his mom had taken hers. He mentioned this in his suicide note. Iver wrote that he was hoping to find her and be reunited.

People who knew Iver and Bruno wondered, "Can anyone ever recover from finding one's best friend hanging dead from a tree?" Sure enough, Iver's death sparked a chain of "copycat suicides." In the weeks to come, four kids in the town took their lives by hanging themselves from tree branches. Bruno was not one of them—yet.

Time passed, and Bruno kept on growing. He had become a known stoner who made extra money by selling weed to friends. He was beginning to feel a certain sense of independence. In high school, he became very tall. The workouts he did started paying off, and he developed a body that looked as if it had been chiseled by the gods. Bruno once told me, "Do you know why I'm getting so well built? 'Cuz now I can kick my dad's ass." We both laughed.

Over time, Bruno's cockiness grew as large as his muscles; yet, at heart, he was a teddy bear. He kept protecting the weak and confronting the bullies. Circumstances brought Bruno and my daughter back together. Shenandoah had been dating a young man who had too many "issues." Bruno and the young man were friends, but Bruno made it clear that he did not approve of the way he treated Shenandoah. Within a few months, Bruno and Shenandoah entered a serious relationship and decided it was in her best interest to leave the young man she had been dating, who had turned out to be a severely abusive, violent, and angry teen who threatened daily to kill Shenandoah.

Shenandoah and Bruno fell deeply in love. Their lives together were filled with joy and laughter. He was over six feet tall, and she was just a tiny mouse. They discovered things about one another that were very personal. Bruno had marks on his back from a chair his dad had used to strike him. Shenandoah's dad had a mental illness and had put the family through a great deal of turmoil. Both had invisible scars that they did not mention to others.

Eventually, Bruno was expelled from high school for selling drugs. Neither parent could cope with the situation, so they sent him to live in a trailer with his grandpa in a small town, distant from Shenandoah and his other friends. The two young people did not give up. They found ways to continue seeing each other, which mostly involved Shenandoah's driving long hours whenever she could.

Bruno's insecurities grew. His grandpa was an angry, mean man who had become a recluse after his wife left him. Shenandoah quickly deduced where Bruno's father had learned to be so violent. This insight was very disturbing for Bruno, as he feared he might eventually follow the family pattern.

Remarkably, Grandpa and Bruno bonded. However, Grandpa could be very abusive, and one night, Shenandoah, who was visiting, found herself caught in the middle of a violent fight. After things calmed down, she had a mature conversation with Grandpa, expressing how violence and verbal abuse were not part of her upbringing. She had lived a very gentle life with her mom and brother, even though life had had its challenges.

By this time, Bruno's parents were divorced. He made several requests to move in with his mother so that he could be closer to my daughter, but she rejected the idea. When Bruno and Shenandoah turned eighteen, they selected colleges within a five-hour commute from each other. Bruno's parents were not supportive, and he did not know how to manage his money. He liked to buy clothes and shoes and gifts for Shenandoah.

But then the couple's relationship began to change. Bruno had spells of moodiness and depression. Sometimes he became intolerant and even bullied others, reminding Shenandoah of her prior relationship. After many struggles, discussions, and attempts to reconcile, they finally separated. A year passed. Both had moved on, but they kept in contact. Bruno was not dating anyone seriously, but Shenandoah was.

On a Sunday morning, at 7:00 a.m., my telephone rang. To my surprise, it was Bruno. He said that he wanted to stop by and say hello. Bruno told me that he had a puppy that he wanted me to meet. I immediately invited him to the house. He arrived looking as if he had been crying. He was not as well developed and fit as I remembered him. He had changed a great deal in a year.

We focused on his new puppy. Bruno was very proud of him, and I was very proud of Bruno! But the whole time we spoke, I could feel that something was wrong. I kept looking at him. There was a glow around him, a light around his head. It went from shoulder to shoulder. He was crying. Something was off. I could feel it.

Each time I tried to mention my eerie feeling, I could not. It was as if an invisible force or presence was there, gently caressing my lips and muting my voice. I wanted to ask whether everything was okay, but I could not. So I asked why he was in town. With a smile, Bruno replied, "It's both my parents' birthdays. My dad already had his, and Mom's is coming up; so I decided to surprise them."

I still felt unsettled. As our conversation went on, he expressed how beautiful I looked. He kept saying I looked like an angel and how he could now see where my daughter got her beauty from. He expressed his gratitude for all that I had done for him over the years and how I had always accepted him. He said he was not able to see and accept my kindness before, but now he could. Eventually, it was time for him to head home, and we texted every step of his drive until he reached his destination. I immediately texted my daughter to tell her about the sudden and surprising visit.

My texting with Bruno continued for the next two days. Within that time, Bruno was communicating with my daughter, asking her to meet for coffee or lunch. She declined the requests, feeling it was not appropriate because she was now in another relationship. She proposed a time when all three of them could meet.

Tuesday was a busy day, but I texted Bruno early evening to check in. He did not reply. At 9:49 p.m., on Tuesday, April 10, my phone rang. It was my daughter. I had a sinking premonition. "Mom . . . Mooommmmmm . . . Bruno killed himself. . . . Bruno killed himself." No words can express the pain we felt. It tore us wide open. My frustration at not being near my daughter at this most crucial time intensified my pain.

Earlier that afternoon, Bruno had texted his parents: "Sorry I was not good enough." At that moment, he hiked to the top of a hill and shot himself in the head. He was found by the police after his location was finally tracked from his phone. They arrived too late.

Bruno's mom used this tragic event to create a GoFundMe page to collect money because she could not work. His dad was forced to face his own demons. They never held a service, a memorial, or any sort of ceremony for those of us left behind. It took them months to acknowledge Bruno's death with an obituary in our local newspaper. The community, Bruno's peers, and his friends never had a chance to grieve together. Instead, they all remained in a state of shock, slowly pushing the nightmare to a hidden side of their hearts.

I often wonder what might have happened if my daughter had met him for coffee or lunch that day. Would he have shot her first and taken her with him? Or would he have just said an indirect goodbye, as he did with me? I will never know.

Takeaway Points

- Sometimes a friend or loved one has an intuitive hunch about a prospective suicide but does not put the pieces together.
- Bullying often involves physical abuse, emotional abuse, or both. They can be deadly, especially in combination.
- Even after a person seems strong enough to overcome bullying, its scars may linger.

CHAPTER NINETEEN

Bullying and the Vulnerable

Any type of bullying is harmful; in some cases, it has led to suicide. While parents typically worry that spending too much time using digital technology is harmful, rigorous research has debunked this concern.[1] Bullying, however, which is far more harmful to adolescents, is too often dismissed with such comments as "Kids will be kids" or "A little teasing will toughen them up."

Channing Smith Was Vulnerable

Channing Smith was a sixteen-year-old high school junior. One September evening, he worked his shift at Burger King, came home, and went to bed. It had been a normal enough day, one would have thought. But his father discovered Channing's dead body the next morning. What had happened?

Two other high school students had discovered Channing's romantic correspondence with another male student and images of the two together on a cell phone. They posted what they found on social media. This was traumatic to Channing, who had told very few people about his sexual orientation. There had been no previous taunting, teasing, or bullying. However, for a vulnerable person at risk for suicide, one episode of "outing" can be a death sentence. Indeed, sexual-minority students are three times as likely both to contemplate suicide and to attempt it.[2]

This tragic story may remind you that many adolescents—their brains not yet fully developed and their social skills still in the formative process—can be extremely vulnerable. An incident that a mature person might shrug off or laugh about can feel catastrophic to a teenager. Likewise, some aggressive adolescents may not yet have developed the emotional maturity to realize that their acts of bullying could have deadly consequences.

The school's art class created artwork in various media to commemorate Channing's death. The pop singer Billy Ray Cyrus sang "Amazing Grace" at one of the memorial services. But none of this could reunite Channing with his grieving friends and family.

Nikki Matlocks Was Vulnerable

A happier story was related by Nikki Matlocks. After breaking up with her first love at the age of eighteen, Nikki was bombarded by negative messages on social media from friends of her ex-boyfriend. One urged Nikki to kill herself. She took an overdose of medication, from which she recovered. Fortunately, Nikki was just about to start her university classes. In this new environment, she made new friends and was free from any sort of bullying. In retrospect, she observed that cyberbullying "made me a kinder, stronger person." It also prepared her for her future career as a mental health advocate who helps others cope with bullying.

Nikki has tweeted her story to thousands of people around the world. One of the tweets asked, "Why do I have to be dead before I get help from mental health?" This question elicited numerous sympathetic replies from other young people.

Emily Drouet Was Vulnerable

Emily Drouet, another eighteen-year-old, did not fare as well. Emily's ex-boyfriend Angus launched a nonstop campaign of abuse against her, calling Emily a "slut," a "freak," and other derogatory terms. He also parodied a school antibullying video, twisting the words to insult Emily. The physical part of the abuse included choking Emily, striking her, and slamming her head against a desk, which brought him to the attention of the local sheriff's office. Angus received no jail time nor a fine. He was only sentenced to 180 hours of unpaid work in the sheriff's court. His school took more direct action by expelling him. But this was too little, too late.

Emily killed herself by taking poison. Her mother told local reporters that the family has been haunted by Emily's death every day for the past three years. She added that, when she was alive, Emily felt unable to escape; "If she'd felt able to run, we'd still have her." The autopsy revealed that Emily's body was covered with bruises that were not self-inflicted. So why did she not escape? Emily had discussed Angus's abuse with a university staff member, who urged her to file a formal complaint. But Emily refused because she "didn't want to get Angus into trouble." She told a friend that she felt that she deserved the abuse because of her arguments with Angus.

Bullying Has Both Short-Term and Long-Term Effects

Bullying in U.S. schools affects at least one in every three children, including those who witness the act. Long-term effects of bullying include anxiety, depression, conduct disorders, thoughts about suicide, and substance abuse, including alcohol, prescription drugs, and illegal drugs.[3] For Channing and Emily, the tragic effects of bullying were short-term. They did not live long enough to experience long-term effects.

Sexual violence can be either a short-term or a long-term effect of bullying. A study published in 2012 involved nearly fourteen hundred middle school girls and boys in a Midwestern state. Using a variety of measures, including pencil-and-paper tests, 12 percent of the group was identified as bully perpetrators. One out of three boys and one out of four girls admitted making negative sexual comments about other students. Five percent of boys and 7 percent of girls admitted spreading sexual rumors, and 4 percent of boys and 2 percent of girls said that they had pulled at someone's clothing. Along with bullying, teasing others about their sexual orientation predicted severe sexual molestation over time. Given the overlap among bullying, homophobic teasing, and sexual violence, prevention programs need to consider these links.[4]

Cyberbullying Can Be Fatal

Bullies can hide behind false names online or enlist their friends to join an attack and never be caught. Large numbers of U.S. teenagers say they have been bullied online. Spurred by European reports of cyberbullying, a teacher of linguistic studies at Belgium's Ghent University trained a machine's learning algorithm to spot and block words and phrases associated with bullying on the social site AskFM.com. This algorithm blocked two out of three insults in almost 114,000 posts, a rate more accurate than a simple keyword search.

Based on "neural signatures," a different machine-learning algorithm was developed by researchers at Carnegie-Mellon University in Pittsburgh. It was able to identify those who were having suicidal thoughts with 91 percent accuracy. In this study, thirty-four participants were asked to think of thirty specific concepts relating to positive or negative aspects of life and death while their brains were scanned using a functional magnetic resonance imaging, or fMRI, machine. One aspect of the study compared nine people who had made a suicide attempt and still harbored suicidal thoughts with eight who had not. All were asked to think about "death," "being carefree," and a number of other topics. The computer was able to discriminate between the two groups with 94 percent accuracy.[5]

What should be done? In September 2019, the alternative newspaper *San Francisco Weekly* published a lawyer's response to a woman's concern about cyberbullying suffered by her daughter; she had asked whether the school should take action. C. B. Jones, the lawyer, responded in a way that illuminates one state's response to this problem. Here is a portion of his response:

> You are right to be concerned. . . . Your daughter's school should have notified all families of the school's reporting and investigation process. Any student, parent, guardian, or other individual who learns of school-related discrimination, harassment, intimidation, or bullying should immediately contact the school's principal or other staff member. Any school employee who learns of cyberbullying is also required to report the activity to the school principal, who must in turn notify the district compliance officer and inform the target students of their right to file a formal written complaint with the District Office of Equity. Cyberbullying victims are encouraged to save and print relevant electronic and digital messages for aid in investigation of the matter. Complainants' names will be held confidential to the extent possible, and district policy prohibits any form of retaliation against any individual who files such a complaint.[6]

Mihaly Csikszentmihalyi and Reed Larson have identified violence, sex, and drugs as the three problems usually associated with adolescence.[7] We have made the case that bullying is itself a form of violence and that it is often associated with sexual assault and substance abuse. We have also reminded our readers that the teenage brain is a "work in progress," vulnerable to peer pressure, to electronic media, and to potentially toxic substances. As we have seen, bullying can be directed against a classmate, a romantic partner, or a virtual stranger.[8]

Even one life lost to bullying is too many. Apart from the pain inflicted on the surviving family and friends, vulnerable teens often have outstanding artistic, technical, and other creative propensities that are worth cultivating, saving, and—in many cases—rescuing.[9]

Takeaway Points

- Bullying, including cyberbullying, can have both short-term and long-term effects that can be devastating.
- Some victims of bullying have committed suicide or contemplated doing so.
- Preventive actions can be taken by schools and state legislatures, even though their effectiveness has yet to be demonstrated.

Notes

1. Denworth, L. (2019). The kids are all right. *Scientific American, 321*(5), 44–49.

2. West, E. P. (2019, October 1). A teen died by suicide after being outed online. *Nashville Tennessean* (online).

3. Smokowski, P. R., & Kopasz, K. H. (2005). Bullying in school: An overview of types, effects, family characteristics, and intervention strategies. *Children and Schools, 27,* 101–110.

4. Robinson, J. P., & Espelage, D. L. (2012). Bullying explains only part of LGBTQ-heterosexual risk disparities: Implications for policy and practice. *Educational Researcher, 41,* 309–319.

5. Griffiths, S. (2019, February 11). Can this technology put an end to bullying? *Machine Minds* (online).

6. Doan, C. B. (2019, September 26). What responsibility do schools carry for cyberbullying? *San Francisco Weekly,* p. 6.

7. Csikszentmihalyi, M., & Larson, R. (1984). *Being adolescent: Conflict and growth in the teenage years.* New York: Basic Books.

8. Espelage, D. L., Basil, K. C., & Hamburger, M. E. (2012). Bullying perpetration and subsequent sexual violence perpetration among middle school students. *Journal of Adolescent Health, 50,* 60–65.

9. Snyder, R. B., Kupchik, A., & Kovacs, M. S. (2016). *Improving communication to combat bullying.* Atlanta, GA: Cartoon Network.

CHAPTER TWENTY

Bullies, Victims, and Bystanders

Bullying is intentional, unwanted, threatening, and aggressive behavior that occurs in relationships with unequal power. One person may be smaller than the abuser, or weaker, or poorer, or perceived as "strange." Bullies do not threaten people who are larger, stronger, richer, or more popular than they are.[1] Bullying is not only characterized by an imbalance of power but also by deliberate and repetitive attempts to cause harm.[2]

Bullying is unfortunately widespread. According to the U.S. Department of Education, one out of every four students between the ages of twelve and eighteen reports being bullied at school. An even larger number have been *bystanders* to bullying as members of a peer audience. Half of high school students and one-third of younger students report being cyberbullied.

Most young people who are bullied do not engage in self-harm, and the percentage of those who are bullied has not increased in recent years and may even have decreased. That is the good news. The bad news is that suicidal behavior is of special concern to those who lack support from their schools or their families, the usual buffers against self-harm.

Adults may encounter bullying at work or in their communities. Cyberbullies use computers, media, and social networks to bully others. Abusers of any age seem to have an uncanny knack for sensing who can defend themselves and who cannot. The easy targets are those who are vulnerable, frail, or "different" in some way, whether by ethnic background, economic status, sexual preference, or something else. Bullies abuse people who are disabled, who are overweight or underweight, or who attend a place of worship outside the community's mainstream.

Bullying has serious long-term negative consequences for bullies as well as for victims and bystanders. Some victims become bullies themselves as a coping strategy. Other consequences include anxiety, depression, substance abuse, and delinquent behavior.[3] Bullying tends to escalate; what starts as an interaction between individuals or small groups of unequal power may evolve into a peer group phenomenon involving cliques and gang wars. Bystanders play an important role in bullying; without an audience, the bully's intent may not materialize. Of course, there are some bullies who do not need an audience; they obtain perverse pleasure simply from seeing the results of their actions.

The Bullying System

In the Middle Ages, a "bully boy" was a swashbuckling figure who protected the weak and the vulnerable. Over the centuries, the definition was reversed to mean one who hurt people for no good reason. Both definitions leave out the victims and the audience; without bystanders, most bullies derive little satisfaction from their malevolence. The social interaction of all three players is essential to understanding the context in which bullying occurs and to constructing effective prevention programs.

Psychiatrist Stuart Twemlow and psychologist Frank Sacco present a social systems perspective.[4] They see bullying as an interpersonal and large-group process that humiliates or even injures a victim in the presence of an audience. A casual insult or demeaning remark, while regrettable, is not bullying. Instead, bullying involves a clear intention to humiliate a victim. Child bullies push, shove, threaten, and name-call. The victim is often called a "sissy," "gay," or a "whore," and in an earlier era, "moron," "dummy," "fag," "queer," "tart," "kike," "nigger," "Polack," and "Chink" were common. Does reading those hateful names make you uneasy? Now, imagine they are hurled at you, day after day, and no one helps you.

Twemlow and Sacco see *shame* as playing a key role in bullying. Bullies are often ashamed of some personal quality of their own, real or imagined. To improve their status and enhance their identity, they belittle and degrade others, externalizing the ridicule they fear and hoping to gain respect. This drama is played out in far too many schools at every point on the socioeconomic spectrum. Schools that emphasize competitions and scholastic achievement are fertile arenas for social bullying.

School administrators are often baffled when bullying is reported. They usually punish the bully or mediate between the bully and victim, although there is no evidence that either action produces positive results. Sometimes teachers find themselves playing one role or the other. A coach might bully members of her team, thinking it will spur achievement. A teacher may become a victim of a student clique whose members deliberately flout disciplinary rules, daring him to take action. Parents may bully a school administrator to allow their child to retake a college entrance exam in hopes of producing a higher grade.

These roles may be played out in other settings. A bully may be a victim of parental bullying at home; a victim may bully siblings; or a bystander may become an active bully or victim in the neighborhood setting. People can become stuck in one role and unconsciously gravitate toward other members of the triad long after they leave school. Twemlow and Sacco's perspective has debunked several fallacies about bullying:

- Bullying is a normal part of growing up.
- Bullying is found only among children and adolescents.
- Bullying is always physical in nature.
- Bullying is worse among boys than among girls.
- Bullying happens only in poor schools in low-income neighborhoods.
- Bullying involves only a victimizer and a victim.

In William Golding's classic 1954 novel *Lord of the Flies*, a group of boys, survivors of an airplane crash, create their own societies. Two of the boys, Simon, an epileptic, and an overweight boy nicknamed "Piggy" are bullied by some of the older boys. Many of the bystanders, who could have stopped the bullying, begin to sympathize with the bullies. First Simon and then "Piggy" are killed, and only the arrival of a rescue ship prevents further mayhem. When the boys are rescued, they resume their everyday lives as if the ghastly cruelty and violence had never occurred.

The Lord of the Flies is a work of fiction. However, there are eerie parallels to historical events. Ordinary Germans participated in the murder of millions of Jews, Slavs, homosexuals, mentally challenged individuals, those with criminal records, and other "undesirables." Many of them returned to their families following a day of running the gas chambers. Recalling our reading of evolutionary psychology, we might ask, How does human evolution account for this contradiction?

Early humans evolved to be both cooperative and competitive, depending on the context and the desired outcome. Cooperation led to successful hunting expeditions, sharing of food, and group protection against animal predators and human enemies. Competition led to securing more desirable mates, obtaining resources for one's family, and protecting oneself and one's family from competitors both within the tribe and outside. Historian of science and popular skeptic Michael Shermer concluded, "We evolved to be moral but have the capacity to be immoral some of the time in some circumstances with some people. Which direction any one of us takes in any given situation will depend on a complex array of variables."[5] He added that the news media focus on acts of violence and immorality, largely ignoring the kind, generous, and benevolent actions that occur every day.

Two classic studies demonstrate the malleability of moral decisions. At Yale University, many years ago, Stanley Milgram presented his research participants with a "learning experiment" in which they supposedly tested the memory of other participants. Those "other participants" were actually decoys who were part of the research staff. The participants were told to give the decoy participants an electric shock every time they made a mistake. The decoy participants, of course, made several "mistakes" and received "shocks," which were also not real. There were several categories of "shocks," with one labeled "DANGER: 450 volts." Those "shocks" were administered by 65 percent of the actual participants, and 100 percent administered at least one "Strong Shock, 135 volts." If two of Milgram's staff members were present and urged stronger shocks, the participants were more likely to comply. Milgram expressed astonishment, interpreting the results as the impact of "obedience to authority."[6]

At Stanford University, Philip Zimbardo conducted a study with another set of student volunteers. He created a mock prison in which research participants were randomly assigned to be "prisoners" or "guards." The guards were given uniforms, clubs, whistles, and sunglasses. The prisoners were forced to stand naked and then were sprayed for lice, given identical uniforms, and assigned to live in small cells. Within a few days, the students played their roles only too well, transforming into authoritative, violent guards or demoralized, impassive prisoners. The experiment was to have lasted for two weeks, but Zimbardo ended it in half that time.[7] He probably made the right decision; as previously noted, if bullying behavior persists in school settings, it may recur in adulthood, in one form or another.

In 1960, a decade before Zimbardo conducted his prison experiment, one of us (Krippner) was a program director for a YMCA camp in rural Wisconsin. Each week, he and his staff announced a theme day, sometimes a Roman Day for which campers wore togas made of their bed sheets or a Backwards Day for which campers wore their clothes backward and ended the day with breakfast. When campers awakened on Communist Day, they found the American flag had been replaced by a red banner and that a rigid set of rules would be enforced. Three of the older campers, who had been designated "the Red Guards," promptly imprisoned any camper who broke a rule.

The staff was astonished at how quickly the Red Guards adapted to their new roles. To prevent overt violence, the guards were neither muscular nor of an imposing height. Even though the "prison" was an area only marked off by a slender rope, no prisoner attempted to escape. Indeed, they became surprisingly submissive. When a preplanned "revolution" overthrew the Red

Guards at the end of the day, the staff breathed a sigh of relief. Communist Day never became a theme again.

In 2007, Zimbardo published *The Lucifer Effect*, in which he reviewed what he had learned during the prison experiment and subsequent investigations. He also defended his prison research in the face of subsequent criticism. More importantly, Zimbardo cited numerous examples regarding how time and place can impact people's moral and immoral behaviors. In light of the media tendency to highlight the evil and destructive, he called for the celebration of heroic acts that bolster human connections and that can be performed by anyone. Some writers have described the "banality of evil." Zimbardo wrote of the "banality of heroism," the choices that are readily available.[8] Zimbardo's sentiments are in accord with system scientist David Loye's careful reading of Darwin's last works. While acknowledging the role played by both conflict and cooperation in evolution, Darwin ultimately concluded that the improvement of one organism supports the improvement of another.[9]

Pioneering psychotherapist Albert Ellis emphasized unconditional acceptance of oneself, of others, and of life. He never called a *person* evil or wicked, but he had no hesitation in using negative labels to describe *behavior* that was life-denying rather than life-enhancing. Ellis, an anthropologist as well as a psychologist, was well aware of human complexity and the impact of context on one's behavior. Although an atheist, Ellis would probably have agreed with Jesus's remark when a woman was sentenced to death by stoning for adultery: "He who is without sin among you, let him cast the first stone."

Takeaway Points

- Bullying usually involves bullies, victims, and bystanders; it can have long-lasting effects on all three.
- To write off bullying as a normal aspect of development is to ignore the harm it can inflict and its role in suicidal behavior.

Notes

1. Smokowski, P. R., & Kopasz, K. H. (2005). Bullying in school: An overview of types, effects, family characteristics, and intervention strategies. *Children & Schools, 27*, 101–110.

2. Meyers, L. (2016). Fertile grounds for bullying. *Counseling Today, 58*(1), 26–35.

3. Snyder, R. B. (2013). *The 5 simple truths of raising kids and how to deal with modern problems facing your tweens and teens.* New York: DemosHEALTH.

4. Twemlow, S. W., & Sacco, F. C. (2012). *Preventing bullying and school violence*. Washington, DC: American Psychiatric Publishing.

5. Shermer, M. (2004). *The science of good and evil: Why people cheat, gossip, care, share, and follow the Golden Rule* (p. 74). New York: Henry Holt and Company.

6. Milgram, S. (1969). *Obedience to authority: An experimental view*. New York: Harper Row.

7. Zimbardo, P. (1991). *The psychology of attitude change and social influence*. New York: McGraw-Hill.

8. Zimbardo, P. (2007). *The Lucifer Effect: Understanding how good people turn evil*. New York: Random House.

9. Loye, D. (2010). *Darwin's lost theory: Bridge to a better world*. Carmel, CA: Benjamin Franklin Press.

CHAPTER TWENTY-ONE

Preventing Bullying

Hundreds of programs have been designed to curb bullying and school violence in the United States, England, Norway, Finland, and other countries. Stuart Twemlow and psychologist Frank Sacco carefully evaluated these efforts and concluded that their effectiveness was "disappointing." They acknowledged that evaluation is difficult. One perspective sees the bully as a relatively rare, emotionally disturbed individual with antisocial traits who is heading for a life of crime. Another perspective conceptualizes offenders as fairly ordinary students who engage in antisocial behavior but do not see themselves as bullies, nor do their peers, parents, or schools. However, by their sheer numbers, these latter individuals cause much more damage than those in the disturbed group.

Economic factors influence types of bullying. The emphasis on scholastic achievement in affluent neighborhoods can underlie bullying by an unexpected group—parents. Twemlow and Sacco described a twelfth-grade girl who attempted suicide after being berated by her father for bringing home an assignment on which she had received a 95 percent grade. Instead of congratulating his daughter, the father said, "If you had done what I told you, you would have gotten 98 percent."[1] Twemlow and Sacco pointed out that less-than-superior academic achievement in high-income neighborhoods is often seen as a negative reflection on the family and thus a motive for parental bullying, while simply getting a high school diploma can be a source of pride for many low-income families. Cliques, which by definition are created by excluding others, also play a role in a bullying culture. Upper-class cliques are almost always composed of fellow students, while lower-class cliques can include dropouts and members from other schools. This resembles what, among other species, especially birds, is sometimes called the "pecking order."

On the other hand, Twemlow and Sacco have shown that attachment to one's school or community can serve as a life-saving buffer when a child's family attachment is weak or absent. By the time a child enters school, family attachment will have succeeded, partially succeeded, or failed. However, some enterprising girls and boys create a bond with their school or their neighborhood that serves as a sound basis for their future development. Schools that provide safe, peaceful, and stimulating environments can take over significant parental functions. This, of course, is not their official role, but becoming a de facto parent can provide opportunities for intellectual, social, and physical growth that a child may find nowhere else. How often do we read about individuals who credit that one special teacher or staffer for changing their lives?

Some adults exhibit bullying behaviors without realizing it. A school coach may shout at student athletes in the hope that it will inspire better performance. Fans attending an athletic event may use abusive language when the opposing team enters the playing field. A school board may shame citizens into making financial contributions to improve school facilities. Police officers demonstrating survival tactics to a group of students may make "arrests" of those boys and girls who fail to comply with instructions because they did not understand them. One sad result is that students who have been bullied by adults may envy the power of the bullies and copy them when interacting with younger siblings.

These inappropriate activities are examples of what Twemlow and Sacco call *dissociation*, a splitting off from one's own better nature, a separation from a social group, or a departure from a consensual code of ethics. This fragmentation needs to be identified; the dissociated fragments need to be reconnected to the larger self or system; and those adults capable of bullying need to be identified, educated, and encouraged to mend fractured relationships.

The Twemlow and Sacco Model for Preventing Bullying

In an earlier chapter, we noted Twemlow and Sacco's emphasis on the *bystander* (a person who is present but neither bullies nor intervenes) as an integral part of most bullying incidents. Sometimes these bystanders are sympathetic to the bully or even join the gang or clique headed by the bully. Other times, they ignore the problem or intervene ineffectively. An adult may unwittingly use similar methods, such as physical punishment, to chastise the bully. This is not very helpful. In addition, school administrators often underestimate the frequency of bullying behavior and inadvertently become bystanders who fail to intervene.[2]

A systems approach to prevention is needed, encompassing the aggressor, the target, and the bystanders, who may play an important part in this process, whether they are teachers, school staff, students, parents, or volunteers. They can move from being passive bystanders to becoming active problem-solvers. They may have unsuspected leadership potential; students thought of as meek, mild, and passive may suddenly take command, displaying skills of mediating, collaborating, and peacemaking that surprise everyone.

For example, one of us (Krippner) knew Mary Jo, a reserved student who showed little interest in the female cliques at her school. But in a classroom role-playing exercise, she listened to both sides of an argument, reflected the position that each clique was taking, and engineered a satisfactory resolution. From that point on, she was called upon to mediate rivalries and competitions that threatened to disrupt student interactions. Her prowess earned her the title of "the peacemaker," and much to her own surprise, her latent skills became appreciated by both the student body and the faculty.

Sometimes a professionally trained mental health worker will be called upon for a limited intervention, but if the fractured system is going to be repaired, the process needs to involve working from within the system itself. A team within the system created by the professional could continue the repair work, or a few leaders within the system could emerge.

A school in Jamaica was identified by national authorities for its high degree of violence. A police officer became an *active* bystander by composing a song, "Tuck Your Shirt In," which became a reggae chant. This triggered a bevy of songs, chants, and jokes with the same theme. Becoming "tidy" became a school-wide craze, as formerly unkempt bullies took on positive leadership roles. Within a matter of weeks, school violence had decreased, and positive student behavior had increased. Since their systems model was introduced in the 1990s, several projects led by Twemlow and Sacco, like this one in Jamaica, have succeeded in reducing bullying in schools and other institutions.[3]

What Works—And What Doesn't

After examining the evidence, R. B. Snyder pointed out what *not* to do in dealing with bullying. Harshly punishing the bully alienates bystanders and does not prevent future incidents. (It may even motivate the bully to retaliate, bullying the victim even more, out of sight of others.) Teaching the bullied to fight back perpetuates the idea that fighting is acceptable. Mediation is unfair because the victim did nothing wrong and has nothing to concede.[4]

Snyder's recommendations for *effective* prevention are comprehensive and require a serious investment of time by others:

- Show bystanders they can do something.
- Reassure victims that they do not deserve the treatment and get their ideas on what to do.
- Help victims rehearse what to say when menaced.
- Practice role-playing in schools, being sure to reverse roles so that everyone can imagine what it might be like to be bullied and to be the bully.

- Improve the social skills of victims and bullies to help them form and maintain healthy relationships.

Another antibullying specialist, Signe Whitson, has published eight "keys" for teachers and parents:

1. Know bullying when you see it. Bullying is not the same as rude or immature behavior. It is a deliberate attempt to hurt someone.
2. Stop bullying when you see it. Use such phrases as, "It is not okay to say that to someone in my classroom." "Sending that kind of text about a classmate is unacceptable. That cannot happen again."
3. Establish positive relationships with students in the class, especially those who are likely to be bullies or their victims.
4. Deal directly with cyberbullying. Stop it immediately.
5. Turn bystanders into buddies. Bullying could easily be stopped by people who would otherwise be passive observers.
6. Reach out to bullies, not to condemn them but to educate and understand them.
7. Build students' social and emotional skills.
8. Keep the conversation going. After resolving one serious bullying incident, realize that your work is not over.[5]

Whitson suggested how teachers can respond when they see one child bullying another: use short and direct statements when the teacher has students' full attention. Whitson added, "The benefit of brief statements like these is that they don't humiliate or alienate anyone. Instead, they let everyone know the teacher is paying attention, and they send a strong signal that bullying won't be tolerated."

These orientations to the prevention of bullying all call for taking prompt action, making clear policy statements, combating passivity on the part of bystanders, and engaging in activity that will enhance social and emotional skills of all concerned. Ultimately, experts agree that there must be a long-term commitment to creating safe communities.

Takeaway Points

- Stereotypes of bullies do not fully capture the range of people who may engage in bullying behavior.
- Bullying may be supported or passively condoned by individuals, groups, or institutions. These other people must be engaged in the antibullying efforts, which must be system-wide, consistent, nonpunitive, and long-term.

Notes

1. Twemlow, S. W., & Sacco, F. C. (2012). *Preventing bullying and school violence* (p. 18). Washington, DC: American Psychiatric Publishing.

2. Bradshaw, C. P., Sawyer, A. L., & O'Brennan, L. M. (2007). Bullying and peer victimization at school: Perceptual differences between students and school staff. *School Psychology Review, 36,* 361–382.

3. Twemlow, S. W., & Sacco, F. C. (1996). Peacekeeping and peacemaking: The conceptual foundations of a plan to reduce violence and improve the quality of life in a midsized community in Jamaica. *Psychiatry, 59,* 156–174.

4. Snyder, R. B. (2013). *5 simple truths of raising kids.* New York: Demos Health.

5. Whitson, S. (2014, October 25). Eight keys to end bullying. *Daily Good* (online).

Depression, Anxiety, and PTSD

CHAPTER TWENTY-TWO

The Three Dangers

Depression and anxiety, frequent precursors to suicidal behavior, are the two major symptoms, or "tracks," of a third condition, post-traumatic stress disorder (PTSD). In this chapter, we explain all three, showing in subsequent chapters how they can be treated.

Understanding Depression

Loosely speaking, *depression* is a mood that comes and goes, an aspect of the human condition, a sadness or loss of energy resulting from loss, grief, or disappointment. Depression becomes a disorder when a person is extremely sad, pessimistic, despondent, listless, and unable to bounce back or to resume ordinary activities.

For those who have never experienced depression and are baffled by its severity, we include this haunting description by novelist William Styron about his own experience:

> The pain is unrelenting, and what makes the condition intolerable is the foreknowledge that no remedy will come—not in a day, an hour, a month, or a minute. If there is mild relief, one knows that it is only temporary; more pain will follow. It is hopelessness even more than pain that crushes the soul. So the decision-making of daily life involves not, as in normal affairs, shifting from one annoying situation to another less annoying—or from discomfort to relative comfort, or from boredom to activity—but moving from pain to pain. One does not abandon, even briefly, one's bed of nails, but is attached to it wherever one goes.[1]

Several contemporary models (that is, depictions or theories) are currently used by mental health professionals to explain depression.[2]

1. *Aggression turned inward.* Many of the early psychoanalysts believed that when people repressed their anger, the suppressed energy from these feelings ultimately evoked depression.

2. *Object loss.* Object loss refers to traumatic separation from significant objects of attachment, such as a parent.

3. *Loss of self-esteem.* When individuals fail or are not respected, they may feel that they have lost standing, status, roles, identities, and values, and depression sets in.

4. *Negative thoughts and feelings.* Aaron Beck, and Albert Ellis before him, found that people become depressed if they focus on negative thoughts that they are helpless, unworthy, or useless.[3]

5. *Reinforcement.* If individuals are not positively rewarded for their actions by those in their social environment, the lack of reward may evoke boredom, despair, and absence of pleasure.

6. *Learned helplessness.* This term describes people who have been thwarted so many times that they no longer even try. Trauma that cannot be escaped can also trigger learned helplessness.[4]

7. *Psychobiology.* Modern psychobiologists study links between experiences and behaviors to central nervous system and endocrine system functions.

Like other disorders, depression has predisposing factors, initiating (triggering) factors, and maintaining factors.

1. *Heredity.* One's genetic inheritance may play a role in major depressive disorders.

2. *Development.* Parents with mood disorders are often in conflicts that may stunt their children's development. Lack of attachment can lead to an early onset of depression.[5] In Elizabeth Wurtzel's autobiography, *Prozac Nation*, she describes the link between her parents' arguments and the emotional debility that propelled her to use antidepressant medication.[6]

3. *Temperament.* A person's temperament is largely inherited but also partly learned. Prolonged sleep deprivation or other sleep disturbances, fear, and protracted emotional arousal can alter temperament.

4. *Critical life events.* Depression is common in families experiencing separation, divorce, or economic stress.

5. *External biological stressors.* Some physical diseases are known to initiate or contribute to depression, especially if they are severe. Legal and illegal drugs may also play a pivotal role in the onset of depression, while continued use may prolong and reinforce it.

Anxiety

Like sadness, fear is a normal human mood that subsides when the threat passes. But anxiety is more than a passing fear. It is a long-standing, relentless sense of being under threat. Fear reacts to a perceived imminent threat, but anxiety anticipates a future threat. Existential philosopher and author Colin Wilson described his experience of anxiety:

> Anxiety hormones began to trickle into my bloodstream, and my heartbeat accelerated. . . . I tried making a frontal assault and suppressing the panic feeling by sheer will power. This proved to be a mistake. My face became hot, and I felt a dangerous tightness across the chest, while my heartbeat increased to a point that terrified me. . . . Like nausea, it came in waves, and between each wave there was a brief feeling of calm and relief. . . . There was a vicious-circle effect; the anxiety produced panic, the panic produced further anxiety, so the original fear was compounded by a fear *of* fear.[7]

Wilson clearly distinguished the original fear, an actual threat, from further anxiety, the "fear of fear." This is *anticipatory anxiety*, and it is very real.

Anxiety is found in phobias (such as agoraphobia, the fear of open spaces), social anxiety (as in selective mutism, when people fear to speak in social settings), and separation anxiety (as when a child's attachment to a caretaker seems to be threatened). A panic attack is an unexpected episode of intense anxiety, whether it is justified or not. One's autonomic nervous system goes into high gear, causing rapid breathing, nausea, chest pains, trembling, fear, or fainting.

We have listed the predisposing factors of depression, most of which can also be applied to anxiety. The Depression and Anxiety Association of America states that there is no evidence that one condition causes the other. However, it is possible to experience both depression and anxiety at the same time. This often occurs when someone experiences PTSD, which we will now consider.

Post-Traumatic Stress Disorder

Trauma takes many forms: violence or threat of violence, sudden injury, combat, and assault. Traumatic experiences can be sudden and obvious, or they can be cumulative, such as what happens to people who work in dangerous jobs: for example, police officers, psychiatric hospital workers, emergency medical technicians, and other first responders. In either case, these experiences may lead to a serious condition, post-traumatic stress disorder (PTSD).[8] PTSD develops along two separate tracks. One involves anxiety, fear conditioning, hypervigilance, and intrusive thoughts. The other is characterized by depression, emotional numbness, helplessness, and loss of hope. Both tracks may involve flashbacks and the avoidance of contact with any situation associated with the traumatizing event.[9]

Those two tracks can be identified and treated separately or together. If PTSD is not addressed promptly, it becomes increasingly complicated as additional symptoms develop, build on themselves, and influence each other. Commonly, people attempt to bounce back following the traumatizing event, trying to resume their ordinary lives. They may want to avoid a costly stay in a hospital or the time and expense of psychotherapy. But the symptoms may become especially distressing after a month or so, even though some people try to ignore them. You may remember Fred, from the first chapter of this book, who was able to handle his PTSD for decades. It was only after he retired that the disorder wreaked havoc and took its toll.

In 2019, the American Psychological Association (APA) issued its guidelines for the treatment of depression, emphasizing "evidence-based" treatments that often combine psychotherapy and medication. The authors noted that fewer than 1 percent of children and adolescents who live with depression receive treatment, but they found insufficient evidence to recommend a specific treatment for children. For adolescents, the panel recommended cognitive behavioral therapy (CBT) or interpersonal therapy, a brief intervention that focuses on improving a client's relationships. Prozac was the recommended medication, although there was insufficient evidence to indicate it was better than psychotherapy.

For adults, there was support for various types of cognitive behavioral therapy, psychodynamic therapy, interpersonal psychotherapy, and supportive psychotherapy, which is practically oriented and combines elements of the other recommended interventions. If medication is used, the panel recommended "second-generation" antidepressants. For older adults, the panel urged group therapy and a combination of interpersonal psychotherapy and second-generation antidepressants.[10]

Which is more useful, psychotherapy or medication? A systematic review published in 2019 concluded that both are helpful, but there is insufficient evidence to conclude which is more effective.[11] Both reduce the symptoms of PTSD, but few studies examined *improvements* in quality of life, or "posttraumatic growth."[12] This would include changes in quality of life, improved resilience, the development of meaning and values, and the increase in happiness, joy, and the ability to appreciate simple events, such as sunsets, the smell of freshly prepared food, the color and scent of flowers, and the sounds of children at play.

Researchers have identified a cluster of nerves that appear to be related to chronic pain and emotional trauma. Called the *stellate ganglion*, the nerve group is located on the right side of the spine, at the last vertebra of the neck, and seems related to the fight-or-flight response. Deadening the ganglion with an anesthetic was found to relieve such PTSD symptoms as anxiety, depression, and insomnia among patients in some military medical centers. The stellate ganglion block has a few temporary side effects, such as redness and droopiness of the eyes, a flushed face, and a hoarse voice. The healing effects last for several months or even a year or more. The cost ranges from $2,000 to $3,000, but because only a few treatments are needed each year, it is much less expensive than constant therapies. Patients have been able to return to work after a few days, increasing the economic benefits. The stellate ganglion block could ease the pain for thousands of veterans and save lives currently being lost to suicide.[13]

War has triggered trauma in millions of people, both combatants and civilians, who face injury or death, the deaths of comrades or family, the need to defend themselves (under orders, in the case of soldiers), loss of homes, and the complete disruption of their everyday lives. Combatants are directed to kill and destroy, in some cases resulting in the "moral injury" that we have discussed. The psychological effects of war acquired various names over the years: soldier's heart, shell shock, combat fatigue, and, since the Vietnam War, PTSD. No matter the name, suicide is an all too frequent outcome for many combat veterans.

The following chapters of this section will explore some of the dimensions of suicide among veterans, whether or not they engaged in combat.

Takeaway Points

- Depression, a common part of life, becomes a disorder when it cripples ordinary functioning and enjoyment.
- Likewise, anxiety is a distorted version of fear that can interfere with job performance and social relationships.
- When depression and anxiety co-occur, as in PTSD, they create a particularly distressing state, one that can lead to suicidal behavior.

Notes

1. Styron, W. (2010). *Darkness visible: A memoir of madness*. New York: Open Road Media.
2. Deacon, B. J. (2013). The biomedical model of mental disorders: A critical analysis of its validity, utility, and its effects on psychotherapy research. *Clinical Psychology Review, 33,* 846–867.

3. Beck, A. J. (1972). *Depression: Causes and treatment.* Philadelphia: University of Pennsylvania Press.

4. Mikulincer, M. (1994). *Human learned helplessness: A coping perspective.* New York: Springer.

5. Sweezy, A. (Ed.). (2017). *Innovative elaborations in internal family systems.* New York: Routledge.

6. Wurtzel, E. (1994). *Prozac nation: Young and depressed in America.* Boston: Houghton Mifflin.

7. Wilson, C. (1978). *Mysteries* (p. 24). New York: G. P. Putnam's Sons.

8. Hilton, N. Z., Ham, E., Rodrigues, N. D., et al. (2019, December 4). Contribution of critical events and chronic stressors to PTSD symptoms among psychiatric workers. *Psychiatric Services, 71*(3), 221–227.

9. Neld, D. (2019, December 21). We just got closer to understanding how PTSD starts to develop in the mind. *Science Alerts: Health* (online).

10. American Psychological Association. (2019). *The clinical practice guidelines for the treatment of depression across three age cohorts.* Washington, DC: American Psychological Association.

11. Sonis, J. (2019, December 19). Which is more effective for treating PTSD: Medication, or psychotherapy? *University of North Carolina Health Care Blog Post.* http://news.unchealthcare.org/som-vital-signs/2020/feb-27/which-is-more-effective-for-treating-ptsd-medication-or-psychotherapy.

12. Guzman, M., & Padros, F. (2018, September 6). Promoting post-traumatic growth after PTSD. *Psychology Today* (online).

13. Mulvaney, S. W., Lynch, J. H., Hickey, M. J., et al. (2014). Stellate ganglion block used to treat symptoms associated with combat-related post-traumatic stress disorder: A case series of 166 patients. *Military Medicine, 179*, 1133–1140.

CHAPTER TWENTY-THREE

Treating Depression

Fortunately, we know a lot about depression and the ways people can forestall or resolve it, sometimes without professional treatment. Exercise has long been known to prevent and lift depression because vigorous movement stimulates health-giving changes in blood flow and oxygen supply. Cognitive therapy is a focused, short-term approach that teaches people how to identify negative thoughts and replace them with healthy ones. In our chapters on rational emotive behavioral therapy (REBT), you will learn more about this. For some people, antidepressant medications work well, at least temporarily.

Internal Family Systems Therapy

An emerging therapy developed by Richard Schwartz seems promising. Internal Family Systems (IFS) therapy identifies and addresses the "subpersonalities" that coexist within each person's psyche, rather like an "internal family." (Chaos theorists call some subpersonalities "chaotic attractors," while Jungian psychotherapists call them "complexes.") They are caused by wounds inflicted by painful or traumatic emotional experiences. Other subpersonalities, developed to protect people from their wounded parts, are often at war with each other and with the core self. IFS attempts to heal the client's wounded parts, creating balance and harmony. Depression is one of the disorders for which IFS practitioners claim to have produced positive effects.

The wounded subpersonalities are referred to as "exiles," the "managers" who try to keep the "exiles" under control, and the "firefighters" who distract the core self from the exiles when they are released. Without the firefighters, the risk of suicide would increase. The managers, which may take the form of eating disorders and substance abuse, need to be healed and transformed. The IFS practitioner attempts to modify the extreme activities of the subpersonalities, strengthen the core self, and coordinate all these parts with the core self in charge. No subpersonality can be addressed without permission of the managers. Each subpersonality has its own agenda; attempting to change it prematurely could remove a valuable defense and increase the risk of suicide.[1]

The concept of subpersonalities has a venerable history in psychotherapy, notably in Roberto Assagioli's development of psychosynthesis and in Gestalt therapy. Because of the devastation wreaked by depression, IFS therapy is one of many promising interventions that deserves serious attention.

Clinical Practice Guidelines for Depression

In 2019, the APA issued its *Clinical Practice Guideline for the Treatment of Depression across Three Age Cohorts*.[2] The handbook provides research-based recommendations for treating depressive disorders, including major depression, depression that does not meet criteria for a full diagnosis, and persistent depressive disorder of children, adolescents, adults, and older adults. The goal was to create a comprehensive handbook comparing the efficacy of different types of treatments in different patient populations. The panel members considered four factors:

1. The overall strength of the evidence
2. The balance of a treatment's benefits versus its harms
3. Client values and preferences
4. Applicability of the treatment

Children

The APA guidelines noted that depression is less common in children than in adults. Boys and girls are affected equally, but after adolescence, young women are twice as likely as young men to develop depressive disorders. The depression rate among marginalized populations, such as ethnic or sexual minorities, may be significantly higher. Fewer than 1 percent of children and adolescents with depression receive outpatient treatment. Depression affects people in different ways, so it is impossible to make a generalization as to treatment.

Adolescents

For adolescents, the panel found sufficient evidence to recommend CBT or interpersonal therapy as the initial treatment. Interpersonal therapy attempts to clarify the client's interactions with significant others, including the therapist. The therapist helps the client explore current and past experiences related to relationships and environmental influences.

For clinicians considering pharmacotherapy, the handbook recommended fluoxetine (Prozac) over other medications. There was not enough evidence to determine the comparative effectiveness of fluoxetine versus psychotherapy. The panel recommended against the use of clomipramine, imipramine, mirtazapine, paroxetine, and venlafaxine because of the increased suicide risk in young people taking these drugs.

Adults

Among adults, women are almost twice as likely as men to experience depression, with a lifetime prevalence of major depression of 21 percent among women compared to 12 percent among men. For the initial treatment of depression among adults, the handbook recommends either psychotherapy or second-generation antidepressants, including selective serotonin reuptake inhibitors (SSRIs) and serotonin-norepinephrine reuptake inhibitors (SNRIs). The second-generation antidepressants are considered more effective than the earlier first-generation antidepressants, but they all alter the levels of designated neurotransmitters available at receptor sites in the brain.

There was support for CBT and mindfulness-based cognitive therapy, interpersonal therapy, psychodynamic therapies, and supportive therapies. In mindfulness-based cognitive therapy, thoughts and feelings are experienced freely as they arrive and are then discussed with the therapist. Psychodynamic therapies focus on drives and other internal forces that shape behavior. Supportive therapies search for a client's relationship patterns both inside and outside of the therapeutic process. For clinicians considering combining treatments, the panel recommended combining CBT or supportive therapies with a second-generation antidepressant.

About 3 percent of older adults experience depression, especially if there is an associated medical condition. These clients generally prefer psychotherapeutic and psychosocial interventions to medication. The panel members recommended group CBT or group "life review" treatment, the latter of which recalls and analyzes past experiences for the purpose of arriving at a meaningful life story. When considering combined treatment, the panel recommended a combination of second-generation antidepressants and interpersonal psychotherapy.

Notably, there are risks associated with fluoxetine, described in such books as *Prozac Nation: Young and Depressed in America*, Elizabeth Wurtzel's first-person account of her struggles with both depression and the side effects of this medication.[3] Psychiatrist Peter Breggin has been outspoken in his opposition to what often seem to be indiscriminate prescriptions of Prozac and other antidepressants. Breggin has described the struggle he has observed among his patients, notably helplessness in the face of feeling unworthy. When he asked his clients how medication can help resolve this struggle, he found no solid answer.[4]

Takeaway Points

- Many treatments for depression exist. It is important to find the one that works for each individual.
- The American Psychological Association's *Clinical Practice Guideline for the Treatment of Depression across Three Age Cohorts* provides research-based recommendations.

Notes

1. Sweezy, A. (Ed.). (2017). *Innovative elaborations in Internal Family Systems.* New York: Routledge.

2. American Psychological Association. (2019). *The clinical practice guideline for the treatment of depression across three age cohorts.* Washington, DC: American Psychological Association.

3. Wurtzel, E. (1994). *Prozac nation: Young and depressed in America.* Boston: Houghton Mifflin.

4. Breggin, P., & Breggin, G. R. (2014). *Talking back to Prozac* (2nd ed.). New York: Open Road Media.

CHAPTER TWENTY-FOUR

Deconstructing Anxiety: A New Way of Dealing with Suicidality

A person considering suicide faces deep existential questions: "Is there meaning to existence?" "Does my life have value?" "Is there a purpose in suffering that is worth enduring for a better future?" Anxiety, one cause of suicidality, can be deconstructed by addressing these questions at a fundamental level, thereby providing the direct experience that suffering is the result of faulty assumptions, irrational beliefs, and dysfunctional personal myths.

Deconstructing anxiety was developed by psychologist Todd Pressman, who was baffled by his depressed clients and their chronic suffering. Over the years, he developed a treatment that appeared to resolve the root causes of suffering for most of his clients.[1]

Fear and Fulfillment: Two Drives in Conflict

In the deconstructing anxiety method, fear and fulfillment are positioned as the two great drives in human experience. A person's first impulse is for fulfillment, but children learn to restrain it as they experience disapproval or punishment. They alter, postpone, or bury their quest for fulfillment until they feel safe, oscillating between these two poles and using fear as one strategy for trying to secure fulfillment. But when life becomes a morass of too many problems and too little fulfillment, some people question whether it is worth living.

As the fundamental obstacle to fulfillment, fear is understood as the true source of any suffering, including suicidal depression. Any problem, upset, or grievance can be traced to a fear. The great revelation in deconstructing anxiety is that when fear is properly deconstructed, it transforms, giving way to fulfillment. In exposing the fear, *facing* rather than *avoiding* it, people find that the feared event simply does not play out as they had imagined. Either they encounter a problem they can deal with (rather than the ruinous experience they had anticipated), or they discover that there is no problem. One study showed that beliefs *about* worry were more important than the feared thing itself.[2] In both these ways, deconstructing and facing fear revealed it to be an illusion, a mirage that disintegrated once it was faced.

Finding the Core Fear

What does *facing fear* actually mean? And why are the best exposure therapy efforts successful in resolving anxiety only about half the time they are used?[3]

The deconstructing anxiety model holds that people must find and face the *correct* fear. As infants move through the world, their understanding of that world begins to include *fear blueprints* as a strategy for securing fulfillment. They may start out in a state of relative fulfillment, but sooner or later, they have their first encounter with danger or loss: perhaps mother takes too long to respond to their cries or father expresses irritation at their clumsiness. This signals the arrival of the *core fear*, their fundamental interpretation of how the world can threaten them. In many cases, this is the fear of abandonment, a loss of attachment that can last a lifetime and impact an individual's capacity to make and sustain relationships.

For example, the youngest infants whose mothers leave the room do not realize they will return; they may conclude that their lifeline to survival has vanished. Pressman discovered that there are five core fears:

1. Fear of abandonment
2. Fear of loss of identity
3. Fear of loss of meaning
4. Fear of loss of purpose
5. Fear of death

Once the core fear is established, people begin to filter many of their experiences through it. They become vigilant for signs, suggesting that the problem, or some version of it, might return. In our example, the children may become highly sensitized any time their mothers (or others they depend on) make a move to leave or otherwise withdraw. These children may develop separation anxiety. The core fear, or one of its derivatives, becomes the lens through which people interpret *every* difficult experience. For this reason, when people thoroughly deconstruct a problem, Pressman concluded, they will uncover the core fear at its root.

The Chief Defense

Making sense out of the dangers of life is helpful, but it has its own disadvantages. When mothers leave the room, infants may spontaneously begin screaming. As the mothers rush back to see what's wrong, the infants discover that they have some agency over their fear after all—they have found a solution! The impact of this discovery is profound. They now have a strategy (scream and protest) for making themselves safe. Or a toddler finds that screaming makes mother angry and decides to be a "good girl" and never upset mother again. Such a basic strategy becomes the *chief defense* to respond to the core fear. Over time, growing children evolve, making new adaptations of the chief defense.

All Defenses Backfire

However, this strategy for securing fulfillment eventually backfires: by defending against a situation, people tell themselves that there is something real to defend against, that the situation truly is threatening. The chief defense concretizes the core fear, making it a map for life. Failing to gain a guarantee of safety, they repeat the defensive effort all the more earnestly. Suicidal patients have become so entrenched in this strategy that they sacrifice fulfillment to protect against threats that may not even exist. Eventually, it can be hard for them to find life worth living.

Digging for Gold: Finding the Core Fear

Luckily, this model suggests a way out: clients must dismantle the chief defense to have an exposure to the core fear (the true fear generating their problems) and discover it is not real. They set themselves free by recognizing there is nothing to defend against.

To accomplish this, they must first identify their core fear and chief defense. The deconstructing anxiety method provides a surprisingly powerful, effective, and quick process for uncovering one's core fear; this is called "digging for gold." People begin by writing down, at the top left of a page (or discussing with the therapist) any presenting problem in a short, single phrase: "My husband will leave me if I speak up for myself," "I know I'm going to fail this course," or "My parents will kill me if they find out I had sex with my boyfriend."

One of three questions is then asked:

1. "Why is that upsetting to me?"
2. "What am I afraid will happen next?"
3. "What am I afraid I will miss or lose?"

They write down their answer at the top right of the page on the same line as the problem. One of the same three questions is asked about this *new* problem, and the process of deconstruction continues until the core fear is reached.

Discovering one's core fear is highly significant, often accompanied by powerful catharses, insights, and flashbacks regarding the major decisions made throughout one's life. It also reveals a fundamental truth about what has been causing one's suffering. Performing the exercise with a variety of problems, one makes the remarkable discovery that the same core fear is at the root of them all.

Finding the Chief Defense

After identifying the core fear, clients must find their chief defense against that fear. The deconstructing anxiety method offers a variety of techniques for this, asking, "What do I do to protect myself from the core fear?" There will be a variety of answers, but the chief defense is the distilled answer beneath them all. For instance, individuals with a core fear of losing their identities may become overly responsible and people pleasers. The chief defense underneath may be to make certain no one thinks they are "bad" people. Someone else with a core fear of abandonment may become dependent but also fall into depression. Both are ways of mitigating the pain of being unwillingly alone. Indeed, depression is a defense that tries to minimize pain by shutting it down and avoiding the problem. Those whose core fear is loss of meaning may fill their schedule with constant busyness and set up standards of perfectionism, attempting to feel important and full rather than devoid of meaning.

The Master Key to Resolving Fear

It is usually not enough to simply encourage someone to "resist" the chief defense. Instead, they must identify the precise moment and mechanism by which the defense is applied—when and where they push against, run from, or otherwise manipulate their fear—and practice doing the opposite in as many ways as they can imagine.

The nuts and bolts of the deconstructing anxiety method, then, are these exercises for doing the opposite. There are three primary techniques: "the Alchemist," "the Witness," and "the Warrior's Stance." A fourth is called

"Letting Go the Resistance to Resistance." In brief, each of these locates the precise moment in consciousness when defensiveness is applied and allows people to expose themselves safely to their fear without deploying the defense. Once they have done so thoroughly, leaving all traces of defensiveness behind, the illusion causing their fear disperses, and they are set free.

Janet

Janet (a pseudonym) was a forty-five-year-old woman who sought Pressman's help for severe anxiety, including panic attacks and depression. Coming from a difficult background, she had recently suffered a serious car accident that left her with constant physical pain and severe post-traumatic stress. The combination of pain, PTSD, and her preexisting anxiety and depression had overwhelmed her. After developing a rapport with Pressman, she confessed that she was considering taking her life. This is how they performed the digging for gold exercise:

> Janet: I'm exhausted from trying to take care of everyone and everything. It brings me pain and nothing but problems.
>
> Pressman: I understand. And why is that upsetting to you?
>
> Janet: I don't know if I can keep it up much longer.
>
> Pressman: Why is that thought upsetting to you?
>
> Janet: If I can't keep it up, my family will think that I am a bad person.
>
> Pressman: If they do, what are you afraid will happen?
>
> Janet: They won't want to be bothered with me.
>
> Pressman: Why is *that* upsetting to you?
>
> Janet: I'll be left alone.
>
> Pressman: And what are you afraid will happen after that?
>
> Janet: I'll feel worthless.
>
> Pressman: If you feel worthless, what are afraid you will miss or lose?
>
> Janet: If I'm worthless, there's no point to anything. No love. No reason for staying alive.
>
> Pressman: If that were so, what are you afraid you would miss or lose?
>
> Janet: Everything. That's who I am. I'll lose me.

Janet's core fear was losing her identity, and her chief defense was to become a caretaker, incessantly taking care of others' needs at her own expense. She recalled the origins of this defense. Although they meant well, her parents continually rewarded her for being "good." Their other children had created significant problems, and Janet watched as her parents began to distance themselves from them. This observation inspired her solution: she would be good, becoming the person her parents wanted to win and keep their approval. But her parents were too busy with their other children to really notice her efforts. So she tried harder and harder to earn their recognition. By the time she came to Pressman, she was burnt out from a lifetime of sacrifice and self-denial.

First, they employed the Warrior's Stance, physically freezing whenever her compulsion to take care of others arose. Once she gained some facility with this, she discovered anger for the first time in her life—anger at those who had taken her good deeds for granted and anger at those who took advantage of her self-sacrifice.

Then Janet recognized that, while it was a step in the right direction, her anger was also a defense. In the Witness, she learned to embrace it with infinite space, creating a deep relaxation and ease. This worked well to ease her physical pain and went a long way to giving her real hope for the future.

With the Alchemist, she had a truly transformative experience. At first, she realized that she was afraid to truly let go of her anger: "If I do, they'll think they can get away with it and take advantage of me again." She visualized living through her fear of being taken advantage of (and losing her identity) for longer and longer periods of time. Eventually, she imagined living through it for "millions of years" without trying to escape or defend against the experience. With this realization, Janet became very quiet and still.

When Pressman asked what was happening, she whispered in a voice filled with awe and surprise, "I've come out the other side. I've moved all the way through the fear, and I see that it's just a thought!" She added, "This whole time, my whole life, really, I thought I had to take care of others no matter how unhappy it made me, and that, if I didn't, I wouldn't have any value. I see now that I made that up, that it was just a thought. And I see this is true for everything in my life. We make up what we're afraid of. There's really nothing stopping us from being happy. It's all a free choice!"

From that moment, her anxiety and depression lifted. She became more effective in choosing how she spent her time and how she related with others, and she was able to translate more quickly any old-style thoughts that came up into those promoting fulfillment and authenticity.[4]

Takeaway Points

- Insight into the core fear at the root of any problem yields the potential to resolve that fear effectively. Anything less will provide only partial or temporary relief.

- Defensiveness is the source of suffering, not what we are defending against. Understanding this reveals a pathway to freedom.

- Discovering and confronting the core fear frees us to choose a new response in any circumstance that confronts us.

Notes

1. Pressman, T. (2019). *Deconstructing anxiety: The journey from fear to fulfillment.* Lanham, MD: Rowman & Littlefield.

2. Borkovec, T. T., Hazlett-Stevens, H., & Diaz, M. L. (1999). The role of positive beliefs about worry in generalized anxiety disorder and its treatment. *Clinical Psychology and Psychotherapy, 6,* 126–138.

3. Hofmann, S. G., & Smits, J. A. (2008). Cognitive-behavioral therapy for adult anxiety disorders: A meta-analysis of randomized placebo-controlled trials. *Journal of Clinical Psychiatry, 69,* 621–632.

4. Pressman, T. (2020, January). Deconstructing anxiety. *Counseling Today,* pp. 40–44.

CHAPTER TWENTY-FIVE

Evaluating Treatments for PTSD

In 2017, the APA adopted a policy statement titled *Clinical Practice Guidelines for the Treatment of Posttraumatic Stress Disorder (PTSD) in Adults*. The guidelines were designed to provide recommendations on psychological and pharmacological treatments for PTSD.[1] The authors were health care professionals from psychology, psychiatry, social work, and family medicine as well as community members and PTSD survivors. They focused on two outcomes: reducing symptoms and avoiding adverse events (including suicide) related to PTSD.

The panel used the APA's definitions in the fifth edition of its *Diagnostic and Statistical Manual of Mental Disorders (DSM-5)*, which describes four clusters of symptoms: intrusive and recurring memories of the trauma, avoidance of situations related to the trauma, numbing or negative changes in thoughts and emotions relating to the trauma, and changes in reactivity and arousal, such as startle responses and hyperarousal.

Recommended and Suggested Psychotherapies

Since PTSD has received attention from many quarters of the psychotherapy profession, various treatments have been proposed. After assessing these, the panel "strongly recommended" the use of cognitive behavioral therapy (CBT), cognitive processing therapy (CPT), cognitive therapy (CT), and prolonged exposure therapy (PET). It "suggested" the use of brief eclectic psychotherapy (BEP), eye movement desensitization and reprocessing (EMDR), and narrative exposure therapy (NET). The panel's key recommendation was for prolonged exposure therapy (PET) or for a combination of PET and one of the cognitive therapies. Let's review each of these in turn.

Cognitive Therapies

All the cognitive therapies date back to the rational emotive behavior therapy (REBT) developed by psychologist Albert Ellis, who began offering training seminars on REBT in 1956. A decade later, psychiatrist Aaron Beck developed cognitive therapy (CT), the first psychotherapy to undergo rigorous clinical testing. Both Ellis and Beck based their programs on the "cognitive model": the way people *perceive* situations influences the way they think, feel, and behave.[2] Both Ellis and Beck began their careers as psychoanalysts, but they became dissatisfied because too much time was spent discussing clients' histories rather than focusing on current life issues. Beck incorporated breathing exercises into CT, and Ellis recommended meditation for many of his clients.

Cognitive behavioral therapy (CBT) is an umbrella term for a variety of practices that share common elements, namely, cognitive, behavioral, or a combination. When Beck's work with CT became widely known, many behavior therapists incorporated cognitive techniques into their practice.

Cognitive processing therapy (CPT) is a specific type of CBT that has been deliberately geared to help clients with PTSD. Special attention is paid to automatic thoughts that may be maintaining the PTSD symptoms. Clients are asked to write an essay about the traumatizing event and how it has shaped their lives, along with detailed impact statements about how their lives have been affected. Once clients know how to spot PTSD symptoms, they can take actions to block or transform the thoughts. CPT can be delivered individually or in group settings.

Prolonged Exposure Therapy

Prolonged exposure therapy (PET), developed by psychologist Edna Foa to treat PTSD, anxiety, and depression, involves two core components: imaginal (imagined) exposure and in vivo (real-life) exposure.[3] The first consists of retelling the traumatic experience to the therapist, thereby *exposing* the client to the stimulus. This is done several times in as much detail as possible. In the second type, frightening stimuli related to the trauma are listed in order of degree, from least (such as hearing a loud noise) to most (such as seeing a bomb explode and kill someone). The client is exposed to each stimulus until it is no longer frightening and then moves to the next one. By the time the whole list has been treated, the client has become *desensitized* to the stimulus.

Exposure is combined with emotional processing and additional writing assignments. Clients are urged to participate in enjoyable activities so that their days are not filled with prolonged exposures to unpleasant stimuli. This is especially important for clients exhibiting emotional numbing or depression. Foa and her associates claimed that PET instills confidence, a sense of mastery, stress reduction, coping strategies, and the ability to distinguish safe from risky activities.

Eye Movement Desensitization and Reprocessing

Eye movement desensitization and reprocessing (EMDR) was originally designed to help clients cope with traumatic memories, but it is now used for a broader range of problems. EMDR therapists believe this method helps a person access and process adverse life experiences, bringing them to an adaptive resolution. Therapist-directed lateral eye movements are the most frequently employed external stimuli, but hand tapping and audio stimuli are sometimes used. Francine Shapiro, who developed EMDR, hypothesized that any of these stimuli enabled clients to access traumatic memory networks in the brain. The memories that laid the groundwork for the current distress are "desensitized" and then "reprocessed," forging new links with more adaptive memories and information sources. Imagined scenarios of future events are incorporated to enable clients to acquire the motivations and skills they need.[4] EMDR therapy is said to resolve the traumatic memories, allowing natural recovery to take place in a few sessions.

Narrative Exposure Therapy

Narrative exposure therapy (NET) is a treatment for trauma-related disorders, particularly for people, including refugees, affected by multiple or continual traumas, such as cultural, political, or social upheavals. NET is particularly adaptable for use with small groups. With a therapist's help, clients establish a chronological narrative of their lives, concentrating on their traumatic experiences but including positive experiences as well. This process contextualizes the network of sensory, emotional, and cognitive memories, refining the trauma into a coherent story. Clients relate the narrative, describing their emotions, thoughts, sensory information, and body reactions without losing their orientation to the present.

What may formerly have been disconnected episodes are now seen as an integrated, coherent whole that can be imbued with meaning. NET claims to differ from other treatments by focusing on recognizing and creating an account of what happened. This is done in a way that affirms clients' self-respect. At the end of treatment, clients are given a written biography.

Implications for Treatment

The community members of the APA panel stressed the importance of the alliance between psychotherapists and clients, the psychotherapists' knowledge about PTSD, and their sensitivity to cultural and social differences. They also favored a personalized approach to psychotherapy and the psychotherapist's ability to offer pertinent information and coping skills. The panel did not find evidence of serious harm associated with any of its recommended psychotherapies.

Suggested Medications

The evidence supporting medication was not as strong as the evidence supporting psychotherapy; thus, no medication received a "recommendation." The suggested medications were found to have a "small magnitude of benefit" for reducing PTSD symptoms in contrast to the "medium to large magnitude of benefit" found for the recommended psychotherapies. It also noted that there were fewer known harms for psychological treatment than for medical treatments.

Paroxetine, sertraline, and fluoxetine are all selective serotonin reuptake inhibitors (SSRIs) thought to act by blocking the reuptake of serotonin into serotonin-containing neurons in the brain, increasing the availability of this substance, often called the "happiness neurotransmitter." When SSRIs have a positive effect, clients feel calmer and more optimistic, and they report feelings of well-being.

Selective serotonin-norepinephrine uptake inhibitors (SNRIs) such as venlafaxine not only increase the amount of serotonin available but also norepinephrine. Norepinephrine is an "action neurotransmitter" that helps the brain focus attention on a given task and mobilizes the system to initiate an activity. Critics of SSRIs and SNRIs allege that their overuse has been linked to suicide and violence.[5] The possible hazards of antidepressants, which are discussed in other chapters of this book, are reflected in the panel's decision to "suggest" but not "recommend" them.

The Panel's Conclusions

The panel concluded its report by emphasizing the urgency of the problem. Unresolved PTSD symptoms can become chronic and emerge across one's life span, causing suffering to the primary victim and to loved ones as well.

The panel noted several limitations in the investigations they studied. Clients' quality of life was infrequently studied or reported, nor was the degree of functional impairment (the ability to complete daily tasks). Most studies excluded clients with suicidality or substance abuse, even though these conditions are often comorbid, appearing along with PTSD. Dissociation was also not studied, despite the fact that *DSM-5* includes a dissociation subtype. There was little discussion regarding client preferences, even though there is considerable evidence that clients who receive their personal choice of treatment are 50 percent less likely to drop out of treatment and 60 percent more likely to demonstrate improvement.[6] There was also a "researcher allegiance" effect; greater improvement from PTSD is observed for treatments for which the researcher has an allegiance or identification. Some investigators studied a treatment they had developed or modified.

In 2019, the APA published a summary of the guidelines in its flagship journal *American Psychologist*.[7] While its use of *DSM-5* can be criticized as supporting a medical model of PTSD, it includes a cautionary statement on medication and advocates psychological therapy.

Another Analysis

The APA team evaluated studies using a meta-analysis, a statistical procedure in which the results of several studies are combined, producing a single result. Psychologists at the University of Basel, Switzerland, and the University of Freiburg, Germany, conducted a meta-analysis of PTSD studies published between 1960 and 2018. Comparing psychological to pharmacological treatments, and examining combination approaches, the team divided the studies into those studying short-term effects and those studying long-term effects.

The short-term results showed very few differences among the treatments, but long-term studies gave the edge to psychotherapy, with combined treatments producing the best results. However, the small number of clients treated and the different ways of charting results mean the findings are preliminary. Even so, the team advised that its results appeared not to support the use of medication as the initial treatment for PTSD.

Takeaway Points

- The American Psychological Association's clinical guidelines for treating PTSD were based on a comprehensive review of published research studies. The guidelines recommended several types of psychotherapy and suggested several medications.
- The APA study and a similar investigation at the University of Basel found more support for psychotherapy than for medication. However, the difference was not clear-cut, and more comparisons need to be made.

Notes

1. Courtois, C. A., Sonis, J., Brown, L. S., et al. (2019). *Clinical practice guidelines for the treatment of posttraumatic stress disorder (PTSD) in adults.* Washington, DC: American Psychological Association.

2. Wylie, M. S. (2014, December 26). How Aaron Beck and Albert Ellis started a psychotherapy revolution. *Psychotherapy Newsletter.*

3. Foa, E. B., McLean, C. P., Capaldi, S., & Rosenfeld, D. (2013). Prolonged exposure vs. supportive counseling for sexual abuse-related PTSD in adolescent girls: A randomized clinical trial. *Journal of the American Medical Association, 310,* 2650–2657.

4. Shapiro, F. (2018). *Eye movement desensitization and reprocessing (EMDR): Basic principles, protocols, and procedures* (3rd ed.). New York: Guilford Press.

5. Naulati, E. G. (2018). *Saving talk therapy.* Boston: Beacon Press.

6. American Psychological Association. (2019). Summary of the clinical practice guidelines for the treatment of posttraumatic stress disorder (PTSD) in adults. *American Psychologist, 74,* 596–607.

7. Merz, J., Schwartzer, G., & Gerger, H. (2019, June 12). Comparative efficacy and acceptability of pharmacological /psychotherapeutic and combination treatments in adults with posttraumatic stress disorder: A network meta-analysis. *Journal of the American Medical Association, Psychiatry, 76*(9), 904–913.

THOSE WHO SURVIVED: BOBBY GREY

He did not even remember trying to kill himself. When he woke up in the intensive care unit, he thought he had been in a car accident. They had to bring him a mirror so he could see the red weal around his neck.

Bobby Grey had spent four years in the Marines, including combat in Iraq. When a suicide bomber attacked his base, he suffered a concussion and a mild traumatic brain injury. He survived because two others saw the truck bomb approaching and tried to abort the attack.

"They basically sacrificed themselves for thirty-some Marines," he says. "And then, me and another buddy of mine, we actually had to put two of them in their body bags ourselves. That's the kind of stuff that really weighed on me, even years after leaving the Marine Corps."[1]

Discharged in 2007, Bobby experienced classic signs of PTSD: poor sleep, irritability, depression, and intense mood swings. He even physically attacked a relative who made an insensitive comment. His wife frequently urged him to get help, but this only made him angrier.

"She knew something was going on, but I was ignorant and had too much of an ego to admit it," Bobby says. "I was like, 'Woman, stop. You're making me think I'm crazy when there's nothing wrong. Just leave me alone.'" Bobby recalls that he and others looked down on PTSD. "There was this stigma with having PTSD, like you're somehow less of a man," he says. "I didn't want that label on me, so I didn't talk about it."

Denying it did not help. On Memorial Day 2013, after a fight with his wife, he stormed out of the house. Bobby then sent her a text message: "I love you. I always will. I'm sorry."

Some instinct told her to run to the backyard, where she saw him hanging from the magnolia tree. Her screams brought a neighbor and a ladder. They got him down, gave him CPR, and called 911. After ten days in a medically induced coma, he awoke.

It took another year for Bobby to decide to stop hiding. A friend helped him make a video about his PTSD, including the suicide attempt. They posted it on YouTube. "I did that video, and it's been great strides ever since," he says. Sharing his story became a mission. He's spoken at schools and churches and testified before Congress on behalf of the Armed Forces Foundation. His most important audience is fellow veterans and active military personnel; he shows them in person that it is possible to open up, share one's pain, and emerge ready to live.

Bobby believes God gave him this second chance at life so he could fight the scourge of PTSD. "There's no other explanation for it," he says. "I've been put in the hells of war and life for a reason, and that's something I had to understand: Why am I still alive? I mean, there are guys who hung themselves who never came out of the coma or had the quality of life that I have, so I'd be stupid not to use this second chance to share my testimony and try to stop this thing."

Bobby found meaning in his life. Although he is not totally free of struggle, he has a lot to live for. He is one of those who survived.

Note

1. This and other quotations are taken from Jimmy Tomlin (2019, December 15), The wounded warrior: Bobby Grey's PTSD nearly killed him—now it's helping others. High Point Enterprise. https://hpenews.com/news/12889/the-wounded-warrior-bobby -greys-ptsd-nearly-killed-him-now-its-helping-others. See also Bobby and Kia Grey's *Soldier's Kiss: A PTSD Documentary.*

SECTION VI

Other Groups at Risk

CHAPTER TWENTY-SIX

Suicide on the Land: The Farmer's Dilemma

Hank was a prominent rancher in Colorado Springs who was working to bring environmental ideas into the ranching community: preserving land rather than depleting it, using water wisely, and rotating the cattle from one pasture to another to let the grassland recover. He knew his stuff and worked to spread the word. A reporter wrote,

> While Hank stood on the crumbling [creek] bank, giving an impassioned speech about the watershed protection group that he'd helped to organize, telling me about holding ponds, landscaped greenways and the virtues of permeable parking lots covered in gravel, I lost track of his words. And I thought: "This guy's going to be governor of Colorado someday."[1]

Alas, the ruthless pressures of Big Ag, the exhausting work of protecting his land, falling cattle prices, and the county's plan to build a highway right through his ranch drained Hank's energy, intelligence, and love of his family beyond endurance. At the age of forty-three, he took his own life.

Hank was just one of many farmers who have given up the hope of saving the land that may have been in their families for generations. This is not a new development. Farm Aid started in 1985 with a series of concerts to benefit farmers who were at risk of losing everything. The group continues as a nonprofit, working to save family farms. Yet, the problems have increased; farmers' net income has dropped 50 percent since 2013, according to Farm Aid. Trade wars with China and other countries make it harder to sell their grain. Climate change makes weather especially unpredictable, even calamitous, ruining the crops that farmers have worked all year to raise.

According to the Farm Bureau, the rates of bankruptcy and loan delinquency are rising.[2] Tracking suicide rates from 1992 to 2010, researchers found that 230 farmers and their employees committed suicide—averaging one every month.[3]

Help Is on the Way

Help is coming in the forms of suicide hotlines in rural areas, support groups, funding for counseling, and public awareness programs. The U.S. Department of Agriculture created the Farm and Ranch Stress Assistance Network to expand these services and a pilot program to train some of its workers to help farmers in extreme distress and make mental health referrals for them.[4]

Courageous and caring individuals are also providing assistance to at-risk individuals. Psychologist Michael Rosmann of Harlan, Iowa, has a unique insight into this dilemma because he is also a fourth-generation farmer. Farmers and their family members, knowing his background, call or e-mail him to report their struggles. Rosmann has observed that the calls have become more frequent each year, sometimes amounting to a dozen every week.

The wife of one farmer, Matt, observed that one day he "wasn't himself." He reached out to Rosmann for help, but it was too late; Matt took his life on the same day. Ten years later, his widow keeps going to Rosmann for support because, she reflects, "He listens. I think that's his secret. He listens, and people need that."

Rosmann attributes farm suicides to many factors, but the main one is the low prices obtained for their products and the politics of trade, interactions that most farmers in his neighborhood have had no prior experience in negotiating. The resulting uncertainty makes coping difficult because both prices and politics may suddenly change, even within a single day. Social isolation, which often prevents them from turning to others for advice, is itself a factor in rural suicide.[5]

Dick Tyler's Story

The suicide rate is 45 percent higher in rural areas than in large urban areas, and Montana has the highest suicide rate for farmers in the United States. The city of Billings is in the middle of the breadbasket of the state, and Dick Tyler was born on a nearby farm. Like most farmers, Dick Tyler toiled alone, took risks, and relied on personal judgments. But the very traits that contribute to the success of farmers may work against them when they are struggling financially and emotionally. They often take financial risks and make judgment calls without having adequate information. Admitting to depression is often seen as a weakness, and seeking professional help can be a stigma.

Dick took his son, Randall, with him to the fields; the boy could identify the owner of each field and was steering a truck between bales of hay by the age of six. He remembers his father's advice: "Gotta keep moving. Gotta take care of the farm, keep it active, do what you think is right."

Montana is part of the gun culture. Two out of three suicides in Montana are carried out with firearms, in contrast with one of two for the United States as a whole (67% versus 50%). Montana is also home to a large military veteran community and many Native American reservations; suicide rates are high in both groups. As we have noted elsewhere in this book, the suicide rate in high-altitude areas is high; seven of the top ten states for suicide are in the Mountain States. This is the farmers' dilemma; they may love working the land, but there are both geographical and social dangers embedded in their chosen life.

Dick Tyler also had a rare hereditary eye disease and dreaded going blind. After his cornea transplant, he was hospitalized for gastrointestinal problems. Ten days after his surgery, and shortly after he had made an appointment with a specialist, he was dead. But instead of using one of his two guns, Tyler drowned himself in the farm's reservoir.

Tyler's daughter, Daria, directs student health services at Montana State University, but even she did not see it coming. She had been trained to spot depression and suicidal ideation in her students, so just imagine the guilt she must feel. That is true for her brother, Randall, as well, who had seen his father successfully cope with a number of other crises. Dick's wife, Lenore, expressed her grief in a poem, part of which reads as follows:

> Rest well, my love
> In heaven above
> This farm is kept well
> As I do tell
> This land of the sand
> Is cared for by loving hearts and hands.

The poem ends with the blessing that Dick Tyler is now "free from all harm."[6]

Tyler's family shared their experiences and feelings with reporters and neighbors, hoping that his story would save others. They became advocates for other farmers in crisis, urging them to seek help from family members, friends, and mental health practitioners. As we have often observed in this book, suicides are frequently unpredictable. Yet, there are signs that can be wake-up calls, and there is value to listening without judgment to a person who is feeling depressed. A good listener may save a life.

Phil Revisited

You may remember Phil, whom you met in chapter 1. Phil was raised on a farm in a bucolic setting in the American Midwest. But Phil was bullied to death by his father, Curt, who constantly berated him for "not being a man." At the same time, Curt was also abusing his wife, Phil's mother, Dora. She was scolded for not being "tough" enough with Phil, for not having meals ready on time, and for spending too much money on clothes for herself and the children. Dora would accompany her husband and the rest of the family to church with heavy makeup disguising the bruises Curt had inflicted the previous night.

After Phil's death, Curt began to date a younger woman and eventually demanded a divorce. Dora was only too happy to agree, despite the fact that divorce was heavily criticized at that time, even when the wife was being assaulted. Church members had ignored the obvious physical abuse that Curt was inflicting on Dora, but they lost no time in criticizing her once they heard about the divorce. This is not unusual in rural communities, where internal and familial struggles are often tightly held secrets.

All three of the suicides discussed in this chapter occurred in rural areas. Despite the satisfaction that many people take in working the land, farmers are an at-risk group, joining fishing and forestry as the occupations with the highest suicide rates.

You Can Help Farmers with Your Food Choices

Three other rays of hope are helping farmers, and one of us (Riebel) has described how you can be part of it.[7] In recent years, the concepts of farm-to-table and Community Supported Agriculture (CSA) have taken hold. In CSA, individuals and families "join" a farm! That does not mean that they go out to the fields to work; they share the risks and rewards of farming. They subscribe to regular deliveries of whatever "their" farm has produced and harvested. The farmers have stable income without having to pay a middleman. Some farms even invite their customers to harvest festivals on their land.

Farm-to-table is a more general term that reminds people where their food comes from. Many restaurants have adopted the term to show that they source their raw materials responsibly—they want their diners to know it.

Finally, many people have realized that food grown without pesticides is healthier for them, their children, and the land, air, and water everyone shares. The organic sector of the food economy has grown exponentially for decades, and even large manufacturers now include organic offerings among their products. Farmers who move from chemical to organic farming face a challenging transition period; while the chemicals are gradually fading, the land is not yet ready to be certified organic. So besides buying organic, if you see food labeled "transitional," you can help by purchasing it, knowing you are participating in growing a healthier food economy.

Takeaway Points

- Life on the land can be gratifying in many ways, but the social isolation and unpredictability of farming may contribute to thoughts of suicide.
- In many parts of the country, stereotypes and stigmas prevent at-risk people from seeking help from family members, friends, and mental health professionals.
- Groups such Farm Aid recognize both the value and the vulnerability of farmers.
- Respect the vital work farmers do and support farm-to-table agriculture and organic offerings in your region.

Notes

1. Schlosser, E. (2001). *Fast food nation* (p. 135). Boston: Houghton Mifflin.
2. Farm Bureau. (2019, July 31). Farm loan delinquencies and bankruptcies are rising. https://www.fb.org/market-intel/farm-loan-delinquencies-and-bankruptcies-are-rising.
3. Ringgenberg, W., Peek-Asa, C., Donham, K., et al. (2018). Trends and characteristics of occupational suicide and homicide in farmers and agriculture workers, 1992–2010. *Journal of Rural Health, 34*, 246–253.
4. U.S. Department of Agriculture. (2020, April 23). Farm and Ranch Stress Assistance Network (FRSAN). https://nifa.usda.gov/funding-opportunity/farm-and-ranch-stress-assistance-network.
5. Policastra, J., Maass, A., & Knap, T. (2019, September 4). Suicide on the farm: How one man is trying to save lives. WAFB9 (online).
6. Ravitz, J. (2019, August 21). A daughter mourns her dad. A son keeps his farm alive. *CNN* (online).
7. Riebel, L. K. (2012). *The green foodprint: Food choices for healthy people and a healthy planet*. Lafayette, CA: Print and Pixel Books.

CHAPTER TWENTY-SEVEN

Spirit Sickness and Soul Loss

Early humans evolved to survive, not to discover truth—scientific forms of inquiry came much later. If early humans believed that eating a foul-tasting herb would cure a malady, they would give it a try. The herb might not contain medicinal properties, but many people would get well anyway. Those who got well, responding to what is now called the *placebo effect*, passed on their genes to future generations. Those who did not survive had no opportunity to pass anything on, unless they had already had offspring. It was millennia before researchers discovered the power of the placebo effect. The word *placebo* comes from the Latin "I will please." And this is exactly what sick people did when given a remedy or asked to participate in a ritual that would prolong their lives. They tried to please the person who gave them the remedy or arranged the ritual.

Yet, people were curious about the world around them and what caused things to happen. Every culture we know has evolved stories to explain creation, or that oddly shaped rock, or why childbirth is so painful. The drive to explain is a double-edged tool, leading to understanding but also to incorrect ideas and the invention of gods to explain why things happen.

Popular usage of the word *myth* is derogatory, implying falsehood and superstition. However, we have used this word from an anthropological perspective to refer to attempts to explain the world. Native storytellers used both metaphor and symbolism to tell stories about the creation and destruction of the universe, the beginning and end of societies, and the birth, death, and possible rebirth of individuals.

French anthropologist Lucien Lévy-Bruhl used the term *participation mystique* to describe how native peoples interact with the natural world. Lévy-Bruhl was influenced by the sociological work of Émile Durkheim, using the term *group ideas* to describe such phenomena as cultural myths. In his book *How Natives Think*, Lévy-Bruhl suggested that such myths are not opposed to logical thinking but combined with group ideas that Western writers would consider irrational and superstitious.[1] Levy-Bruhl cautioned that Westerners ignore these nonlinear, "romantic" ways of thinking at their peril, as they represent a resource that can complement analytic methods.

What can be described as the "metaphoric mind" is primordial, seen in ancient myths, rituals, and art. It has not gone away. Science itself often operates through metaphors. Freud thought of libidinal energy as a hydraulic system, recent psychotherapies borrow the computer analogy to explain and alleviate human problems, and the process of evolution has been compared to a tree (though it is more accurately conceived of as a bush).

Gregory Cajete has proposed that this type of mind evolved before early humans developed language. Then the holistic perspective of the metaphoric mind was categorized and labeled until it eventually receded into the unconscious.[2] Yet, the metaphoric mind continues to operate, remaining dormant until the conscious, rational mind calls upon its special skills for help. Then it emerges in creative play, artistic production, contemplative meditation, imaginative reverie, community rituals, campfire stories, and nighttime dreams.

The past few decades have seen a renaissance in Native American ceremonial practices, especially with the Sun Dance, the Gourd Dance, and rituals using peyote and other vision-evoking plants. Shamans used several methods of disciplined inquiry in their search for medicinal substances, including trial and error, self-administration of likely substances, and keen observation, especially when monitoring the effects of a medicine over time.

Shamans and Their Journeys

You may remember that Durkheim identified four types of suicide, including *anomic suicide*, which results from feelings of not belonging or losing one's personal direction.[3] Wolfgang Jilek, a Canadian psychiatrist, has used the term *anomic depression* to describe a malaise associated with feelings of discouragement, defeat, a low self-image, and existential frustration, or anomie.[4]

The tribes in the Pacific Northwest studied by Jilek referred to the condition as *spirit sickness*, and other tribes have used various terms, including *soul loss*. A person with such a diagnosis is at risk for suicide because of profound spiritual problems. To heal the spirit and retrieve the soul, Native American practitioners developed a variety of interventions, including sweat lodges, community rituals, herbal tinctures, and "journeying." The journey is led by the tribal shamans, who are highly trained native healers with these three characteristics:

1. They have been socially sanctioned; their community has given them that title and the accompanying role. Unlike most physicians in the Western world, shamans do not make a rational decision to choose this vocation and

then undergo the required training. They are "called" in some way, such as in nighttime dreams or daytime visions, but their community needs to verify that call and provide the means to follow it.

2.   They can access information in ways that are not ordinarily available to other members of their community.[5] Sometimes a tribal member will pray for a loved one who, following the prayer, makes a remarkable recovery. Another tribal member may have a memorable dream that comes true. Shamans claim that they can perform each of these "journeys" at will or on demand.

3.   Shamans use the information they obtain to help or heal members of their community. No one can claim the title of "shaman" (or whatever term is used by a tribe) without having a community to which he or she is responsible. It can even be a "virtual community" connected by the internet or social media.

The Shamanic Journey of Fawn Journeyhawk

Spiritual sickness and soul loss may lead to suicide. Shamans have a variety of interventions to prevent these deaths. Some cultures hold that people have more than one soul; *soul retrieval* consists of bringing back the lost soul so that the afflicted persons can regain their balance and equilibrium. Other cultures believe that the soul meandered away during a dream, so there needs to be a subsequent dream that will enable retrieval. Ceremonies may be performed to retrieve the errant soul, such as burning incense, going on a special diet, or participating in magic rituals.

In one type of shamanic journeying, the shaman makes a trip to the locale of the client's missing soul. The soul may have been lost due to a sickness, disappeared as the result of a curse, or slipped away while its owner performed an act that was immoral, such as violating a tribal taboo or hurting a defenseless child.

Fernando (a pseudonym), a suicidal Vietnam War veteran with PTSD, came to consult a well-known healer, Fawn Journeyhawk, at her center in Arizona, who discussed her case with one of us (Krippner). Fernando's sleep was marred by nightmares in which he relived the moment when he killed every member of a Vietnamese family because he believed they were carrying firearms. When he discovered that they were simply transporting groceries, it was too late. Following several days of preparation, Fawn "took a journey" to Vietnam, where she begged the spirits of that family for forgiveness. Apparently, Fawn was successful because the veteran's nightmares declined dramatically. Fernando's dreams no longer replayed the tragic event. Instead, they used symbols and metaphors—a collection of dollars swept to their destruction by a flood, a group of animals shot by overly zealous hunters, or a small house ravaged by a flamethrower. These symbols and metaphors aided Fernando's emotional processing. Within a few months, he was sleeping well and had no further thoughts of suicide.

Fawn Journeyhawk, who spent most of her life in Arizona, was of Shawnee and Cree ancestry. As a child, she reported vivid dreams to her parents and performed spontaneous healing ceremonies for friends and relatives when they became indisposed. Concerned about this bizarre behavior, a social worker took Fawn to a psychiatrist. The psychiatrist gave Fawn a diagnosis of "clinical depression with schizophrenic tendencies" and put her on medication. The medication inhibited Fawn's dreams but induced a drug dependency that took years to overcome.

Once she was no longer taking medication, Fawn began recalling her dreams. This time, the dreams served a teaching purpose. Indian spirits Red Tomahawk Halfmoon and Stormy Winds taught her how to shamanize, and she soon had people from various parts of the state arriving at her "medicine lodge" for assistance. Because of her own history, Fawn was especially adept in working with drug addicts, substance abusers, and alcoholics, many of them at risk for suicide.

Fawn was aware of the allure that both drug addiction and suicide cast on their potential victims. She described the "spirit" of cocaine as a glamorous, enticing woman dressed in black. The "spirit" of heroin (and other opiates), which could be either male or female, is "strong, selfish, and demanding" and difficult to escape. Alcohol's "spirit" is low class and cheap. Alcohol's allure is due to its banality; people tend to think this entity is "just like me," failing to see what harm it can do. Indeed, Fawn felt that alcohol is one of two drugs that can be used in moderation, the other being marijuana. As for nicotine, this "spirit" is the most addictive of all. It can be of either gender and shift its shape so that it resembles the user or someone close to the user and lures people into taking nicotine. By the time the disguise is discovered, it is too late.

In treating addicts, Fawn called upon White Owl, an ally from the spirit world. Fawn would ask her client to prepare for healing by fasting and praying for several days. When Fawn went on her journey, she was accompanied by White Owl. She would adopt her warrior stance and fight the alluring spirit for the possession of her client's soul. Fawn and White Owl would then take the client's soul to a crystal cave, where more healing would take place. Afterward, Fawn's client was given daily instructions on how to keep the soul intact because losing it again would make it even more difficult to get back.

Ricki (pseudonym) reached Fawn's medicine lodge at a low point in her life. In discussing the case with one of us (Krippner), Fawn noted that Ricki was suffering from a chronic sinus condition and was barely able to breathe. No physician had been able to provide even temporary relief. Ricki was so miserable that she had contemplated suicide. Fawn advised her to discuss her thoughts of suicide frankly. Once there, it became obvious to Ricki and Fawn that killing herself would cut short the lessons she needed to learn in this life. To start all over again was too heavy a burden for Ricki to contemplate, so she began to work with Fawn on her health. Following a week of fasting and taking herbal medicine, Ricki journeyed with Fawn to the crystal cave. When they returned, Fawn gave her some actual crystals for her to contemplate between sessions. After four meetings with Fawn, Ricki's sinuses were clear. She commented, "No one who I have seen for counseling has been able to delineate and pull back the armor as effectively as Fawn was able to do."

In 2018, Fawn passed on while in a California hospice. Visitors reported seeing a double rainbow when she died. Caretakers of Fawn's Arizona medicine lodge also independently reported seeing a double rainbow. These unusual experiences may be doubted by many people who hear about them, but they are seen as auspicious signs and outcomes by members of indigenous communities.

Takeaway Points

- Group ideas and cultural myths play an important role in suicidality, sometimes promoting suicide and sometimes preventing it.
- Shamans are socially designated tribal healers who can access useful information in unique ways, such as journeying.
- *Soul loss* and *spirit sickness* are terms used by shamans to describe people whose spiritual problems have put them at risk for suicide. Shamanic interventions for these maladies may have relevance for other groups of suicidal people.

Notes

1. Lévy-Bruhl, L. (1926). *How natives think.* Chicago: University of Chicago Press. (Original work published 1910)

2. Durkheim, E. (1951). *Suicide: A study in sociology.* Glencoe, IL: Free Press. (Original work published in French, 1897)

3. Cajete, G. (2000). *Native science: Natural laws of interdependence.* Santa Fe, NM: Clear Light.

4. Jilek, W. G. (1982). *Indian healing: Shamanism ceremonialism in the Pacific Northwest today.* Blaine, WA: Hancock House.

5. Lewis, I. M. (2003). *Ecstatic religion: A study of shamanism and spirit possession* (2nd ed.). New York: Routledge.

CHAPTER TWENTY-EIGHT

Suicide among Indigenous Peoples

Indigenous peoples have suffered the onslaughts of colonization, slavery, exploitation, and the loss of their lands, and not just in the United States. Here we tell the story of a tragedy in South America.

The Guarani are indigenous people who live in the southern part of South America, spanning parts of Paraguay, Argentina, Brazil, and Uruguay. The rich cultural mythology of the Guarani has served as source material for contemporary music, novels, poetry, films, and even an opera. Namandu, the mythic "first father," is seen as the arbiter of all creation and destruction and of a pantheon of deities, both benevolent and malevolent. Plants, minerals, humans, and other animals are seen as alive and interchangeable; butterflies and glowworms, for example, are reincarnated humans. The rainforest is especially sacred, particularly the area surrounding the famed Iguassu Falls.

The Ones from the Jungle

The Guarani first encountered the Spanish invaders in 1537, when the Spanish conquistador Gonzalo de Mendoza traversed what is today Paraguay and southern Brazil. The Spanish conquerors initiated a policy of intermarriage and the practice of slavery; both institutions worked to the benefit of the Spaniards. Jesuit missionaries came to convert the Indians to Catholicism. Those who accepted the new religion were dubbed *Guarani*, the people from the Spanish province of Guayra. Those who opposed it were referred to as *Cagua*, or "the ones from the jungle," a pejorative term.

The Jesuits did what they could to protect the Guarani, opposing slavery and founding a college in Asunción, today's capital city of Paraguay. They also founded several missions, but these were regularly raided during Mass by slave traders, who carried off many of the parishioners. Within a few years, only a few thousand tribal members remained out of some one hundred thousand who had lived in the area before the Spanish invasion. Nonetheless, a strong bond between the Jesuits and the Guarani had been established.

In 1767, the tides of history shifted again; the Jesuits, including their missions, were expelled from Spanish territory. The Guarani wrote the governor of Buenos Aires to protest the edict, but they were unsuccessful. Most Guaranis returned to the countryside, but some stayed in urban environments and became "civilized Indians." Many of them participated in the formation of Brazil as an empire and later as a nation. These accounts served as the basis for a spectacularly photographed 1986 film, *The Mission*.

The Jesuit legacy was long-lasting; in the area of the former missions, the educational attainment remains high 250 years later, average income is higher, and adaptation to new technologies is more rapid.[1] There are Guarani settlements in Bolivia, Uruguay, Argentina, Brazil, and Paraguay, where the native Guarani language is widely spoken, a legacy of the intermarriage policy from the 1530s.

Ecologists from various countries have supported the preservation of nature, with mixed results. The nonprofit Survival International states on its website, "We exist to prevent the annihilation of tribal peoples and to give them a platform to speak to the world so they can bear witness to the genocidal violence, slavery and racism they face on a daily basis." This is especially the case in Brazil, where generations of legislators have attempted to protect the rainforests; unfortunately, generations of plantation owners and loggers have ruthlessly exploited the natural wealth that abounds in Guarani lands. This greed can become a death sentence for the Guarani who try to protect their land and culture.

A Death Sentence in More Ways Than One

Indigenous peoples may feel that their relationship with nature is broken when they are separated from their land. In addition to undermining their spiritual base, the loss of their land disrupts the social structure of the community, with deplorable consequences. Besides suicide, these indigenous people have high rates of homicide, spousal abuse, alcoholism, and drug addiction.[2] All too often, tribal leaders who speak out against the theft of their land are beaten, tortured, or murdered. In 2014, according to Survival International, Marcos Vernon, a Guarani leader, exclaimed, "This here is my life, my soul. If you take me away from this land, you take my life." Shortly after making this statement, Vernon was murdered as he attempted to lead his tribe back to its homeland.

The newsletter *Survival International*, published by the organization of the same name, reported in its October 2013 issue a Guarani campaign requesting that their ancestral land be mapped and returned to them. The territory stolen from the Guarani-Kaiowá (one branch of the Guarani) is frequently used for sugarcane production. Some of the resulting sugar is used to make alcohol, which triggers its own type of slavery.[3] In its May 2016 issue, *Survival International* published a follow-up story revealing that a Brazilian judge had ordered a small Guarani community to permanently move off the land that had been theirs for hundreds of years but had been seized without compensation in the 1970s by wealthy plantation owners.

Survival International cited Tonico Benites Guarani, a community leader and anthropologist, who stated of the loss of ancestral lands, "It will be a death sentence." He observed that over one thousand Guarani, most of them young, had killed themselves during the past decade. He also observed that the tribe had lost about 95 percent of its ancestral land to biofuel producers, sugarcane and soya plantations, and other industries over the years.

Tonico explained, "So many young Guarani people commit suicide. It's around one a week. The time comes when you have had enough of waiting. You work yourself up with hope, then the courts dash your hopes. Your family suffers with hunger and malnutrition, the despair increases, there is no security, no hope."

Tonico continued, "The root of the problem is the loss of the land. Our culture does not allow violence, but the ranchers will kill us rather than give it back." Brutal evictions of the Guarani have continued for the past few decades, with loggers and ranchers hiring gunfighters, the police and armed forces bringing in tanks and helicopters, and the courts usually siding with the rich farmers. According to Tonico, "Our young people's only choice is to work with pitiful wages in atrocious conditions in the sugarcane plantations. If we cannot plant, what is our future? We suffer from racism and discrimination. Until 1988 indigenous peoples in Brazil were not considered human beings in the constitution. This created racism and prejudice. It suggested Indians could be killed, that they were a free target."

Officials estimate that there are presently about forty-seven thousand Guarani in Brazil and a few thousand more in Argentina, Bolivia, and Paraguay. The Guarani have their own language and culture, with variations from region to region. In Brazil, most of them live by the highways or on tiny patches of land surrounded by cattle ranches and plantations.[4]

A Personal Encounter

In 2011, one of us (Krippner) had a personal encounter with Dom João Guarani, a shaman for the Eastern Guarani tribe. Following an international conference in Curitiba, Brazil, Krippner was invited to participate in a sacred ceremony held on Guarani land in a dome constructed from twigs and animal skins. Seated around a small fire, the dozen participants witnessed a remarkable dance performed by three statuesque women while accompanied by drums. Following the dance, Dom João produced a huge pipe, filled it with a smoking mixture, inhaled deeply, and passed it on to Krippner, who repeated the procedure.

Following two more mixtures and three cups of various brews, Dom João asked members of the group to offer a prayer. Krippner prayed that the Guarani youth find some alternative means of protesting the takeover of their land. He noted that the loggers, farmers, and ranchers benefited from the suicides, and most of the rest of the world did not even know about them. He urged that nonviolent alternatives to suicide be developed and implemented.

Dom João expressed surprise, asking Krippner how he knew about the suicides. Krippner responded that he was a member of the Rainforest Action Network (RAN) and that a Guarani leader had addressed the group in San Francisco, providing details of the suicides. RAN initiated a global program to focus attention on the ranchers who had broken the law, hoping international attention would bring them to account.[5]

Final Thoughts

Sociologist Émile Durkheim placed the suicides of these young tribal members in his "altruistic" category, as they comprise a form of protest. But they also remind us of the fifth category we proposed: moral wounding. Having lost their homeland and all it means to them, and seeing the futility of trying to get justice, the young people are morally wounded and would rather die than continue. The loss of these vibrant young women and men is a tragedy for the earth, which needs commitment and wisdom to halt the destruction of the planet and its inhabitants, human and nonhuman alike.

Efforts to protect indigenous peoples are being made by individuals, nonprofit organizations, and even governments. Will they be enough to save the last of the earth's native peoples?

Takeaway Points

- Suicide has many causes, some of which are enmeshed with national and international politics and economic interests.
- Moral wounding and altruistic suicide can result in the loss of young people whose potential for leadership is badly needed in today's world.

Notes

1. Corry, S. (2011). *Tribal peoples for tomorrow's world: A guide by Stephen Corry*. Alcester, UK: Freeman Press.

2. Caicedo, F. V. (2017). The mission: Human capital transmission, economic persistence, and culture in South America. *Quarterly Journal of Economics, 134*, 507–556.

3. Vidal, J. (2016, May 18). Brazil's Guarani Indians killing themselves over loss of ancestral lands. *The Guardian* (online).

4. Ibid.

5. Krippner, S. (2006). We know how. In S. M. S. Jones & S. Krippner (Eds.), *The shamanic powers of Rolling Thunder* (pp. 107–112). Rochester, VT: Bear.

CHAPTER TWENTY-NINE

Children, the Elderly, and the Sleep-Deprived

In this chapter, we describe some other groups at risk, groups that are often neglected. The attention given to teenage suicide and to the high rate of suicide among middle-aged men means that children and the elderly are frequently overlooked. Sleep deprivation can increase suicide vulnerability for anyone and deserves the emphasis we have given it.

Children

Who would have thought that children would think of killing themselves, much less do it? But the suicide rate among American children has tripled in the last ten years, becoming their second leading cause of death.[1] Such grim statistics do not refer to teenagers but to *children* as young as five years old, including a deplorable increase among black children.[2] True, these deaths occur at a rate only 2 percent that of teens, but they represent an appalling reflection on our society.

What can contribute to such despair in individuals so young? One team of researchers studied suicidality in over eleven thousand children. They found that the rate of suicidality and self-injury was much higher than they expected, and 75 percent of the at-risk children's parents or caregivers were unaware of their children's desolation, or perhaps unwilling to mention it. Conflict within the family and insufficient parental monitoring were key factors linked to those cases of suicidality.[3] Racism and economic hardship have been mentioned, and as we have seen, bullying can be severe and unremitting and can take place in a setting children are forced to be in day after day, year after year—school.

The Other Two Groups

Three basic conditions impact suicide-prone people: getting older, not getting enough sleep, and not making enough money to sustain themselves. We remind our readers that George Bailey, in the classic movie *It's a Wonderful Life*, had a horrible realization: "I'm worth more dead than alive." Thomas Joiner's psychological theory of suicide holds that people will not kill themselves unless they have the desire to die and the ability to do so.[4] We discussed poverty in chapter 5, so we turn our attention here to aging and sleep disorders.

Taking One's Life at the End of Life

Even in our youth-obsessed culture, life beyond sixty can be vibrant and fulfilling. Unfortunately, this is not true for everyone. For those experiencing health problems, deaths of friends and relatives, financial stress, lack of work identity, and other losses, the prospect of ending it all may have considerable allure. Even nursing homes are not guaranteed protection. A recent study found that the rate of suicide in nursing homes was similar to that in the general population.[5]

Belonging simultaneously to two at-risk groups is especially hazardous. Some older veterans, who may be long past their service years, commit suicide even when they have access to health care. One study found that VA health care workers did assess their patients' rates of depression and suicidal ideation, but they failed to ask the older vets (over age fifty) about two crucial factors: impulsivity and access to firearms. The older veterans were also less likely to receive mental health referrals than their younger peers. The study concluded that interventions from primary care for reaching older patients at risk for suicide have the potential to improve prevention efforts in this population.[6]

This group is also more likely to experience loneliness, which has been found to have a negative impact on people's lives. Over the years, the number of people who live alone and who become socially isolated has increased. Evidence shows that, for older citizens, physical and mental health are compromised by loneliness, which can lead to depression, dementia progression, hypertension, heart disease, and stroke.[7]

Longing for the Big Sleep

Anyone who has struggled with a serious sleep problem, whether from stress, a new baby, anxiety, or economic worry, knows that it can be more than exhausting: it can be dangerous. When one of the many sleep disorders deprives a person of sufficient sleep, it ranks as a genuine hazard. Major accidents such as the Three Mile Island nuclear meltdown and the *Exxon Valdez* oil spill have been partly attributed to employees' sleep deprivation, as have some serious health problems. In our context, the danger is to the individual's will to live.

Unwanted wakefulness leaves one prey to an endless round of terrible fears and regrets, physical exhaustion, and helplessness and frustration that can turn to anger. This pushes sleep even further away. There is evidence that insomnia contributes to suicide among older adults. Fortunately, such approaches as cognitive behavioral treatment for insomnia carry considerably less stigma than seeking help for depression or anxiety. Addressing insomnia from this perspective can be a useful entry point in convincing people to get help.[8]

The National Sleep Foundation states that sleep disorders are closely linked to PTSD, notably repetitive nightmares, which is why we emphasize the treatment of nightmares for PTSD sufferers.

Criticizing the *Diagnostic and Statistical Manual*

Sleep apnea can be treated medically, but PTSD requires a more holistic approach. In 2019, two clinical psychologists, J. C. Norcross and B. E. Wampold, voiced a strong objection to the American Psychiatric Association's *Diagnostic and Statistical Manual*'s (DSM) advocacy of a medical model for the treatment of trauma. They prefer a model based on "evidence-based practice," which uses research evidence, clinical expertise, and client preferences; it emphasizes the therapeutic relationship, adaptations of treatment to the individual client, and the personal characteristics of the therapist. These last three factors have been found to be more important for client improvement than the specific intervention employed, yet they are notably absent from treatments that follow the *DSM*'s medical model.[9]

About the same time, researchers from the University of Liverpool presented a detailed analysis of five key chapters of the psychiatric manual, namely, those on schizophrenia, bipolar disorder, depressive disorders, anxiety disorders, and trauma-related disorders. One of their major findings was that the role of trauma in all five chapters had been underestimated. They also noted the overlap in symptoms from one chapter to another, even though those parts of the manual advocated different decision-making guidelines.

The Liverpool team concluded that *DSM* diagnoses tell the therapist little about specific clients and what treatment they need. One team member stated that the biomedical diagnostic approach in psychiatry does not serve a useful purpose. Another team member advocated "thinking beyond diagnoses and considering other explanations of mental distress, such as trauma and the adverse effects of life experiences."[10]

In 2017, an international group of fifty psychotherapists claimed that the *DSM* was marred by "fundamental shortcomings." They suggested that the manual be replaced by an alternative diagnostic system that would provide continuums of severity and understanding of what the problems have in common. For example, social anxiety disorder, or shyness, would be placed on a continuum ranging from people who experience a mild discomfort when asked to give a public talk or in other social situations to those who are fearful in most social interactions. Many people are shy at parties and other gatherings, but they are not considered to have a "disorder" because they function well in other social settings.[11]

There are excellent guidelines for treating PTSD that are holistic and humanistic in nature, incorporating medication into the treatment when it can serve a specific purpose.[12] Hence, we can appreciate the criticisms that have been made of the *DSM* while acknowledging its usefulness and its brave attempt to make sense of the chaotic world of mental illness.

Takeaway Points

- Suicide is often an outcome of problems associated with age, sleep, and income.
- The *Diagnostic and Statistical Manual* is an important development in classifying mental disorders, but it is not without its critics.

Notes

1. Curtin, S. C., & Heron, M. (2019, October). *Death rates due to suicide and homicide among persons aged 10–24: United States, 2000–2017* (NCHS Data Brief No. 352). National Center for Health Statistics.

2. Bridge, J. A., Asti, L., Horowitz, L. M., et al. (2015, May 18). Suicide trends among elementary school-aged children in the United States from 1993 to 2012. *Journal of the American Medical Association Pediatrics, 169*(7), 673–677.

3. DeVille, D. C., Whalen, D., Breslin, F. J., et al. (2020). Prevalence and family-related factors associated with suicidal ideation, suicide attempts, and self-injury in children aged 9 to 10 years. *JAMA Network Open, 3*(2), e1920956.

4. Joiner, T. (2005). *Why people die of suicide*. Cambridge, MA: Harvard University Press.

5. Baker, M., & Aleecia, J. (2019, April 12). A desperate place in the end: Seniors in long-term care turning to suicide. *Kaiser Health News* (online)

6. Simons, K., Van Orden, K., Conner, K. R., & Bagge, C. (2019). Age differences in suicide risk screening and management prior to suicide attempts. *American Journal of Geriatric Psychiatry, 27*(6), 604–608.

7. Ong, A. D., Uchino, B. N., & Wethington, E. (2016). Loneliness and health in older adults: A mini-review and synthesis. *Gerontology, 62*, 443–449.

8. Bishop, T. M., Simons, K. V., King, D. A., & Pigeon, W. R. (2016). Sleep and suicide in older adults: An opportunity for intervention. *Clinical Therapeutics, 38,* 2332–2339.

9. Norcross, J. C., & Wampold, B. E. (2019). Relationships and responsiveness in the psychological treatment of trauma: The tragedy of the APA Clinical Practice Guidelines. *Psychotherapy, 56,* 391–399.

10. Allsopp, K., Reed, J., Corcoran, R., & Kinderman, P. (2019). Heterogeneity in psychiatric diagnostic classification. *Psychiatric Research, 279,* 15–22.

11. Kotov, R., Krueger, R., Watson, D., et al. (2017). The hierarchical taxonomy of psychopathology (HiTOP): A dimensional alternative to traditional nosologies. *Journal of Abnormal Psychology, 126,* 454–477.

12. Courtois, C. A., Sonis, J., Brown, L. S., et al. (2019). Clinical practice guidelines for the treatment of posttraumatic stress disorder (PTSD) in adults. *American Psychologist, 74,* 596–607.

SECTION VII

How Professionals Understand Suicide

CHAPTER THIRTY

Two Views of Suicide from Evolutionary Psychology

Evolutionary psychologists apply the theory of evolution to human behavior to explain why certain actions and traits seem to come untaught. When early humans faced challenges, they developed ways of solving those problems. Over time, the genetic bases for the traits that led to these successful solutions were passed on to succeeding generations. This is not to say that a trait evolved to perform a specific task. Some random mutations proved to be highly adaptive, fostering survival. Mutations irrelevant to survival were not adaptive and usually did not make the cut for genetic transmission.

We found some fascinating ideas in an unexpected place: an undergraduate senior thesis.[1] Zachary Catanzarite observed that almost all the research on suicide primarily studied individuals, families, and cultural groups rather than the human species as a whole or other forms of life. Catanzarite suggests that suicide is, in fact, one way that humanity's evolutionary heritage interacts with contemporary environments. He argues that it is not the behavior but rather the social environment that is maladaptive.

We have observed the same throughout this book: people who have experienced combat, sexual molestation, or bullying desperately attempt to cope with abnormal events. Once they return to civilian life, reflect on the consequences of their abuse, or find that no one will help them, they realize that life may never seem normal again. For some, this realization leads to hopelessness and despair that may be severe enough to override their natural instinct for survival. Self-harm, such as cutting, may represent "rehearsals" for suicide, even though it, too, is contrary to nature.

In summary, Catanzarite proposes that learning to harm oneself is adaptive from an evolutionary point of view. It distracts from the pain caused by abnormal life situations. But for vulnerable people who lacked significant attachments earlier in their lives, this ability is no longer a useful reaction but one that careens wildly, resulting in a fatal outcome.

A parallel is found in programmed cell death (PCD), a well-established process in biology that is responsible for pruning excess neurons, which allows efficient processing of thoughts, emotions, stimuli, and threats. Approximately ten billion cells die in each person by PCD every day. Programmed cell death illustrates how suicidal behavior can be functional for the good of the overall organism. You might remember that "altruistic suicide" was one of Émile Durkheim's proposed sociological categories. Catanzarite uses the same term but takes an evolutionary point of view.

The Pain and Brain Model

Psychotherapist Cas Soper also has used evolutionary psychology to explain suicide. He reviewed many of the same studies that we have examined, noting that no single symptom or set of symptoms has been found to be a reliable predictor of suicide. Suicidologists keep looking for markers that will reliably predict when people will take their own lives. But there is no evidence that there are such markers, and there is no theory that convincingly demonstrates that there should be. Thus, suicide is "predictably unpredictable."[2]

Soper compared current psychological theories about suicide to "folk psychology," the attempts of everyday people to explain behavior, often based on cultural myths. Folk psychology in different parts of the world attributes suicide to evil spirits, curses, or a "divine plan," "fate," or "karma." For Soper, current explanations of suicide seem more like folk psychology than scientific psychology, a skepticism shared by many other researchers.[3,4]

Soper developed what he called his "pain and brain" model: suicide is a by-product of two adaptations: pain (physical, social, or both) and mature human cognition (which can plan and carry out suicide). Pain exists at an emotional, affective level, while defenses exist at an intellectual (brain) level. Pain supplies the motive for suicide, and the brain provides the means.

Deterrence

Soper's pain and brain model holds that conventional medication may ease the pain but dull the brain, sacrificing long-term solutions for short-term relief. And if medication is prescribed without the addition of psychotherapy, the risk of suicide may be increased rather than lessened. A person too lethargic to attempt suicide may be energized by medication and make a successful attempt. A number of research studies point to the real possibility of this tragic outcome.[5]

In concrete terms, suicidal people often lack the level of cognitive functioning needed to seek alternatives. Any slight delay to one's plans may be enough to allow a de-escalation from a suicidal crisis, allowing anti-suicide defenses time to take effect.

Sometimes a practical deterrent is surprisingly simple. In an isolated Canadian village near the Arctic Circle, there were many suicides among teenage boys. The teenagers had entered their closets and tied nooses to the rods to hang themselves. Authorities removed the closet rods from their homes. That town went from having the highest rate of suicide in the region to the town where there were no suicides for four years running. Other simple steps include placing nets under bridges, limiting the size of over-the-counter drug containers, and making swimming lessons mandatory for children.

Young suicide attempters often report that they only spend a few minutes between deciding to kill themselves and making the attempt. The notion that a person bent on suicide will keep trying is not always true. Impulsive suiciders often choose drastic means, such as firearms, hanging, or jumping. Making it more difficult for them to initiate the attempt can save lives.

Takeaway Points

- Evolutionary theory has been used by some psychologists to explain how many common traits helped early humans survive.
- The speculations of evolutionary psychologists have led to practical proposals that can save the lives of suicide-prone people.

Notes

1. Catanzarite, Z. (2002). An evolutionary theory of suicide. Class paper for Evolutionary Psychology, graduate course taught by D. Barrett, New York University.

2. Soper, C. A. (2019). *The evolution of suicide.* Zurich, Switzerland: Springer.

3. Soper, C. A. (2019, July 9). Adaptation to the suicidal niche. *Evolutionary Psychological Science, 5,* 454–471.

4. Franklin, J. C., Nero, J. D., Fox, K. R., et al. (2017). Risk factors for suicidal thoughts and behaviors: A meta-analysis. *Psychological Bulletin, 142,* 187–232.

5. Sharma, T., Guski, L. S., Freund, N., & Gotzshe, P. C. (2016). Suicidality and aggression during antidepressant treatment: Systemic review and meta-analyses based on clinical study reports. *British Medical Journal, 352,* i65.

CHAPTER THIRTY-ONE

Suicide as a Public Health Issue

This chapter will highlight the work of Edwin Shneidman. His contributions to the study of suicide are so important that we ran across his work quite early in our quest to understand why people kill themselves.[1]

The First Clinical Suicidologist

In 1949, Edwin Shneidman, a clinical psychologist, was working for the Los Angeles Veterans Administration when his supervisor asked him to write condolence letters to widows of two veterans who had killed themselves. He searched the Los Angeles County Coroner's Office and discovered a vault of suicide notes, a formative experience that launched his career. Shneidman was a cofounder of the American Association of Suicidology and the Los Angeles Suicide Prevention Center. This center was a pioneering effort, and hundreds of similar centers have used it as their model. The American Psychological Association gave him its Award for Distinguished Contributions in the Public Service.

Shneidman saw suicide as a public health issue and identified the misunderstandings ("fables") that people believe about suicide:

Fable: *People who talk about suicide rarely commit suicide.*

Fact: Eight out of ten people who kill themselves give advance warning of some sort.

Fable: *Suicide happens without warning.*

Fact: Again, eight out of ten people give some type of warning.

Fable: *Suicidal people are fully intent on dying.*

Fact: Most suicidal people are undecided about dying until they make the attempt.

Fable: *Once a person has made a suicide attempt, that person is suicidal forever.*

Fact: People who kill themselves are generally suicidal for a limited time period.

Fable: *Improvement following a suicidal crisis means the suicidal risk is over.*

Fact: Most suicides occur within three months of apparent "improvement," when the individuals have found the energy to act out their intent.

Fable: *Suicide occurs most frequently among the very rich or very poor.*

Fact: Suicide is represented proportionately among all economic brackets.

Fable: *Suicide is inherited and "runs in the family."*

Fact: Suicide represents an individual action, not a family pattern.

Fable: *Suicidal individuals are mentally ill.*

Fact: Suicidal people are desperately unhappy, but most of them are not mentally ill. Less than half have been given a psychiatric diagnosis.

Shneidman did not consider suicide to be a disease or an immoral act but an attempt to seek a solution to a problem, which he called "psychache," or intolerable pain. Psychache is accompanied by hopelessness and helplessness in the face of unmet psychological needs. Shneidman found considerable ambivalence on the part of people who eventually kill themselves. If a therapist or other caring person can reach out to suicide-prone people before they make the final decision, lives may be saved. Shneidman coined the term "suicidologist"—someone who studies suicide professionally.

Ambivalence

Ambivalence toward killing oneself is apparent in the life of Tex, a young man raised in a fundamentalist Christian family. There were constant arguments over his lifestyle, which ran counter to his parents' values. One night, Tex went to his room, exhausted after a recurring argument regarding his sex life, which failed to meet the standards imposed by his parents' church. Tex slashed his wrist with a hunting knife and then realized he had made the wrong decision. He quickly telephoned for help, and an ambulance rushed to his home, saving his life. In retrospect, Tex stated, "Immediately after cutting my wrist, I realized my mistake. The act provided a release of tension, and I realized that things were not as hopeless as they seemed at the time."[2]

Tex's suicide attempt is an example of Shneidman's description of suicide as a behavior that is against one's self-interest, involving the constriction of intention and the inability to see viable alternatives. Suicide is not so much a movement toward death as it is a flight from intolerable emotions. Shneidman would agree with Dabrowski that suicide is complicated and with Durkheim's emphasis on the social conditions that impacted suicide-prone people.[3] For Shneidman, the understanding of suicide is multidimensional and multidisciplinary, involving biology, psychology, sociology, and philosophy.

Shneidman emphasized the role of research in understanding suicide, stating the psychache is not the only factor involved in suicide but is the one we can most readily measure. Indeed, Shneidman constructed a psychological instrument that he thought was able to measure one's degree of psychache. Another research project involved reading the biographical data for thirty people who had been identified as gifted in their youth. Shneidman was able to correctly identify each of the five who committed suicide based on their early life histories.[4]

The Public Health Viewpoint

Positioning suicide as a public health issue is a sensible approach that does not label suicide-prone people as sinful, wicked, or crazy. We agree with Shneidman that suicide is best thought of as a public health issue, not a mental disorder and certainly not a crime. Public health requires the cooperation of scientists, physicians, public officials, and others who work together to support the health of the general populace. Public health addresses such issues as clean water, sanitation, environmental hazards, infectious diseases, and, more recently, mental health.[5]

Recall Shneidman's statement that many people who die by suicide have never been diagnosed as being mentally ill, nor have they manifested pathological symptoms. At one point in history, suicide was conceptualized as a crime, either as a crime against the state, the community, or the Divine. The very term "committed suicide" is a carryover from those days. One does not say that a friend "committed a broken neck."

By the same token, such terms as "a successful suicide" and "a failed suicide attempt" imply that it is something to be achieved. If suicide is to be considered a public health issue, and if the taboo against discussing suicide is to be lifted, the vocabulary needs to change. Jesse Bering, a specialist in communication science, proposes such terms as "she died by suicide," "he took his own life," or simply "he suicided," and we agree that these terms are preferable.[6]

Helping the Helpers

An experienced nurse who works in the intensive care unit of a major urban hospital told us that she and her colleagues had never received training on how to talk to people who arrive after a suicide attempt. She acknowledged, "We don't know what to say to them." And she added that, as people working hard to save lives, nurses are not always sympathetic to those who try to end them.

Sad to say, nurses themselves are at risk. They are experts at taking care of others but possibly put their own needs aside—especially when it comes to asking for help about sensitive topics, such as a colleague's suicide. Further, their hospitals or organizations may feel a need to conceal the decedent's cause of death, leading to a "conspiracy of silence" such that the healing work of sharing and understanding is not even begun.[7] So, we recommend education for *all* health care workers about the risk factors, causes, and treatments for suicidality—and permission to be open about the suicide death of a colleague.

The Economy, the Future, and Public Health

The future of one's vocation can have serious consequences. The fading of certain industries as society changes can be particularly hard on workers. For instance, the important medical publication *Morbidity and Mortality Weekly* found in 2020 that the highest suicide rates occurred among those employed in mining and in oil and gas extraction.[8] While we may rejoice that renewable energy is rising, we should not neglect individuals whose jobs are vanishing. More generally, research cited in this report found that suicide risk is greater if one has less education, lower skills and status, job insecurity, and other job-related factors. The authors concluded, "Industry, labor, and professional associations, as well as employers, and state and local health departments can use this information to focus attention and resources on suicide prevention." Retraining laid-off workers in sustainable professions, such as organic farming and solar panel installation, is a win-win solution.

Finally, we must comment on the reality of environmental destruction, which creates a background of short- and long-term dangers. Hurricanes, tornadoes, droughts, and floods have increased from the climate change that is already occurring. Loss of coastlands, depletion of water resources, changes in crop yields, climate migration, and other slow processes will play out over decades. Younger people will inherit the mess created by the generations that preceded them, bearing the brunt of changes that are not all predictable. Climate change has now been identified as a trauma on its own.[9]

Addressing these massive social issues is beyond the scope of this book, but at least we can urge our readers to be aware of them as risk factors for suicide.

Takeaway Points

- Suicide is best thought of as a public health issue, not as an immoral act or the result of mental illness.

- Ambivalence is common among suicide-prone people and provides therapists an opportunity to save lives.
- People may not be fully aware of their personal myths, even though these beliefs provide a framework for their lives.
- Large social, economic, and environmental forces that are beyond individuals' control may contribute to hopelessness, leading to suicide.

Notes

1. Leenaars, A. A. (2010). Edwin S. Shneidman on suicide. *Suicidology Online, 1,* 4–18.

2. Shneidman, E. S. (1993). Suicide as psychache. *Journal of Nervous and Mental Disease, 111,* 145–147.

3. Shneidman, E. S. (1985). *Definition of suicide.* New York: John Wiley & Sons.

4. Shneidman, E. S. (1971). Perturbation and lethality as precursors of suicide in a gifted group. *Life Threatening Behavior, 1,* 23–45.

5. Hamblin, J. D. (2005). *Science in the early twentieth century: An encyclopedia* (pp. 260–262). Santa Barbara, CA: ABC-CLIO.

6. Bering, J. (2019). *Suicidal: Why we kill ourselves.* Chicago: University of Chicago Press.

7. Davidson, J. E., Accardi, R., Sanchez, C., & Zisook, S. (2020). Nurse suicide: Prevention and grief management. *American Nurse Today, 15*(1), 14–17.

8. Peterson C., Sussell, A., Li, J., Schumacher, P. K., Yeoman, K., & Stone, D. M. (2020). Suicide rates by industry and occupation. *Morbidity and Mortality Weekly, 59*(3), 57–62.

9. Woodbury, Z. (2019). Climate trauma: Toward a new taxonomy of trauma. *Ecopsychology, 11*(1), 1–8.

CHAPTER THIRTY-TWO

The Archetypes of Suicide

Carl Jung, founder of analytical psychology, thought there were mental structures common to all human beings, past, present, and future. He called these structures *archetypes* and believed that they were perennial reservoirs, serving as frames of reference with which people view their world. Their expression varies from one culture to another and from one historical era to another. However, there is an underlying similarity within an archetype that is apparent when one reads folktales and legends from various times and cultures. For example, what Jung called the "Wise Old Man" archetype is manifested in Merlin the Magician in English mythology, the wizard Gandalf in *The Lord of the Rings* trilogy, and Preto Velho, an elderly black slave to whom members of African Brazilian religions pray and seek counsel.

Katherine Best, a Jungian psychoanalyst, revealed what she called the "archetypes of suicide."[1] Like other authors we have cited, Best observed that suicide symbolizes different things to different people. But she saw a similarity: the core archetype of suicide is a *threshold* where one chooses to leave life on one side and enter the field of death on the other. This threshold operates at both conscious and unconscious levels. Many people are unaware of this threshold, and most that are aware are not tempted by suicide's allure. However, at-risk people are quite aware, and for some people, the archetype occupies a major part of their waking thoughts, emotions, and motivations. Like other archetypes, symbols and metaphors of suicide can be found in nighttime dreams.

Guidelines and methods for the prevention of suicide are more readily available than ever before, yet suicide rates have increased worldwide and have reached epidemic proportions in the United States. Moreover, suicide attempts are twenty times more frequent than completed suicides.[2] The complexity of suicide and suicide attempts across ages, social groups, and ethnic groups suggests an undercurrent of unseen factors that archetypal theory attempts to address.

Hillman's Categories

Another psychotherapist, James Hillman, has written about suicide from a Jungian perspective. Hillman's "archetypal psychology" includes four categories of suicides, reminiscent of Durkheim's taxonomy:

1. *Collective suicide* is dying for others or for a cause, such as politically motivated death, the kamikaze pilots of World War II, and assassinations or terrorist bombings in which the assassin dies along with the victim.

2. *Symbolic suicide* involves seeking public reaction through such acts as self-immolation (burning oneself to death in a public place) and other exhibitionistic and voyeuristic suicides, such as killing oneself on a live television broadcast.

3. *Emotional suicide* results from such feelings as shame, guilt, grief, loneliness, or desire for revenge.

4. *Intellectual suicide* adheres to a higher principle, such as the deaths of Socrates, Seneca, early Christian martyrs, and, more recently, hunger strikers.[3]

Hillman agrees that a suicide attempt is often a call for help, but he sees it as a call to someone to help the person die, not to help survive. The intended death may be symbolic, as in helping a part of oneself die, helping a fruitless relationship or project die, or helping a dysfunctional personal myth die.

Hillman's third category includes shame as an impetus for suicide. In ancient Greece, Adios, the dual-natured goddess of both shame and self-respect, was a handmaiden to Athena, the goddess of wisdom. In *The Iliad*, Greek warriors rushed into battle screaming "Adios!"—proclaiming their self-respect as an antidote to shame. Shame also resulted from breaking social agreements, as this resulted in isolation from the group.

Hillman's fourth category (intellectual suicide) brings to mind such Christian martyrs as the fifteen-year-old Pelagia of Antioch, who jumped from a rooftop to avoid sexual assault from a group of Roman soldiers. Apollonia, another Christian maiden ultimately granted sainthood, threw herself into the fire rather than renounce her faith, even after her teeth had been pulled out or bashed. The Japanese tradition of *seppuku* is well known, but samurai wives had their own form of traditional suicide to avoid rape from marauders. In *jigaki*, they cut the arteries of their neck. Before killing themselves, these women tied their knees together so that their bodies would be found in a dignified position when the invaders arrived. When the Christian Vietnamese government persecuted Buddhists in the early 1960s, Thich Quang

Duc burned himself publicly. This resulted in a joint communiqué in which Americans and Vietnamese officials agreed to Buddhist demands. When the U.S.-backed government lost the civil war, the spot of Thich Quang Duc's suicide became a national monument where present-day Vietnamese honor his suicide as a protest against American imperialism.

In Hinduism, suicide was acceptable for elder monks who had no more responsibilities in life. The aged Hindu monks who engaged in *prayopavesa* (death by fasting) did so with the intention of leaving resources for the monks of their communities.[4]

The Place and Time of Suicide

Archetypal field theory acknowledges the "field" in which the suicide or suicide attempt takes place. This field can be internal or external, and it reflects the power of place and time in self-destruction. As a riverbed may dry up for a while, the suicide archetype may remain inactive for an individual for periods of time. But a storm of adverse life circumstances may fill up the riverbed to the point of overflow.

In archetypical field theory, the place of one's suicide makes an important statement. Referred to as "attractor sites," certain locations serve as magnets to attract some at-risk people, such as San Francisco's Golden Gate Bridge, Suicide Forest near Japan's Mount Fujiyama, the Gap in Australia, Nanjing Yangtze River Bridge in China, and England's Beachy Head and Humber Bridge. Each location is marked with warning signs and suicide hotline numbers in attempts to mitigate suicide rates. We cannot determine the success of these signs. In any event, most suicides do not occur in these populated sites; they usually take place in locations that are more convenient.

Time also plays a key role in suicide archetypes. An anniversary, birthday, or a date marking the death of a loved one may be chosen.

Suicidal archetypes are expressed in many ways; a person at risk may collect songs, poetry, artwork, and photographs that augment the allure. Thoughts of suicide dominate his or her waking hours and appear in dreams. The specific method of suicide is thought about, dreamed about, and reinforced by collections of newspaper clippings, sketches, and items on social media. An astute friend or relative may even hear snatches of conversation that are belatedly realized to have been premonitory clues.

The Dreams of Kenneth

Kenneth, suffering from extreme trauma, sought counsel from Alan G. Vaughan, a Jungian psychoanalyst. Kenneth's father had committed suicide after killing the assailant of his best friend, a law enforcement officer. The suicide was traumatizing to Kenneth, as he found no good reason for his father to feel guilty. Kenneth had recurring nightmares, many of them containing the death scene, with his father's body on the floor surrounded by blood.

Kenneth was also taking medication for severe depression and anxiety. However, he could not resume his career as a writer because images of his father invaded his waking thoughts and his dreams. He was estranged from his friends and from his wife, even though she continued to be supportive. Kenneth's father had emigrated from Africa, beginning a "hero's journey" that eventually went terribly wrong.

Vaughan asked Kenneth to keep a daily journal, an activity that helped him reconnect to his career. Kenneth frequently read what he had written to Vaughan, and this eventually enabled Kenneth to return to work. Kenneth also read his dreams to the psychoanalyst. Here is a dream that was especially valuable:

> A friend from college and I go to my father's apartment. I open the door with my key, and we call out his name and look for him in the apartment. The phone rings, and it is my mother, who says she is worried about him and that she has been calling him for days, since Wednesday. That is when I realize he is dead; I suddenly see that he is on the kitchen floor, partially hidden, in front of the stove. My friend goes over to look and says, "Your father is dead." But, suddenly, my father gets up. I scream in horror and shout, "He's alive!" into the telephone. My father comes over to me and takes my hand, and we go into the living room, where he sits on the arm of a chair. He is about to say something. I put the back of my hand gently against the side of his face. I want to feel that human warmth and kindness of his flesh. Then I realize that he's going to keep doing this. He's going to keep doing this. He's going to keep on killing himself and coming back to life. Then I woke up, frightened.[5]

Vaughan asked Kenneth for his associations to the dream. Kenneth recalled touching his father during the funeral, and it was like "touching death." Kenneth described his friend as being "real" and "gruff." In the aftermath of his father's death, his friend represented both the reality and reason needed to manage the tragedy. The dream indicated that Kenneth had begun to incorporate those same qualities into his own psyche. For the first time, Kenneth began to discuss the warmth and kindness he had felt from his father. Many thoughts and feelings emerged that had been masked by his post-traumatic stress disorder (PTSD).

Vaughan was reminded of the archetypal death of Osiris by the hand of his brother Set in Egyptian mythology. This story about murder and resilience is a rough parallel to the death of Kenneth's father. Vaughan observed that Kenneth's ego had been shattered, fragmented, and depressed. Kenneth felt no healthy connection to feeling, which is represented in the myth by the female goddess Isis. Once Kenneth made a connection to the warmth and kindness of his father, resurrection was possible. In the Egyptian myth, this was brought about by the birth of Horus, the hawk-headed god of the sun.

Vaughan reflected, "This myth pointed to deep archetypal level of tragedy encountered by the patient's psyche and to the cure found in the illness. . . . The myth offered a lesson on how the tragedy of murder is . . . transformed into manageable human experience and symbolized in a higher spiritual consciousness." Jung often sent his patients to libraries to seek possible mythological correlates to their own life issues. Those readers who want a fuller account of Kenneth's dreams and Vaughan's analysis will find them in the book listed in the notes section below, which presents several therapeutic approaches to PTSD dreams and nightmares.

Takeaway Points

- Jung's concept of archetypes is helpful in understanding both conscious and unconscious aspects of suicide.
- Archetypal field theory explores the time, place, and other aspects of the "field" in which suicides and suicide attempts take place.
- Archetypal themes often appear in the dreams and nightmares of traumatized people.

Notes

1. Best, K. (2013). *The archetype of suicide.* Sarasota, FL: Runaway Press.

2. U.S. Department of Health and Human Services. (2012). *National strategy for suicide prevention: Goals and objectives for action.* Rockville, MD: U.S. Public Health Service.

3. Hillman, J. (1997). *Suicide and the soul.* Woodstock, NY: Spring Publications.

4. Wessley, S. (2014). Preventing suicide: Are the best barriers physical or philosophical? *Lancet, 383,* 861–862.

5. Vaughan, A. G. (2016). Jungian dreamwork. In J. E. Lewis & S. Krippner (Eds.), *Working with dreams and PTSD nightmares: 14 approaches for psychotherapists and counselors* (pp. 1–21). Santa Barbara, CA: Praeger.

CHAPTER THIRTY-THREE

Why Mythology Is Personal

In contemporary usage, the word *myth* often refers to a false belief or fanciful story. Originally, though, traditional myths explained natural events and human origins. Seasons come and go, an oddly shaped mountain has a story, and humans were created at the whim or plan of invisible beings. Science has replaced these with more accurate facts about life, but personal and cultural myths remain, with unconscious underpinnings, metaphors, and images. For example, many Americans believe in an outdated myth called "progress," in which we are both heirs and heroes.

A personal myth is a story or image that powerfully resonates within a person and may even direct his or her death. From chapter 1, you may remember Carlton, who walked into a lake to unite with his mother. Finn choreographed his suicide around his blazing red sports car. Each of these ways of death represented a highly personal myth or image.

The thwarting of passionate love may lead real people to kill themselves. The joint suicides in 40 BCE of Marc Antony of Rome and Cleopatra VII of Egypt have been immortalized in art, cinema, and opera. In 1889, Prince Rudolf of Austria and Baroness Mary Vetsera were in love; however, he was already married, and his father forbade him to ask for an annulment. The lovers died in an apparent murder-suicide in Mayerling, a hunting lodge. A century later, the 1997 suicide of Nirvana vocalist Kurt Cobain shocked millions of his fans. Could a personal myth have been involved? It was rumored that he wanted to join rock musicians who had died at aged twenty-seven: Jimi Hendrix, Janis Joplin, Jim Morrison, and Brian Jones.

Mythic Narratives

Personal myths are complexes of images, beliefs, emotions, values, and priorities coalesced around a common theme. They may be expressed via symbols (images with deeper meanings), stories, explanations, rationales for behavior, and aspirations. They may express a wish to experience something greater than oneself—a divinity, nature, or humankind as a whole.

In his autobiography, Jung announced, "I have now undertaken, in my eighty-third year, to tell my personal myth,"[1] a statement that reflected his longstanding recognition that individuals create and maintain mythological belief systems. Jung was not alone in this idea. Existential psychotherapist Rollo May argued that contemporary psychotherapy "is almost entirely concerned . . . with the problem of the individual's search for myths."[2] Sigmund Freud made use of myths, most memorably the Oedipus myth but also in his proposal that "Eros," the survival drive, was opposed by "Thanatos," a hypothesized drive to extinction that may culminate in suicide. In his classic book *Persuasion and Healing*, Jerome Frank (1973) points out that all schools of psychotherapy bolster clients' sense of mastery by providing them with a "myth" that explains their symptoms and how to resolve them in rituals that involve evocative imagery.[3]

For many individuals and groups, Jungian psychology offers, as psychoanalyst James Hillman put it, a contemporary "form of traditional mythology."[4] In a culture left with few collectively sanctioned values or moral absolutes, members of Western industrialized societies have few forms of finding meaning other than prearranged religious or secular structures or formulating their own personal myths through education, creative work, or psychotherapy.

Myth may also have meaning beyond daily life. According to Joseph Campbell, myths are metaphors for what lies behind the visible world, explaining the "invisible plane" that underlies the visible. Campbell emphasized that myths teach people to identify not with the body but with the consciousness, for which the body is a vehicle. At the same time, Campbell also believed that myths emerge from the body and are created in part to explain such bodily mysteries as childbirth, puberty, menstruation, menopause, sickness, and death.[5]

Perhaps the resurgence of tribalism around the world, in the forms of racism and hostility to outsiders, represents a personal and collective myth: "I belong to the best group, and we will protect our special identity by any means necessary." If so, perhaps understanding this deep level of human meaning can suggest ways to dilute this deeply dangerous collective myth via a counter-myth, such as David Korten's concept of the "Great Turning," which renowned environmental educator and activist Joanna Macy calls "the essential adventure of our time: the shift from the Industrial Growth Society to a life-sustaining civilization" (https://www.ecoliteracy.org/article/great-turning).

Personal myths do not focus on trivial matters; instead, they involve life and death issues. They are the loom on which people weave the raw materials of daily experience into a coherent story. They provide a framework by which people make sense of their lives. A young woman convinced that she is destined to become the next Marilyn Monroe is harboring a personal myth. Parents who tell their sons, "All boys in our family become doctors or lawyers," are expressing a family myth. An ethnic myth is expressed by a community that rejects minority individuals' applications for housing on the grounds that they are not "our kind of people."

Some people kill themselves at dramatic locations, perhaps to embellish their personal myths. Shortly after California's Golden Gate Bridge opened in 1937, a World War I veteran jumped off it to his death. He had been receiving treatment for "shell shock," now referred to as post-traumatic stress disorder (PTSD). About two thousand people have ended their lives this way; the exact number is uncertain because the current quickly carries bodies off to sea.

A leap from the Golden Gate Bridge almost always ensures death. One of the few survivors limped to his automobile and drove himself to a hospital for emergency treatment. He represents the ambivalence Shneidman noted, which also appears in those who are talked out of jumping. Very few of the survivors tried again, perhaps because the incident gave them a new personal myth. One survivor remarked that he suddenly appreciated the "miracle of life." It was like "watching a bird fly—everything is more meaningful when you are close to losing it. I embraced a feeling of unity with all things and a newness with all people. After my psychic rebirth I could also feel for everyone's pain."[6]

Andrew's Personal Mythology Took His Life

One of the most poignant cases known to one of us (Krippner) was Andrew (pseudonym), who was adopted by a childless couple when he was a few days old. His parents were delighted to finally have a child and treated him with much love and care. But Andrew seemed incapable of returning their love and had difficulty relating to his parents or classmates. The school nurse suggested that Andrew was probably autistic. Andrew's parents had provided piano lessons for him, and this became his most notable talent. He spent hours composing music and enjoyed playing whenever someone asked him to perform.

Andrew met a young woman, Lois, who shared his interests in music. Her parents were uncomfortable with Andrew because he lacked common social skills. To their dismay, the couple spent nights together at the home where Andrew lived. Andrew could communicate with Lois quite well on a nonverbal level, making sexual activity enjoyable for them both.

Eventually, Andrew shared his personal myth with Lois. His birth parents were from another planet and had left him at a hospital so that he could learn about life on Earth. When the time came, they would call him back home. Lois was alarmed at this revelation, especially the predetermined end. When she suggested that he might like to see a counselor or therapist, Andrew brusquely dismissed the idea, and Lois did not try again or tell anyone.

Andrew showed Lois his special place, a grove of trees where he said his birth parents would communicate with him. On one of their visits, a rattlesnake crossed their path. Andrew picked it up with a stick. Lois was terrified but Andrew seemed nonchalant, eventually releasing the snake. He said he had no fear of death because his faraway birth parents would determine the best time for him to "return home."

Andrew composed a piece of music for Lois, one for family friends, and another for his adoptive parents. They gathered to hear him perform. The music was exquisite and brought tears to their eyes. Even the pet dogs seemed to appreciate the music. Andrew took this occasion to give away his most cherished possessions: a collection of stones, a collection of shells, and a hand-carved staff for Lois. They were delighted with Andrew's generosity, not knowing that this act sometimes precedes a suicide attempt.

One of Andrew's neighbors had been a hunter and still owned a rifle. One morning, he was surprised when the rifle was missing. The couple went into the woods and found Andrew's body. He had found the rifle, taken it to his special place, put the barrel into his mouth, and pulled the trigger. Andrew left a note for Lois, thanking her for her love, but his birth parents had called him home.

A Group Myth That Encouraged Suicide

Andrew never received a psychiatric diagnosis, but his personal mythology resembles that of the Heaven's Gate cult of San Diego, California. Founded in 1974, the group was led by Marshall Applewhite and Bonnie Nettles. In their personal myth, they had been given "high-level minds" and were chosen to fulfill biblical prophecies. They spoke to local church groups, telling their audiences that they would be killed and then restored to life to travel in a spaceship to a distant destination. The couple recruited a few people to join the "crew" that would accompany them on their journey.

In 1975, the group sold their possessions, said farewell to loved ones, and disappeared from public view. They recruited new members, preaching a new religion, "Sheiaism." Nettles died in 1985, and Applegate revised the doctrine to include an oncoming comet as a sign that their transformation was impending. In 1997, thirty-nine members gathered in a mansion they called "the Monastery," took phenobarbital mixed with applesauce, and washed it down with vodka. They were dressed in identical black shirts and sweatpants. They placed plastic bags around their heads to induce asphyxiation and ensure death. By the time the bodies were discovered, they had started to decompose and had to be cremated.

The group's myth held that Earth was about to be "recycled," so they should leave as soon as possible. This belief system was so compelling to two former members of the group that they committed suicide in the same way, believing that space aliens would resurrect them. A personal or collective myth can be so important to some people that they will literally die for it.

Personal Mythology and Psychotherapy

For individuals, psychotherapy takes place within the context of their culture's broader mythological framework, ideology, and competing visions of reality. For example, one of the great embarrassments for the psychotherapy establishment is the hand it unwittingly lent in suppressing the brewing discontent among women in the late 1950s and early 1960s. By framing the complaints of their female clients as their own intrapsychic problems, therapists served as a repressive force in their lives. But a mythic conflict was unfolding. The myth of the woman-servant was being rejected, and the myth of the warrior woman emerged. In a related vein, we might say that gay liberation came too late to save Finn. His good looks, artistic talents, and social skills were lost because his sexual orientation was rejected by the culture of the early 1960s.

We have mentioned that Jung's term "archetype" refers to the images humanity uses to address these common concerns—symbols that appear in dreams, fantasy, art, and other expressions of the psyche. As the individual, the family, or the group searches for meaning, archetypes (which are said to reside in the collective unconscious) become the raw material for the narratives that become "myths."[7] Psychotherapist Anthony Stevens takes Jung at his word—that archetypes are biologically based (and socially canalized)—and reformulates them in terms of neuropsychological processes. Drawing from research on the brain's subcortical structures and hemispheric asymmetry, and from investigations of naturally occurring mental imagery (especially nighttime dreaming), Stevens concludes that "from the viewpoint of modern neurology, Jung's work stands as a brilliant vindication of and belief in the value of intuitive knowledge."[8]

This framework fits within the emerging area of *narrative psychology*, which treats narrative as an organizing metaphor for human activity. People are both authors and actors in their own personal dramas. The narrative expression of myths need not be written; it may be pictorial, oral, or expressed in dance, pantomime, or sculpture. The emerging field of expressive arts embodies the value of using these art forms to fulfill one's creativity.

Using narrative in psychotherapy enhances both awareness and responsibility, as it teaches clients to redefine themselves and reconstruct their life stories, and it shows them how to take a hermeneutic, meaning-oriented approach to personal experience. For these reasons, T. R. Sarbin nominates narrative as a "root metaphor" for psychology and psychotherapy.[9]

Purpose is part of narrative and has real-life consequences. A long-term study of some seven thousand U.S. adults between the ages of fifty-one and sixty-one defined "life purpose" as "a self-organizing life aim that stimulates goals." The men and women who lacked a strong life purpose were more than twice as likely to die of any cause, specifically of cardiovascular diseases, than those who had a purpose. There were no significant differences of gender, economics, education, or ethnicity. Life purpose was found to be more important than exercising regularly or avoiding tobacco and alcohol. Facing and resolving the existential issues in one's life seems to be a recipe for longevity—and understanding one's personal mythology is part of that quest.

Takeaway Points

- It is important that therapists recognize their own guiding mythology and the mythologies of their clients.
- Many suicides take the form of rituals that are often the explicit, observable manifestation of a personal myth that has lost its power to instill hope.

Notes

1. Jung, C. G. (1961). *Memories, dreams, reflections*. New York: Random House.

2. May, R. (1991). *The cry for myth* (p. 9). New York: Norton.

3. Frank, J. D. (1973). *Persuasion and healing*. Baltimore, MD: Johns Hopkins University Press.

4. Hillman, J. (1972). *The myth of analysis: Three essays in archetypal psychology* (p. 20). New York: Harper & Row.

5. Campbell, J. (1986). *The inner reaches of outer space: Metaphor as myth and as religion*. New York: Alfred van der Marck.

6. Rosen, D. H. (1975). Suicide survivors: A follow-up study of persons who survived jumping from the Golden Gate and San Francisco-Oakland Bay Bridges. *Western Journal of Medicine, 122*(4), 292.

7. Jung, C. G. (1959). *The archetypes and the collective unconscious*. New York: Pantheon Books.

8. Stevens, A. (1982). *Archetypes* (pp. 273–274). New York: William Morrow.

9. Sarbin, T. R. (1986). The narrative as a root metaphor for psychology. In T. R. Sarbin (Ed.), *Narrative psychology: The storied nature of human conduct* (pp. 3–21). New York: Praeger.

CHAPTER THIRTY-FOUR

The Psychophysiology of Suicide

Brain science has made great strides in the last century, and many of these discoveries have relevance to the understanding of suicide. Electroencephalography (EEG) and magnetoencephalography (MEG) have provided valuable information about activity of the brain's neurons, and chemical changes in those neurons can be mapped with positron-emission tomography (PET) and single-photon emission computed tomography (SPECT). Functional magnetic resonance imaging (fMRI) can detect small increases in the amount of blood flow in the brain. Thus, neurophysiologists can now identify the brain mechanisms associated with the thoughts, emotions, and disorders of suicide-prone people.[1] We highlight brain activity in this book not to devalue or simplify complex human behavior but to describe an important dimension that can lead to deeper understanding. Remember, however, that these studies were not conducted in real-life situations when participants were contemplating suicide.

Neurotransmitters

Neurotransmitters are brain chemicals that facilitate or inhibit signals between neurons. Serotonin, a major neurotransmitter, plays a key role in emotional processing, mood stabilization, pain control, and regulating appetite and sleep. The brains of suicide attempters are generally found to be low in serotonin, especially in the prefrontal area of the brain. Suicide rates are especially high in mountain states such as Montana and Wyoming, where the altitude inhibits the production of serotonin, especially for older men, who represent the fastest-growing risk group in the United States. In a 2016 study of one hundred at-risk people, fifteen attempted suicide, and two did not survive the attempt.[2]

Normally, the body's response to stress is regulated by two hormones: cortisol, which floods the body in response to a stressful event, and oxytocin, which brings cortisol levels back down once the stressor has passed. If these hormones continue to regulate each other, they promote resilience and recovery from trauma. However, this system can break down in response to trauma, leaving the cortisol levels unchecked and the body in a stressed and vulnerable state.

Cortisol triggers the fight-or-flight response to danger. It is released when the body's sympathetic nervous system is aroused. Eye pupils dilate, heart rate increases, and glucose is converted from glycogen, providing quick energy for either fight or flight. When the perceived danger passes, these bodily processes return to normal. When these hormones regulate each other, they promote resilience and can protect against PTSD. Unfortunately, a traumatized person may lack the stamina to either fight or flee, and this puts at-risk people at a disadvantage. They simply "freeze," a term becoming familiar as the third automatic response to danger.

The Brains of Suicidal Children

Aliona Tsypes reviewed the literature in 2019, asking why suicide prevention had not been more effective. Tsypes concluded that key risk factors had been overlooked, especially *anhedonia*, the inability to experience pleasure.[3] Anhedonia has been associated with thoughts about suicide, even without severe depression.[4]

Tsypes and her group studied twenty-three children between the ages of seven and eleven with a history of thinking about suicide and compared them to forty-six similar children who had not reported such thoughts. All the children engaged in a number of simple guessing tasks that were rewarded with small amounts of money for correct guesses and penalized for incorrect guesses while EEG signals were recorded. Most of the children were able to recover from their losses and enjoy the rewards for their successes. But those with a history of thoughts about suicide did not recover easily from their losses and failed to enjoy their successes. These responses were not closely associated with measures of depression, anxiety, or psychopathology, but they were especially notable among children whose parents had made suicide attempts.

These results reflect the perspective of two other suicidologists, Maurizio Pompili and Gianluca Serafini, who discussed the interplay between neurophysiological abnormalities, genetic factors, and stressful childhood events in suicide. These factors suggest an *epigenetic effect*, the impact of stressful experiences on gene expression, which can be transmitted to future generations.[5] We, the authors of this book, see epigenetics as an emerging discipline that can play an important role in suicide science.[6]

Tsypes, who was a graduate student when she designed this pioneering research, has provided another innovative contribution to suicide science, notably an investigation of nonsuicidal self-injury. Tsypes and her team compared nineteen children with self-injury histories with thirty-eight children with no such history; all participants were between the ages of seven and eleven. Again, they engaged in guessing tasks while brain wave activity was being monitored by the EEG. Those children with self-injury histories displayed significantly greater negative reactions to losses than other children, as measured by the EEGs, and these differences were not closely associated with their histories of psychopathology or current symptoms.[7] Both of these studies point out an avenue for suicide prevention; perhaps providing opportunities for enjoyment and pleasure, with a minimum of failure risk, could save lives. Bringing more fun and happiness into the lives of these at-risk children would go deeper into their existential condition than any type of medication.

Takeaway Points

- In general, the brains of suicide-prone children and adults often display differences from other people's brains, especially in regard to serotonin and cortisol.

- The findings of brain science can be used to better understand suicide and, perhaps, to devise preventive measures.

Notes

1. Mann, J. J., Oquendo, M., Underwood, M. D., & Arango, V. (1999). The neurobiology of suicide risk: A review for the clinician. *Journal of Clinical Psychiatry, 60* (Supplement 2), 7–11.

2. Oquendo, M. A., Golfalug, J., Sullivan, G. M., et al. (2016). Positron emission tomographic imaging of the serotonergic system and prediction of risk and lethality of future suicidal behavior. *JAMA Psychiatry, 73,* 1048–1055.

3. Tsypes, A., Owens, M., & Gibbs, B. E. (2019). Blunted neural reward responsiveness in children with recent suicidal ideation. *Clinical Psychological Science, 7,* 1–11.

4. Ducasse, D., Loas, G., Dassa, D., et al. (2018). Anhedonia is associated with suicidal ideation independently of depression: A meta-analysis. *Depression and Anxiety, 35,* 382–392.

5. Pompili, M., & Serafini, G. (2013). The neurophysiology of suicide. In D. Lester & J. L. Rogers (Eds.), *Suicide: A global issue* (pp. 85–101). Santa Barbara, CA: Praeger.

6. Krippner, S., & Barrett, D. (2019). Transgenerational trauma: The role of epigenetics. *Journal of Mind and Behavior, 40,* 53–62.

7. Tsypes, A., Owens, M., Hajcak, G., & Gibb, B. E. (2018). Neural reward responsiveness in children who engage in nonsuicidal self-injury: An ERP study. *Journal of Child Psychology and Psychiatry, 59*(13), 1289–1297.

CHAPTER THIRTY-FIVE

The Rational Emotive Approach to Suicidal Thoughts

When hope is gone; when the heart feels heavy; when depression, despondency, or rage dominate; when people see no way of improving what they perceive as "a life not worth living," they may attempt to end their lives. Sometimes they succeed.

A person who is able to think in rational ways does not choose to end his or her life when negative things occur. Finding a healthy perspective can help a person endure dire circumstances and survive. This can be done either through gaining a realistically optimistic and hopeful perspective or through reaching out to others who can provide help. In this chapter, we show you the first way.

Understanding the connection between beliefs and emotions is the key. It is not circumstances but our *view* of the circumstances that creates our emotional reactions, including despair.

Rational Emotive Behavior Therapy (REBT)

Suicidal people may be consumed by irrational thoughts such as the following:

- I lost my job during a good economy. That proves I'll never work again.
- My sister earns far more than I do, and my parents never let me forget it. I'm obviously inferior to her and worthless.
- Now I have a second illness on top of my chronic one. This must be a punishment for something.

- All the colleges I applied to rejected me. I guess I'm too stupid to even know how stupid I am. No college will ever accept me.

Such irrational thoughts create hopelessness, which may make suicide seem alluring. Psychotherapy can help at-risk individuals resist the allure with various types of cognitive behavioral therapy, which identify and change irrational thoughts. The originator of this method was Albert Ellis, the husband and partner of one of us (Joffe Ellis).[1]

Ellis began his career as a psychoanalyst but was dismayed at its passive nature, so he became more active and directive with his clients. He encouraged his clients to think in sensible, realistic, and life-affirming ways. His approach encompassed reasoning (rational), feelings (emotive), and actions (behavior). REBT vigorously encourages insight, realistic perspectives, reasoning, and logic. The therapist compassionately poses strategic questions that help clients clarify their core beliefs and feelings, discovering distortions and errors. Ellis helped people understand the inseparable interplay between thoughts, emotions, and behaviors and that each person has the power to create his or her own emotional destiny.

Ellis initiated REBT in the late 1950s, and before long it had inspired other "cognitive," "behavioral," and "cognitive behavioral" therapies.[2] Together, they comprise effective evidence-based therapeutic approaches; that is, there is experimental evidence that they work.[3]

Brief REBT is enough for some clients to achieve and maintain substantial transformation within five to twelve sessions, depending on their willingness to take responsibility for thinking in rational ways, learn the tenets of REBT, and apply them on a frequent and regular basis.

Clients with severe emotional disturbances, greater physiological challenges, co-occurring conditions, or poor learning skills are likely to benefit from longer-term therapy or a combination of individual and group REBT therapy. As progress continues, they may attend group therapy to maintain their therapeutic gains or return for individual refresher sessions. REBT has built-in relapse prevention practices: regular self-monitoring, robust application of the disputing methods that had been helpful in the past, and the practice of unconditional self-acceptance, especially in the face of any relapses that may nevertheless occur.

The REBT Therapist

The effective REBT therapist develops rapport with his or her clients, models unconditional acceptance, and warmly acknowledges clients' progress. The therapist reminds clients of REBT tenets, encourages them to take responsibility for their emotions, and continues teaching them the practices for doing so.

Effective REBT therapists also listen well and educate themselves about their clients' culture and religious and nonreligious backgrounds. In addition to print and video material on REBT, the therapist may suggest resources from other approaches or philosophies. The effective therapist stays abreast of current news, inspiring stories, and popular books and movies that support themes being worked on in therapy and that can be recommended to clients.

REBT therapists respect the contribution that appropriate medication can make for some people in creating greater chemical balance in the brain. However, medication alone is not empowering as much as it is relieving. Combined with appropriate medication, REBT reaches underlying causes of despair and can help create lasting change.

The Basic REBT Philosophy

REBT is founded on a keen philosophical insight: it is not events or circumstances that create people's emotional experiences and reactions, but *what they tell themselves* about those events and circumstances. This philosophy was enunciated by the Greek philosopher Epictetus, the Roman philosopher and emperor Marcus Aurelius, and other wise men and women over the centuries.

For example, the end of a romantic relationship could lead to the belief that the situation is awful, life will never be as good again, and there will never be anyone else to fill that empty space in the heart. Such thoughts create unhealthy negative emotions such as depression, hopelessness, despondency, anxiety, and dread, which could then trigger such extreme behaviors as substance abuse, withdrawal, and attempts at suicide. Understandable as these reactions may be, they are the results of mistaking an *emotion* for an unprovable *prediction*: "I will be unhappy forever."

A healthier response would be, "It's a pity this happened, and I'll miss the good times we had together. Yes, I am sad and this hurts. But I can make an effort to meet other fine people. Even if I don't find them right away, I can keep trying, and there are other things in my life that provide meaning and fulfillment. I'll make it a priority to take good care of myself until the sadness fades."

Rational thinking is based on facts and evidence. It creates appropriate and healthy emotions and behaviors, honors preferences rather than demands, encourages flexibility, promotes healthy perspectives, and encourages high frustration tolerance, unconditional acceptance, and not condemning self, others, and life. REBT encourages people to take a constructively critical stance on behaviors but not on their essential selves. They might think, "I made a serious mistake that will impact my life and that of others. But I am still a person with many positive traits and potentials."

By contrast, irrational thinking creates debilitating and unhealthy negative emotions and behaviors. It creates rigid and dogmatic demands, leads to low frustration tolerance, encourages absolutistic attitudes and overgeneralizing, exaggerates facts and includes awfulizing and catastrophizing thoughts, depletes frustration tolerance, and condemns self/others/life when events do not go the way the irrational beliefs demand that they *should* go.

There are three core irrational beliefs that can create unhealthy emotions and lead to detrimental behavior:

1. "I must always do well and be loved and approved by others."
2. "Others must treat me well and act the way that I think they should."
3. "Life must always be fair."

Negative and Positive Emotions

Some emotions are negative but not destructive. That means they are not bad or stupid but rather unpleasant, painful, or simply not enjoyable. Fear in the face of a genuine threat, sadness and grief at the loss of a loved one, and disappointment at the failure of a cherished project are normal and healthy emotions. *Healthy negative emotions*, such as concern, sadness, grief, healthy anger, and regret make it possible to learn from mistakes, contributing to enhancing life and providing wisdom and greater meaning.

Unhealthy negative emotions are based on exaggerated thoughts and do not easily pass. They include self-hatred, anxiety, despondency, hopelessness, depression, rage, guilt, shame, and jealousy. Such unhealthy emotions tend to be present when suicidal thoughts and actions take place.

The Formula for Self-Help

The ABCDE self-help formula provides a clear template for clarifying the connection between an activating event and its consequences. It then provides the means for replacing irrational beliefs with rational ones, thereby creating healthy emotions. The ABCDE formula is as follows:

A. Identify the activating event.
B. Identify consequences of the event, in thoughts, emotions, or behaviors.
C. Beliefs: Identify irrational beliefs (yes, in this framework B follows C!).
D. Dispute the irrational beliefs.
    (i) Realistic disputing—"Where is it written? Where is the evidence?"
    (ii) Logical disputing—"Does it follow that . . .?"

(iii) Pragmatic disputing—"How will it benefit me to maintain this irrational belief?"

E. Effective new philosophies: Healthy, functional, and realistic beliefs replace
the former irrational ones.

Homework is an essential part of REBT. Maintaining therapeutic and
other gains requires ongoing work and practice, work and practice, and work
and practice! Techniques suggested by a therapist, or those selected by an
individual doing self-help, can be chosen from cognitive, emotive, and
behavioral techniques. Techniques that are relevant for preventing suicidal
thoughts and ideas are described in a later chapter.

Unconditional Acceptance

One of the philosophical linchpins of REBT is unconditional acceptance,
which can take three forms:

1. Unconditional self-acceptance (USA);
2. Unconditional other acceptance (UOA); and
3. Unconditional life acceptance (ULA).

Unconditional self-acceptance and adaptive thinking may be the best
defenses against suicidal rumination and actions. Does this mean we strive
to be cheerful at all times? That may be unrealistic for many people coping
with difficult circumstances. It means that when we make a mistake, we do
not confuse the mistake with our essential value. We strive to acknowledge
the mistake, learn from it, and move on.

Unconditional other acceptance (UOA) consists of unconditionally accepting that every human being has worth (despite their flaws and misdeeds). It
does not mean that we accept harmful or even despicable behavior. There are
many people—some reported in the media, others whom we may know in
our personal lives—who have succeeded in experiencing UOA and genu-
inely applied forgiveness of the person or people who wronged them. We
admire people capable of such inspiring forgiveness. One way to aspire to
this virtue is to realize that if we had had the backgrounds of those who act
in despicable ways and their brain chemistry and environmental background, thinking the thoughts they were thinking when doing their evil
actions, then we might have acted in similar ways. This is commonly thought
of as "having empathy" and "walking a mile in the other person's shoes."

For those of us who are not cognitively impaired and who recognize that
we have a choice about our thoughts and attitudes, it is possible to work to

experience UOA more of the time. Attitudes of empathy, compassion, forgiveness, and gratitude strengthen our immune systems, support cardiac health, and prevent high blood pressure and atherosclerosis, among many other physiological benefits. Contrariwise, condemning others' bad behavior from a state of hate and anger contributes to rage and hopelessness that can fuel suicidal ideation and actions.

REBT encourages people to learn and practice forms of meditation and relaxation. It is also important to remain motivated to keep making an effort toward healthy change with realistic expectations. Change may not happen as quickly as one might want. As a result, patience, tolerance for frustration, and endurance are encouraged. Two books that we highly recommend are *Overcoming Destructive Beliefs, Feelings and Emotions* by Albert Ellis and *Rational Emotive Behavior Therapy* by Albert Ellis and Debbie Joffe Ellis.

Conclusion

Core elements of REBT are setting goals, exploring the beliefs contributing to debilitating emotions and unwanted behaviors, ongoing encouragement, and acknowledging gains achieved. To prevent relapses, the therapist uses tolerance, nonjudgment, and acceptance, homework activities, and teaching, reminding, and encouraging clients to make ongoing efforts to accept themselves, unconditionally as worthwhile humans.

The attitudes of compassion and care are implicit and explicit in the theory and philosophy of REBT as well as the call to take productive and practical actions to bring about beneficial change. REBT is more than an effective evidence-based theory and psychotherapeutic modality. It is also a holistic approach and a way of life.

Takeaway Points

- It is not events that make people miserable; it is their perception of those events.
- Rational emotive behavior therapy (REBT) is a holistic, humanistic, and psychotherapeutic intervention that has the potential to prevent at-risk people from killing themselves.
- REBT focuses on unconditional acceptance of oneself, of other people, and of life itself. One may not approve or enjoy a specific person or activity, but acceptance is the initial step in coping with them.

Notes

1. Ellis, A. (1993). Changing rational-emotive therapy (RET) to rational-emotive behavior therapy (REBT). *Behavior Therapy, 16,* 257–256.

2. Wylie, M. S. (2014, December 26). How Aaron Beck and Albert Ellis started a psychotherapy revolution. *Psychotherapy Newsletter.*

3. Gaudiano, B. A. (2008). Cognitive-behavioral therapies: Achievements and challenges. *Evidence-Based Mental Health, 11,* 5–7.

CHAPTER THIRTY-SIX

Beyond the Personal Self: Transpersonal Models

Of the many branches of psychology, humanistic psychology focuses on such positive themes as altruism, compassion, and love. Transpersonal psychology includes humanistic themes and also alterations in consciousness, especially experiences in which one's identity expands to include other people, nature, or the cosmos. These experiences go beyond the personal and include precognitive dreams, extrasensory perceptions, near-death experiences, and out-of-body experiences. Their common theme is that there is more to human life than the individual self, which eminent Buddhist scholar and teacher Alan Watts called "the skin-encapsulated ego."[1]

Western science has for centuries dismissed claims that there are phenomena like these that cannot be felt or explained by material factors, but in the last few decades, serious and disciplined research and reports from reputable individuals have made interest in these matters more acceptable.[2]

Jung's Analytical Psychology

Carl Jung's "analytical psychology" is generally considered the first major transpersonal approach to psychotherapy. Jung stated that one never actually sees an archetype, only the way that it is expressed in a particular time and place. Another basic term in analytical psychology is "collective unconscious," an invisible reservoir common to all humankind that contains the inherited collection of archetypes. It is the deepest and least accessible aspect of the psyche.

To Jung, the term "ego" describes that aspect of the psyche that attempts to maintain a balance between the conscious and unconscious, and "synchronicity" refers to events that seem to be connected in a meaningful way. Jung often referred to analytic psychology as the "care of the soul,"[3] and he emphasized the role of religion and spirituality and that one's purpose is to individuate into his or her true "Self."[4]

Jung included suicide in his collection of archetypes, in that it is a threshold where one chooses to leave life and enter the field of death. He did not approve of it:

> The idea of suicide, understandable as it is, does not seem commendable to me. We live in order to gain the greatest possible amount of spiritual development and self-awareness. As long as life is possible, even if only in a minimal degree, you should hang on to it, in order to scoop it up for the purpose of conscious development. To interrupt life before its time is to bring to a standstill an experiment which we have not set up. We have found ourselves in the midst of it and must carry it through.[5]

Assagioli and Psychosynthesis

Italian psychiatrist Roberto Assagioli explicitly called his approach "transpersonal." He had met Jung and adopted several Jungian concepts, such as the collective unconscious, in his own work. As its name implies, the goal of psychosynthesis is to integrate various aspects of the psyche to manifest their full potential and to integrate diverse aspects of a person into a more expansive-transpersonal whole. Psychosynthesis uses various exercises, such as visualizations, to foster a more integrated consciousness, which ultimately reveals the "transpersonal self."[6]

Assagioli paid special attention to trauma, noting how it can produce "sub-personalities" as defenses against the aftermath of a traumatizing event. He used the term "primal wound" to describe the first split from one's "true self," resulting from early childhood experiences where one incurs the wrath of a parent or caretaker. Just as a part of the body is amputated to prevent an infection from spreading to the rest of the body, traumatized children cut themselves off from what is considered to be especially vulnerable. Unlike an amputation, where the diseased body part is discarded, a valuable aspect of the child's being is suppressed, and therapy often consists of finding and restoring that valuable part of the true self.

A unique application of Assagioli's concepts has been made by the Dutch essayist Luc Sala, who takes the position that identity is not a stable and monolithic structure but a dynamic matrix of identities, some being the result of traumatizing events.[7] Trauma may call forth or even generate "substitute identities," one of which might be the "suicidal person in all of us" that information scientist Jesse Bering has described in his book *Suicidal*.[8] Sometimes the substitute identity serves a useful purpose; withdrawing from one's customary social activities provides time to reflect and recover.

Grof's Holotropic Psychotherapy

Transpersonal psychiatrist Stanislav Grof states that any theory about suicide should address two important questions: why individuals want to kill themselves, violating the powerful dictate of self-preservation, and why they choose a particular means of suicide. In Grof's observations, a person who takes an overdose of tranquilizers or barbiturates would not jump off a cliff or under a train, and a person who uses firearms or weapons would not take drugs, even if they were available.

Grof's work using "holotropic psychotherapy" (interventions that move a client toward completion, wholeness, and transcendence) has convinced him that attempts at suicide typically occur when someone is overwhelmed by powerful unconscious material. He also contends that the birth process that each individual goes through, whether easy or difficult, leaves unconscious imprints on the psyche. Nonviolent suicides typify someone who yearns for the "oceanic consciousness" that existed before the birth process began. These individuals are prone to take overdoses of medication or to walk into a lake or ocean and drown. In some parts of the world, there is no large body of water, so suiciders walk into a desert, overdose on legal or illegal drugs, or enter a bathtub and slit their wrists, actions that dissolve boundaries and facilitate merging with the environment.

An alternative is more violent, as Grof asserts that unconsciousness follows the pattern of the birth process. The pain and suffering experienced while traveling through the birth canal are belatedly mirrored in the form of death: throwing oneself under a train, having a deliberate car accident, cutting one's wrist or throat, using firearms, leaping from a cliff or window, or inhaling toxic fumes. Hanging oneself falls into this category, especially if one's birth process involved a period of suffocation. Ritual suicide, such as seppuku or running amok, falls into this category; when one "runs amok," one enters a public place and begins to kill people indiscriminately, seeming to hope that prompt police action will terminate one's own life or, if not, to use one's weapon for the purpose. In the United States, similar acts have also been called "suicide by cop." Grof hypothesizes that many of the highly publicized mass killings in the United States and elsewhere are disguised suicide attempts and that the allure of suicide reflected a tragic misunderstanding of his clients' birth history. Grof further proposes that many people who are drawn to suicide actually desire "egocide," transforming constriction into expansiveness.

Grof's concept of "spiritual emergency" is a practical application of theory, in that many episodes of unusual behavior are incorrectly diagnosed as psychosis. Spiritual emergencies, if handled properly, can lead to "spiritual emergence" and a more fulfilling life. Treating these episodes as mental illness with suppressive medication interferes with a process that the symptoms are trying to complete. In other times and places, spiritual emergencies have characterized the lives of mystics, saints, shamans, and other people who go on to live greatly enriched lives.[9]

Grof's ideas have made little impact on mainstream practice, although they may be ahead of their time.[10] To his credit, Grof distinguished spiritual emergencies from mental health crises that can be treated in more conventional ways. Grof's research laid the groundwork for including "religious and spiritual problems" in the fourth and subsequent editions of the American Psychiatric Association's *Diagnostic and Statistical Manual* (DSM). His early work with psychedelic psychotherapy spread from transpersonal psychotherapy to more conventional practice.[11]

Can Transpersonal Psychology Explain or Prevent Suicide?

We know that established religious beliefs can either trigger or protect against suicide. It may be that exploring an alleged nonmaterial universe calls some people to leave a troubled existence, yet gives others reasons not to do so. "There are more things in heaven and earth, Horatio, than are dreamed of in your philosophy," Hamlet says to his friend.

Sarah B. Neustadter found that some spiritual ideas, especially those that endorse the existence of other planes of existence, encourage suicide attempts. Here is one suicide note she reported: "Somehow I have to believe that there is some original innocence within that transcends all. . . . I'll be entering back into spirit for another round to fully embody myself [as] the Self." Neustadter commented,

> This sentence indicates a belief in a transcendent realm of spirit that provides an ultimate experience of being or of one's greater self. . . . For the author of this note, the human experience was unduly and inherently painful because it created a sense of separation with his ultimate self and the divine, which caused an aching longing to return to a perceived nondual realm of spirit and bliss.[12]

However, such longings can lead to a *spiritual bypass* in which a person never addresses human-level conflicts and problems. Neustadter warns, "If a therapist takes only an exclusively spiritual or transpersonal approach, there runs a risk of romanticizing, philosophizing, minimizing, or spiritually bypassing the more reality-based, essential, and life or death needs of the client." In Alcoholics Anonymous, a person who engages in such avoidance is known as a "two-stepper," who jumps from admitting the problem to becoming a self-proclaimed expert carrying the message to others without having worked through the intermediate growth steps. In the observation of one of us (Riebel), a serious problem of anorexia was overlooked by a therapist who dwelt on spiritual matters and ignored the client's starvation.

Other consciousness-altering methods, in addition to visualizations, can help people grow beyond the culturally accepted notion that they are isolated entities. Profound shifts in consciousness can occur that burst through the bubble in which people seem separate toward a higher realization that the person is more than just what is bounded within the skin and the familiar identity. To transpersonal psychologists, the personal identity is but a fragment of their holistic-transpersonal selves, so given the proper conditions, a profound alteration to so-called normal perception can offer a glimpse into a more expanded sense of self.

Transpersonal psychotherapist Harris Friedman described his experience in a crisis unit, which often admitted people who had tried to kill themselves. These people in crisis were subjected to hours of intrusive and often irrelevant questions, merely for the sake of completing a standard medical record. Friedman tried to implement transpersonal interventions but found the conventional medical model more resistant to change than he had expected.[13]

Clients who choose a transpersonally oriented psychotherapist are more likely than others to reveal experiences that transcend their socially constructed identities. A conventional psychotherapist might attribute a client's reports of "being at one with the universe" as grandiosity or "ego-inflation," but the transpersonal psychotherapist may regard them as evidence of transpersonal growth or at least the initial step in a process that should not be devalued or terminated prematurely. This is what Friedman encountered when he worked in the crisis center, and his experience has been shared by other therapists with similar transpersonal perspectives. Of course, the fine art consists of distinguishing truly transpersonal inklings from more ordinary (if extreme) responses to life's challenges.

Takeaway Points

- One's familiar identity does not encompass one's entire self. There are levels of consciousness with which many people are unfamiliar but which may nevertheless influence their lives.
- Sincere spiritual longings should not be dismissed or pathologized, nor should real-world concerns be ignored.

Notes

1. Watts, A. (1961). *Psychotherapy East and West*. New York: Random House.

2. Cardeña, E., Lynn, S. J., & Krippner, S. (Eds.). (2000). *Varieties of anomalous experience: Examining the scientific evidence*. Washington, DC: American Psychological Association.

3. Jung, C. G. (1969). Psychoanalysis and the care of souls. *Collected Works of C. G. Jung* (Vol. 1). Princeton, NJ: Princeton University Press. (Originally published in 1928)

4. Jung, C. G. (1960). *Answer to Job*. Cleveland, OH: World Publishing.

5. Adler, G., & Joffe, A. (Eds.). (1973). *Selected letters of C. G. Jung* (Vol. 1). London: Routledge and Kegan Paul.

6. Assagioli, R. (1993). *The act of will*. New York: Penguin. (Originally published in 1973)

7. Sala, L. (2020). *Identity 2.0*. Groesbeck, Netherlands: Artscience.

8. Bering, J. (2018). *Suicidal: Why we will ourselves*. Chicago: University of Chicago Press.

9. Grof, S. (2019). *The way of the psychonaut: Encyclopedia for inner journeys* (Vol. 1). Santa Cruz, CA: MAPS.

10. Viggiano, D. B., & Krippner, S. (2010). The Grofs' model of spiritual emergence: Has it stood the test of time? *International Journal of Transpersonal Studies, 29*, 118–127.

11. Miller, R. M. (2018). *Psychedelic medicine*. Roxbury, VT: Park Street Press.

12. Neustadter, S. B. (2010). Understanding the motivation for suicide from a transpersonal perspective: Research and clinical approaches. *Journal of Transpersonal Psychology, 42*, 61–88. (p. 80).

13. Friedman, H. L. (2010, Summer). From A(uschwitz) to Z(ealot) in a crisis unit: A six-month sojourn in a new practice environment. *Florida Psychologist, 7*, 28.

CHAPTER THIRTY-SEVEN

Systems Approaches to Understanding Suicide

A *system* is a collection of interacting elements that perform a specific set of functions. The respiratory system is composed of several bodily organs that enable breathing. An ecological system is a collection of natural elements that enable trees, animals, water supplies, and other living substances to flourish. A corporation is a system with many individuals, levels, roles, and groups. General systems theory is an attempt to move beyond focusing on separate parts of something in favor of understanding how each part interacts with other parts.[1] In this chapter, we examine suicide from a systems perspective.

Studying Systems Can Predict Suicide

Named after a ninth-century Arab mathematician, an *algorithm* is a step-by-step procedure that organizes existing data into a practical plan. It is useful in computer programming, data processing, and the creation of flow charts. The Columbia Classification Algorithm of Suicide Assessment includes failed suicide attempts, thoughts about suicide, self-injury without suicide intent (such as cutting one's skin or taking a large dose of nonlethal medication), and suicidal behavior (such as holding a knife to one's wrist or putting a rope around one's neck). This algorithm has been far more useful than depending on any single category to assess suicidality.[2]

The Belgian Gilles Jacobs developed an algorithm to spot and block words and phrases associated with bullying on social media sites.[3] Haji Saleem and his Canadian colleagues used algorithms to detect hate speech directed against women, black people, and those who are overweight. English engineer

Dan Muriello and his team have been able to notify local authorities when alarming signs occur on Facebook posts. Maria Liakata, another English researcher, has detected mood changes among suicide-prone people from social media comments. These projects may raise privacy concerns, especially in light of the way that Facebook data have been sold without the knowledge of users. In response, researchers and clinicians developed mobile apps such as Woebot and Wysa, which allow users to talk through their problems and receive responses designed by specialists in cognitive behavioral therapy.

U.S. investigators examined the health records of people who harm themselves and created algorithms that were 92 percent successful in predicting how many of them would attempt suicide during the next seven days. A different group used algorithms and predicted suicide with 91 percent accuracy in another group of people who were having suicidal thoughts. This study used neurological data rather than health records or social media posts. When the members of this group were asked to describe such concepts as "death" and "carefree," the computers were able to discriminate with 94 percent accuracy between those with suicidal thoughts who had made a suicide attempt and those who had not. Of particular interest, shame emotions were activated for the suicidal group but not for the nonsuicidal group.[4]

The U.S. Army's Study to Assess Risks and Resilience in Servicemembers (STARRS) is the largest suicide study ever undertaken; it involved 1.6 million soldiers and identified over four hundred personal characteristics. Those enlisting in the army at age twenty-seven or older were significantly at risk as well as those with nonviolent weapons offenses and those scoring in the upper half on the Armed Forces Qualification Test for feelings of depression, loneliness, helplessness, and hopelessness. Substance abuse and PTSD were risk factors. Those scoring in the top 5 percent of risk factors were responsible for 52 percent of the suicides. Authors of the report urged caution in interpreting the results because the algorithm was only based on sixty-eight suicides. Nonetheless, instead of finding a needle in the proverbial haystack, STARRS has found several needles.[5] This study is particularly important at present, when so many active and former service members are committing suicide.

The Durkheim Project uses data obtained by its volunteer military service members to predict when they are at risk based on their use of social media and their VA records. The resulting algorithm predicted suicide attempts with 65 percent accuracy, a rate generally higher than therapists' estimates. Therapists whose clients have their data stored on the Durkheim Project and have proper permission from the clients can be notified when a client posts something alarming. The client is given a "risk rating" that permits the therapist to make suitable interventions. Membership in the project is voluntary, as it would otherwise be an invasion of privacy. Early results indicate that computerized texts can be usefully applied to suicide research and prevention.[6]

Algorithms are not without their problems. Nonetheless, existing models predicting suicidal behavior have an accuracy rate equal to or exceeding widely accepted risk-prediction tools for other behaviors, rates high enough to guide prevention efforts.[7]

The Wilber Quadrant

Ken Wilber, an American philosopher, titled one of his books *A Theory of Everything*.[8] Wilber has constructed a four-quadrant model of the person (interior and external) and the group (interior and exterior). Below we examine Wilber's four quadrants to see how they apply to suicide.

The Person, Interior and Individual

The commonsense explanation for suicide is that it is a result of a person in pain wishing to stop the torment. This is certainly the case with those who have been bullied or sexually abused and for those who find no meaning in their lives. But some suiciders are not in pain, nor are they agitated or depressed. Perhaps their identity has been challenged, their personal mythology has collapsed, or—speaking from a shamanic perspective—their soul has been lost. A substitute identity has monopolized the individual's attention. An irrational belief and a negative personal myth have taken over. Predisposing conditions such as histories of childhood abuse, poor attachment, and mental illnesses may play a major role.

The Person, Exterior and Individual

Exterior factors can be observed by others. One of the best predictors of suicide is a previous suicide attempt. Suicidologists can also study written documents of at-risk people, and therapists can listen carefully to what transpires in the therapy session, including expressions of hopelessness and helplessness, episodes of depression and anxiety, feelings of social isolation, and observed lethargy and loss of energy. Observers can also notice sudden weight gain or loss, disturbed sleep patterns, increased use of legal and illegal substances, rapid mood changes, and giving away of prized personal possessions.

The Person, Interior and Collective

People can react to their culture's mythology in self-destructive ways, such as becoming martyrs to a cause. A subculture, such as a religious cult, might demand suicide on the part of its members. A powerful archetype from the collective unconscious, such as the martyr archetype, may attain salience. Evolutionary forces may be at play that affect people with low resiliency.

The Person, Exterior and Collective

A downturn in the stock market can provoke suicide for those who have lost everything (or who believe that financial losses are the same as "losing everything"). Yet strangely enough, suicides tend to rise in periods of prosperity as well as economic depression. Slavery and imprisonment can evoke suicidal thoughts among oppressed, imprisoned, and enslaved people. The suicide of a cultural icon can bring about suicidal contagion, and the death of a popular classmate can trigger copycat suicides. Poverty and various social and political structures may marginalize ethnic and sexual minorities.

Ten Cases

Let's look at eight cases that one of us (Krippner) has contributed to this book. Andrew, Carlton, Finn, Fred, Jay, Harry, Mildred, and Phil died at different ages, ranging from seventeen to sixty-five. There were three deaths by firearms, two hangings, one jumping from a height, one overdose, and one drowning. All eight suffered "psychache" in one form or another and probably killed themselves to end the pain.

Attachment issues were evident for Jay, Harry, and Phil. Carlton may have suffered from excessive attachment to his mother. Andrew, Finn, Jay, Harry, Mildred, and Phil seemed to view themselves as outsiders. All but Fred lacked a meaningful purpose in their lives, but once Fred retired and his children left home, he also lost his purpose. None of the eight died from poverty. Andrew and Harry had psychiatric diagnoses, Jay was a heroin addict, and Fred knew that he had PTSD. Maladaptive personal myths and irrational belief systems characterized all eight. From a shamanic perspective, all eight could be seen as suffering from spiritual sickness and soul loss.

Tex and Ming are two additional instances of poor attachment in their younger years. Tex cut his wrists but recovered. Ming contemplated taking poison before engaging in a psychotherapy experience that probably saved her life. For both, a constructive life purpose emerged, and thoughts of suicide never returned.

These cases fall into Durkheim's "anomie" category. Using Hillman's categories, all would have been "emotional suicides." We do not want to dwell too heavily on categories because individual cases vary considerably, but they can help us detect patterns and make useful predictions.

Takeaway Points

- Viewing suicide from a systems perspective allows inclusion of individual and group factors along with their interior and external dimensions.

- Algorithms have been able to predict suicides among different groups, but not perfectly. Their limitations are reminders that suicide is complicated.

Notes

1. Laszlo, A., & Krippner, S. (1998). Systems theories: Their origins, foundations, and developments. In J. S. Jordan (Ed.), *Systems theories and a priori aspects of perception* (pp. 41–74). New York: Elsevier.

2. Posner, K., Oguendo, M. D., Gould, M., et al. (2007). Suicidal events in the FDA's pediatric suicidal risk analysis of anti-depressants. *American Journal of Psychiatry, 164*, 1035–1043.

3. Griffith, S. (2019, February 11). Can this technology put an end to bullying? BBC.com.

4. Mitchell, T. M., Shinkareva, S. V., Carlson, A., et al. (2008). Predicting human brain activity associated with the meaning of nouns. *Science, 320*, 1191–1195.

5. Kessler, R. C., Warner, C. H., Ivany, C., et al. (2015). Predicting U.S. Army suicide after hospitalizations with psychiatric diagnoses in the Army Study to Assess Risk and Resilience in Servicemembers (Army STARRS). *Journal of the American Medical Association, Psychiatry, 72*, 49–57.

6. Paulin, C., Shimer, B., Thompson, R., et al. (2015). Predicting the risk of suicide by analyzing the text of clinical notes. *PLoS ONE*. https://doi.org/10.1371/journal.pone.0085733.

7. Simon, G. E., Shortreed, S. M., & Coley, R. Y. (2019, June 26). Positive predictive values and potential success of suicide prediction models. *JAMA Psychiatry, 76*(8), 868–869.

8. Wilber, K. (2000). *A theory of everything.* Boston: Shambhala.

Those Who Survived: Marla

Marla (not her real name), a woman in her midforties, had received therapy for about ten years, primarily psychoanalytic, for help with anxiety and depression. During that time, after the breakup with her then fiancé, Steve (not his real name), she overdosed on drugs and was committed to a hospital, where she was closely watched for some weeks. She explained her suicide attempt by saying that her fiancé was her "soulmate" and that without him life held no meaning. Marla felt agonizing pain and grief unlike any she had ever experienced before.

Marla eventually came to me (Debbie Joffe Ellis) for help. She is an intelligent woman who welcomed the rational emotive behavior therapy (REBT) approach. Marla made solid efforts to pay attention to her self-defeating thoughts when they arose, to immediately dispute them, and to replace them with healthy, encouraging, and realistically optimistic thoughts.

Marla worked to develop unconditional self-acceptance and to change her belief that her worth depended on others accepting her, especially men in whom she was interested. Rejection was her worst fear. When, on occasion, Marla relapsed into feeling depressed when she was rejected and thinking that she was not "enough," she would pull herself up and return to using the REBT techniques for changing her paralyzing despondency into the healthy feelings of disappointment and sadness. Acknowledged feelings will pass; unquestioned negative beliefs do not.

Three years after the end of her relationship with the man she considered her soulmate, Marla met Steve again on a social network, and a passionate and absorbing relationship ensued. After a few months, he declared his "undying love" for her, and they talked about living together. She felt blissful, confident, and joyful. Then Marla discovered Steve's messages of "undying love" to another woman on his cell phone.

Marla reverted to hopelessness and again contemplated suicide. However, instead of acting impulsively and looking for ways to end her life, she made use of her years of writing daily in her "gratitude journal" and of disputing irrational, self-defeating beliefs. She called me and made an appointment, and we identified the return of her self-condemning thinking and the way she had tied her worth to Steve's love. We discussed the absolutistic thinking that had once again convinced her that she would never be happy. We disputed such thoughts and attitudes and came up with realistic, compassionate, and no-nonsense responses.

We resumed weekly sessions for some months, until she felt grounded and more secure in her ability to hold unconditional self-acceptance and compassion. She began to focus on activities that were uplifting for her and did not involve approval from others—walks in nature, painting, and yoga. Marla resumed writing daily in her gratitude journal.

If Marla had not spent the years practicing REBT, usually on a daily basis, she may have attempted to take her life again when she learned of Steve's infidelity. She realized that REBT needs to be practiced during both good times and challenging times. For her, this practice succeeded.

SECTION VIII

Prevention

CHAPTER THIRTY-EIGHT

Preventing Suicide

Organized attempts to prevent suicide date back to 1958, when the Los Angeles Suicide Prevention Center was opened, followed in 1966 by the National Institute of Mental Health's Center for the Study of Suicide Prevention. Prevention falls into three stages: *primary prevention* means educating the public about a risk, *secondary prevention* identifies those individuals who are at risk, and *tertiary prevention* means treatment of those at risk before they take action. Let's look at how two leading professions recently addressed the serious suicide epidemic.[1]

Contributions from Psychology

Monitor on Psychology, the official trade publication of the American Psychological Association (APA), the world's largest organization of psychologists, published an article on suicide prevention in 2019.[2] The authors noted that suicide remains the tenth leading cause of death in the United States and the second leading cause for those between the ages of ten and thirty-four. However, it also found a positive note, pointing out that scientists have improved ways of identifying those at risk. Using functional magnetic resonance imaging (fMRI) technology, researchers could determine with 91 percent accuracy those who had suicidal *thoughts* and those who did not. Among those who had suicidal thoughts, distinguishing those who had made suicide *attempts* from those who had not was determined with 94 percent accuracy.

Psychologists have searched for evidence-based frameworks to identify suicidal thoughts and behaviors, finding that several versions of cognitive behavioral therapy (CBT) have reduced suicide attempts. A short CBT treatment was able to reduce suicide attempts in the military by about 60 percent, and another version reduced suicide attempts by at-risk adolescents. But the overall suicide rates in the military have not been reduced, presumably because evidence-based interventions have not yet been widely enough used in military settings. Psychological procedures have been used by social workers, emergency room physicians, public health experts, pediatricians, educators, and school counselors, among others.

We saw in an earlier chapter that some professionals view suicide through the lens of public health. Psychologists and their colleagues in other professions have called for a public health approach to suicide prevention. Members of these groups sponsored the American Foundation for Suicide Prevention's first rally on Capitol Hill in 2018.

Furthermore, because firearms account for over half of deaths by suicide and 70 percent of postenlistment veteran deaths, the APA has joined over a dozen other professional groups in calling for legislation to prevent gun violence. The APA also supports the Centers for Disease Control and Prevention's National Center for Injury Prevention and Control and the National Death Reporting System, which tracks both suicides and homicides. The APA sees psychologists, whose education includes statistics, testing, and research, as uniquely qualified to conduct scientific studies and use the results in real-life settings that range from the clinician's office to the legislator's.

Public health approaches to suicide prevention include providing confidential hotlines and other resources. There are numerous accounts from people who say their lives were saved by crisis hotlines, outreach programs, and signs on bridges, all of which interrupted their path toward self-destruction. The National Suicide Prevention Lifeline answered over two million calls in 2018, an increase from the one million calls per year when the lifeline was founded in 2005.

Contributions from Counseling

Another recent article appeared in *Counseling Today*, the official newsletter of the American Counseling Association, the world's largest organization of professional counselors.[3] The authors noted that counseling is both a science and an art; both traditions are needed in suicide prevention. There is considerable solid information on suicide, but applying it to specific individuals requires intuition as well as professional judgment. However, most suicidal people refrain from expressing their despairing thoughts directly and make their suicide plans in secret. Professionally trained counselors need to identify subtle clues and the actual risks they represent and to actively work with those at risk.

Both in-person and at-a-distance counseling rely on empathy and trust for their effectiveness; empathizing with a client's thoughts is not the same as endorsing them, and trained counselors know the difference. Grasping a client's full situation requires time, which may run the risk of allowing the client's suicidality to reach lethal levels. On the other hand, if the counselor takes action too quickly, the client may shut down and not return for future sessions. Clients need to be assured that they will not be "taken away and locked up" if they reveal suicidal thoughts.

A mnemonic, SHORES, reminds counselors what to emphasize when working with suicide-prone clients:

- S. Skills and strategies to cope, such as emotional regulation, adaptive thinking, and engaging in interesting activities.
- H. Hope, including goals for the future and ways to meet those goals.
- O. Objections to suicide, both moral and cultural.
- R. Reasons to live, including responsibilities to family and children. Also, restricting means for suicide, such as taking away firearms, some household products that can be poisonous, and medications.
- E. Engaged care, including finding a meaningful connection with a counselor or other mental health practitioner.
- S. Support, including supportive social environments and relationships, professional and career connections, and volunteer or activist groups.[4]

Clients who have already made a suicide attempt are especially at risk, as are those with certain co-occurring conditions, such as bipolar disorder and substance abuse. Access to lethal means, such as firearms or drugs, elevates the risk. Clients who insist they would never come near a gun may behave irrationally and unpredictably when under stress. Indeed, most clients have not been able to rate their own suicide risk accurately on questionnaires.

The American Counseling Association's Traumatology Interest Network has developed a "Fact Sheet" for counselors to use when they have a suicidal client. The questions need to be modified to suit the individual, but they provide a road map for diagnosis and treatment:

- Are you thinking of hurting yourself?
- How long have you been thinking along these lines?
- Do you have a specific plan?
- Do you have the means to carry out this plan?
- If there anything or anyone that could stop you from carrying out this plan?

Depending on responses to these questions, the counselor can work with the client to one or more of the following:

- Set up a suicide intervention contract; for example, the client will promise to contact the counselor before taking a life-threatening step.

- Provide the client with emergency phone numbers.
- Explore what resources are available, such as family members and friends.
- Develop a plan to limit access to firearms, medications, drugs, etc.
- Increase frequency of counseling sessions, including phone or other electronic conversations.
- Discuss the need for assessing the client's need for medication.
- Assess the need to contact a crisis team, if one is available at a clinic or hospital.
- Consider hospitalization if it is necessary.

Counselors are encouraged to employ evidence-based questionnaires and assessment measures regarding degree of risk. These resources include the Suicide Behaviors Questionnaire (Revised), Images for Suicide Assessment Tool, Columbia-Suicide Severity Rating Scale, and Ask Suicide-Screening and Toolkit, among others. Some counselors make intensive use of these instruments, emphasizing the scientific aspect of their craft. Other counselors bypass questionnaires, relying on the artistic equation of their work.

Bad News and Good News

According to suicidologist Kristine Bertini, in her excellent book *Suicide Prevention*, "If someone decides that they are going to die, they will eventually find a way to kill themselves."[5] That is the bad news. The good news is that for each instance of suicidal thought, there are interventions that can alter the course of action. The key is for the suicidal person to reach out for help or for another concerned person to help propel the suicidal person toward assistance.

Many organizations have websites, available through an internet search, and telephone hotlines. The following numbers were accurate at the time this book was published:

- National Suicide Prevention Hotline, 1-800-273-TALK (8255)
- Stop a Suicide Today, 1-781-239-0071
- The Centre for Suicide Prevention (Canada), 1-833-456-4566
- Parents, Families, and Friends of Lesbians and Gays, 1-202-467-8180
- National Institute of Mental Health, 1-866-615-6464
- The Office of Minority Health, 1-240-453-2882
- The Compassionate Friends, 1-630-990-0010
- National Organization for People of Color against Suicide, 1-800-273-TALK (8255)

- The Dougy Center, 1-503-775-5683
- American Association for Suicidology, 1-202-237-2280

Survivors of Suicide is an independently owned and operated website for those who have lost a loved one to suicide (http://www.survivorsofsuicide .com). Remember that websites and phone numbers may change, organizations may combine or dissolve, and new agencies may be formed.

Takeaway Points

- Although suicide remains a leading cause of death, there are useful interventions available to psychologists and counselors who deal with at-risk clients.
- There are many resources a person may use anonymously and without referral by a professional.

Notes

1. Benson, K. M. (2013). Evidence-based approaches to suicide prevention. In D. Lester & J. R. Rogers (Eds.), *Suicide: A global issue* (pp. 1–25). Santa Barbara, CA: Praeger.

2. Weir, K. (2019, July/August). Better ways to prevent suicide. *Monitor on Psychology*, pp. 38–47.

3. Bray, B. (2019, September). Making it safe to talk about suicidal ideation. *Counseling Today*, pp. 20–26.

4. Cureton, J. L., & Fink, M. (2019). SHORES: A practical mnemonic for suicide prevention factors. *Journal of Counseling and Development, 97*, 325–335.

5. Bertini, K. (2016). *Suicide prevention* (p. 93). Santa Barbara, CA: Praeger/ ABC-CLIO.

CHAPTER THIRTY-NINE

REBT and Suicide Prevention

This chapter demonstrates how to apply rational emotive behavior therapy (REBT) to those debilitating attitudes and emotions that can contribute to suicidal ideation and actions. REBT is not restricted to psychotherapists; just about anyone with some discernment and self-awareness can choose to put these principles to work.[1]

The Goal of REBT

The goal of REBT is to change irrational, dysfunctional beliefs into those that generate positive emotions and behavior. Of course, some beliefs come "factory installed" because we are born into existing cultures. Some myths are shared, and some are individual. Albert Ellis often told his clients that if they constructed an irrational belief, they could deconstruct it. He would tell a client, "What do you think you're telling yourself to make yourself feel this way?" They would then say something like, "I don't like my life." And then he would say, "Yeah, but that thought alone wouldn't induce you to contemplate or attempt desperate actions such as suicide. What else are you telling yourself?" Then clients would say things like, "It shouldn't be the way it is. It's terrible that I failed. I'm no good." Ellis would point out the shoulds, the oughts, and the musts and then encourage the clients to revise or abandon them.

REBT May Make the Difference

The following fictional examples illustrate the dramatic difference that rational thinking can make. Two high school girls are bullied by their peers. One girl thinks, "I can't stand this. This is the worst thing that has ever happened to me. I just want to be happy and popular. And now that clique of bullies has ruined my life. I cannot take the taunts and the teasing anymore. I might as well kill myself."

The other girl thinks, "I can cope with this and get by. I will be graduating in two years, go to college, and will never see those bullies again. In the meantime, I will focus on my studies and regard their taunts as immature attempts to play power games." Both girls experienced similar events, but their views of the events were quite different.

Two soldiers fought side by side in Iraq and learned how to detect terrorists. While patrolling the streets of a small village, they were approached by an Iraqi girl carrying a bundle. Suspecting she was holding a concealed weapon, they opened fire. When they inspected the girl's body, they discovered that she had been carrying a doll, her most cherished possession. Both soldiers suffered shock and remorse. One soldier tells his chaplain, "This was the worst day of my life. I can never forgive myself, and I know that God cannot forgive me either. Life is not worth living, and you cannot convince me otherwise. Do not be surprised if you see my dead body after I blow out my brains and wipe out that grim memory forever."

The other soldier tells the same chaplain a different story. "That was the worst day of my life. I reacted at split-second notice, just as I had been trained to do. I will carry the scars of the experience with me for the rest of my life. I know that horrible things happen in wars and did not know that I would experience one of them firsthand. But I have duties to perform and choose to focus on what I need to do. When I finish my tour of duty, I will go home. One of my first activities will be to volunteer at a local youth center. That might help me cope with my guilt and restore some sense of meaning in my life."

Two young men are sexually abused when they left home to participate in a statewide church conference. They were pleased when one of the staff members took the group sightseeing. He was gregarious, friendly, and well informed on the local tourist attractions. He invited several students to his office, where he had a collection of arrowheads found during the excavation of a nearby mound.

One boy came for a private viewing of the arrowheads and was surprised when the staff member gave him a shot of whiskey and made a toast. The boy was not accustomed to hard liquor and made no resistance when the staff member suggested that they "get naked." On returning home, he thinks to himself, "I must have done something that incited that staff member to molest me. I showed up in shorts and a T-shirt that was so tight it showed off my muscles. And when he suggested we take off our clothes, I didn't object. Worse yet, I enjoyed the experience. That means that I am gay, and I know my parents will kick me out of the house. My life is over. I can never live with the shame and guilt. I know where my father keeps his revolver, and using it will be my only option."

The other boy tells his best friend. "I was so naive that I didn't see the abuse coming. And I was too drunk to offer any resistance. Yeah, the staff member did not use force, and I simply went along with what he was doing. But now I will report him to the church leaders and the police, and that will keep him from messing around with other guys. I won't let that creep ruin my life. I will tell my friends about it so that they won't be naive if they ever get approached."

It is easy to determine which of the high school girls, soldiers, and young men had been thinking rationally after their frightening experiences. If the first of these pairs had practiced REBT, they would have been better equipped to interpret their experiences in less harmful ways.

REBT and Suicidal Clients

Clinical psychologist Robert Harper described the approach he takes when a client brings up the topic of suicide:

> A client contends, let us say, that she is devastated and is thinking of killing herself because her lover has just left her. "Why are you so desperate?" the therapist asks this client. "Because this keeps happening to me. And now that it has happened again, I know that I'll never be able to have a permanent relationship with a man. Especially since I am now forty years old. There are no good men over forty in this damned city. And as soon as people see that I've lost out again, they'll all know I'm hopeless and that I just can't keep any man that I go out with."[2]

Even without REBT training, a listener might realistically point out a few things to this sad woman: (1) just because she has lost another lover hardly means she'll *never* be able to make a permanent relationship; (2) her being older may partly but not wholly handicap her in looking for a partner; (3) in her city, there are very likely to be at least a *few* good men over forty; and (4) people may think she is a difficult person to get along with when they see she has lost this latest lover, but surely not all of them will see her as hopeless. Even if they do, she can choose to work on self-sufficiency, self-acceptance, and not needing approval from others.

These realistic (or empirical) arguments are fine; in fact, some of them are quite good. But it is possible to go deeper. This woman explicitly or implicitly believes that she *must* win and retain a good lover, and if she does not do as she *must*, she is a hopeless, unlovable person. The best disputation challenges the underlying belief or attitude that is at the root of the problem, namely, that she has been such a total failure that she might as well be dead.

A Plumber Prevents a Suicide

On December 2, 2019, the first Monday after Thanksgiving, a man stood on the top of the Brooklyn Bridge as policemen tried to talk him down. Joey Hansen, a twenty-nine-year-old plumber, had left work earlier than usual, got a ride home with his buddy, and saw the man as they drove across the bridge. He immediately asked his friend to stop the car and started talking to the man. "Don't do it, man. It's not worth your life. It's not worth it. Walk back down. You can change anything in your life, bro. You can change anything. Your life is worth more than your problems. Come on, man. Things can change."

Finally, Hansen said, "Turn around. It's not worth it." And then the man turned. "And he looked at me, so that's how I knew he was listening to me," Hansen said. "And it looked to me like he was crying. . . . He turned around and just walked right off the bridge." The NYPD said that with the help of that civilian, officers were able to get the twenty-four-year-old man to come down safely and take him to a hospital for treatment. "If everyone put out just a hand to help, people will grab it. They want help," Hansen said.[3]

Joey Hansen may not have studied REBT, but in his words, attitude, and actions, he was exhibiting REBT's principles brilliantly. He expressed compassion and unconditional acceptance. He showed care not only through his words but also through his action of persistently and patiently talking to the man in distress. He spoke wisely and rationally, putting things in healthy perspective and reminding the man on top of the bridge that his life was worth more than his problems. All those factors combined probably saved that young man's life.

Unique Aspects of REBT

Although REBT has spawned numerous psychotherapeutic modalities, it contains several unique aspects:

1. Emphasizing unconditional acceptance and addressing a person's philosophy of life and living.
2. Emphasizing the importance of vigorous, thorough, and substantial disputing of irrational ideas followed by recognizing their rational counterparts.
3. Offering three distinct forms of disputation: (1) realistic disputing, (2) logical disputing, and (3) pragmatic disputing.
4. Paying attention to the *emotive* element of therapy and well-being. REBT encourages people to acknowledge the *healthy* negative emotions, rather than avoiding or suppressing them, and to avoid debilitating *unhealthy* ones.

Karlyn's Story

Karlyn's story is well known to one of us (Krippner), who met her before the events in this narrative took place. In the early 1980s, Karlyn (not her real name) initiated a torrid romance with a handsome young man from overseas. He refused to use a condom, saying it dulled his erotic sensations. Karlyn took measures to prevent pregnancy but was uneasy about her partner's unprotected sex. However, he reassured her that he was neither a homosexual nor a heroin addict, the two assumed categories of AIDS victims.

Karlyn's partner returned to his own country, leaving her with ecstatic memories. He also left her infected by the human immunodeficiency virus, the agent responsible for acquired immune deficiency syndrome (AIDS). When her physician confirmed the diagnosis, Karlyn was devastated. She decided to kill herself rather than suffer a long and devastating illness.

Karlyn's decision made perfect sense to her, but fortunately she decided to discuss the issue with a therapist, one who had been trained in REBT. Dr. Mitzi asked Karlyn to clearly articulate her reason for ending her life and the means that she would use to do so.

Karlyn had not decided whether she would jump from the Golden Gate Bridge, take an overdose of medication, or slit her wrists. She confessed that she lacked the determination to cut her arteries and had even known someone who had cut her arms the wrong way and survived. Karlyn was terrified of heights and had no access to firearms, so she thought she would store medications until she had accumulated the critical dose.

Dr. Mitzi then asked Karlyn about her family's reaction to her predicament. Karlyn admitted that she had not considered their reaction but realized that they would be devastated. All things considered, she speculated that even dying a slow and painful death might be preferable to inflicting sudden grief on her mother, father, and siblings. Dr. Mitzi also asked Karlyn whether she had investigated anti-AIDS medications. Karlyn assumed that AIDS inevitably led to death and did not realize that innovative treatments were being developed. Dr. Mitzi helped Karlyn enter an experimental program.

We wish this story had a happier ending. A decade after Karlyn's death from AIDS-related complications, there were medications that prolonged the lives of people who were HIV-positive, preventing them from contracting full-blown AIDS. However, Karlyn received considerable support from her family and friends. Her physician was not able to save Karlyn's life, but he was able to prevent a painfully lonely demise. Dr. Mitzi helped Karlyn attain greater acceptance of herself, her former lover, and a world in which countless people died of this epidemic. Had she not seen Dr. Mitzi, Karlyn might have missed some of the most memorable times of her life, though sadly it ended too soon.

Altruism, compassion, and empathy, elements strongly encouraged in REBT, are observed in other animals. For instance, the famed vampire bats of Australia bite into their own flesh to produce blood that feeds their infants. David Loye has resurrected what he calls "Darwin's Lost Theory of Love." Loye found dozens of references to love and compassion in Darwin's books.

The Last Word

Albert Ellis addressed the issue of suicide several times. When discussing suicide as revenge, Ellis reflected that some practitioners of REBT would ask their clients, "Do you think that killing yourself would 'get back' at your offenders? Are you sure? It might be that they don't give a damn and that your suicide would be in vain."

In 1990, Jack Kevorkian was arrested for assisting the death of a patient who said that his physical pain was unbearable. Dr. Kevorkian had assisted dozens of ailing people in terminating their lives and was a longtime advocate of physician-assisted suicide. Ellis relates that when he defended Kevorkian, "My mail became heavy with accusations of how anti-humanistic I was. It seems to me, I said in response, that advocates of assisted suicide were usually quite humanistic, since they allowed would-be suiciders the *choice* of staying alive or not."[5]

Nonetheless, REBT therapists encourage *preventive* action, urging as many people as possible to learn and practice REBT principles before things become truly dire.

Takeaway Points

- REBT affirms people's right to choose whether or not to end their lives.
- REBT can prevent suicide by helping clients consider their rationale for killing themselves and the potential consequences of their actions.

Notes

1. Ellis, A., & Ellis, D. J. (2019). *Rational emotive behavior therapy* (2nd ed.). Washington, DC: American Psychological Association.

2. Ellis, A., & Harper, R. A. (1997). *A guide to rational living* (3rd ed.). Chatsworth, CA: Wilshire Book Company.

3. CBSN New York. (2019, December 2). *Exclusive: Good Samaritan helps talk man off edge of Brooklyn Bridge.* https://newyork.cbslocal.com/2019/12/02/good -samaritan-helps-talk-man-off-brooklyn-bridge.

4. Loye, D. (2000). *Darwin's lost theory of love: A healing vision for the new century.* San Jose, CA: ToExcel.

5. Ellis, A. (2010). *All out: An autobiography.* Amherst, NY: Prometheus Books.

CHAPTER FORTY

Resilience Training and Suicide Prevention: Did It Work?

The U.S. Army ended 2018 with a troubling statistic: the highest number of suicides among active duty personnel in at least six years. In addition, about 15 percent of the soldiers stationed in Afghanistan or Iraq experienced post-traumatic stress disorder (PTSD). These sobering figures led many writers to question the army's "soldier fitness" program that has cost U.S. taxpayers at least $287 million.

The army's program followed dozens of similar programs, which met with varying degrees of success. One problem is the lack of agreement as to the meaning of *resilience*. However, there is general agreement that the term refers to an individual's *ability to adapt to a new situation that has resulted from a "stressor," an experience that produced stress*. People tend to be resilient in some situations but not in others, and in some places but not in others. Those with adverse childhood experiences seem to be less resilient than those whose childhood was generally positive.

Most programs began by explaining the nature and goals of the program. This was followed by skill development; participants were taught to set realistic goals, to engage in self-talk in which they told themselves affirming statements, and to use self-regulation procedures, such as deep breathing. Finally, there was an evaluation of the program's effectiveness. In 2018, Susan Forbes and Deniz Fikretoglu published a review of ninety-two resilience programs; about 60 percent of the participants benefited, depending on the way that outcome was measured. Those who showed the most benefits were those who needed it more compared to those who had already developed coping skills.[1]

The army program was initiated in 2009, when General George W. Casey established the Comprehensive Soldier Fitness (CSF) program to address the challenges faced by the U.S. Army because of persistent conflicts in Iraq and Afghanistan. Instead of focusing on treatment *after* issues arose, Casey wanted to provide *preventive* measures for the soldiers, their families, and civilian employees to teach the life skills needed to cope with adversity and to bounce back stronger than before. In 2012, the name was changed to the Comprehensive Soldier and Family Fitness program.[2]

The Army's Comprehensive Fitness Program

The program addressed family violence, PTSD, sexual assault, substance abuse, and suicide. This was done through a focus on the five dimensions of fitness: physical, emotional, family, social, and spiritual. Three types of instruction were designed: online self-development, training, and evaluation.

Online Self-Development

Online self-development begins when soldiers, family members, and army civilians take the Global Assessment Tool (GAT), a survey intended to assess people's psychological health based on four dimensions of strength: emotional, social, family, and spiritual. The user then enters an online self-development site, ArmyFit, a portal to each of the five dimensions of resilience. Each self-development module is about fifteen minutes in length and is self-paced. There are several modules for each dimension. They include such topics as "building self-resilience," "effective communication," and "blended families."

Training

Training develops a cadre of master resilience trainers (MRTs) through an intensive ten-day course so they can teach other soldiers. Local commanders select the candidates for training from noncommissioned officers, army spouses, and army civilian employees. MRTs teach the performance enhancement aspect of the program, which consists of six mental skills: manual skills, building confidence, attention control, energy management, goal setting, and integrating imagery.

Army chaplain Mike MacKrell had an inside reaction to the MRT training program. Eight years after finishing it, Lieutenant MacKrell observed, "The material provides a basic working model that applies to situations and context we all find ourselves in. It is not a cure-all but a framework for approaching life."

Evaluation

The Army Research Evaluation Team constantly monitors the effectiveness and outcomes of the CFS resilience program. Other internal agencies conduct research on various parts of the program. The army claims that soldiers who completed the program reported higher levels of resilience and psychological health than soldiers who did not complete the program, and soldiers in units that worked with MRTs had fewer diagnoses of substance abuse than soldiers in other units. This was the major measured improvement, but positive changes were also noted in the reduction of anxiety, depression, and PTSD by army and defense contractor evaluators.

Criticism of the Army's Fitness Program

A program that affects the lives of over one million people should be closely examined, but much of the information gleaned was not made available to the public. There has been general agreement welcoming the attention of key segments of the U.S. military to address mental health issues of its personnel, but there has been a wide division of opinion as to how well these programs work, especially the army's program for Comprehensive Soldier and Family Fitness.

Criticism of the Program's Construction

Martin Seligman and his team from the University of Pennsylvania's Positive Psychology Center based the program on an earlier intervention for adolescents suffering from depression or anxiety. This program used cognitive behavioral and social problem-solving skills, and several research studies demonstrated that it had a modest degree of success; however, other studies suggested it worsened outcomes for some people. This program was designed for a nonmilitary group of a different age range, so there was no evidence that it would help soldiers. Moreover, the Pennsylvania team developed the army program in less than a month, and there were no pilot or preliminary studies to detect unforeseen problems. This lack of preparation is puzzling, but the army states that it had to move quickly, given the high suicide rate.

Criticism of the Program's Orientation

There does not seem to be any evidence that the Comprehensive Soldier and Family Fitness program has reduced suicide rates among soldiers. Ray Eidelson and his associates wrote an article for *Psychology Today* about this issue.[3] They fault the program for not paying attention to ethical issues. For example, soldiers trained to "persevere" in the face of adversity might shoot civilians at a roadblock or commit some other action that might come back to haunt them. Trainers appear to lack training in helping soldiers who are experiencing "moral wounding" or engaging in "deep questioning and open exploration of existential issues that often arise for soldiers facing extreme circumstances." One research study using the Global Assessment Scale revealed that female soldiers were less trusting than male soldiers. When this difference was attributed to female soldiers who do not feel fully at ease in the army, Eidelson and his colleagues observed that these women might be aware of the high incidence of sexual abuse against female soldiers or have experienced it themselves.

They also commented on positive psychology's emphasis on human strengths and its attempt to derive something worthwhile from stressful experiences. They doubt that there is scientific evidence linking positive states of mind with health outcomes. Further, positive psychologists seem to overlook the functions that such negative emotions as anger, sorrow, and fear can play in a person's life as well as such social realities as poverty and oppression.

Criticism of "Spiritual Fitness"

Some spiritually oriented groups have claimed that the spiritual fitness aspects of the program are promoted as if they were secular in nature, when they really promote religious beliefs. Seligman, the psychologist whose team developed the program, followed army regulations that defined "spiritual dimension" as "identifying one's purpose, core values, beliefs, identity, and life vision." The regulation goes on to contend that these elements "enable one to build inner strength, make meaning of experiences, behave ethically, persevere through challenges, and be resilient when faced with adversity." It concludes by noting that a person's spirituality "draws upon personal, philosophical, psychological, and/or religious teachings and beliefs." So given how broadly "spiritual" is defined in the program, this criticism may be unwarranted.

On the other hand, some atheists have complained that the Global Assessment Tool (GAT) includes questions that may discriminate against nonbelievers. These groups also are skeptical about the value of remedial training for those who score low on the spiritual fitness part of the GAT. The army replied that soldiers making low scores are invited to look over the Comprehensive Training Modules on spiritual support, rituals, making meaning, and meditation. All were written to reflect diversity, acknowledging that each soldier may define spiritual fitness differently. Furthermore, the army spokespeople noted that working with these modules is voluntary, not compulsory. However, in close-knit situations such as army units, there are few secrets and strong pressures for soldiers to engage in these activities.[4]

Many soldiers have questions about the meaning and worth of life that become more insistent upon returning home. Returning soldiers and members of other armed services deal with loneliness, the possible absence of a community, and the loss of the bond that existed between service members. Eidelson's group was surprised that the program does not seek out veterans who could spend time with soldiers, telling them what they should anticipate when they return to civilian life. In this and other articles, Eidelson and his coauthors conclude that the army's evaluation of their fitness program has "failed the test." By contrast, existential and humanistic psychology emphasize meaning and similar topics that are often in the thoughts of suicide-prone soldiers.

Military Morale and Suicides

In 2015, a military analyst, Raphael Cohen, dismissed the contention that combat stress is the "root cause" of the high suicide rate, noting that there was no evidence for this assumption; the suicide rate for soldiers who did not face combat is actually higher than those who engaged in battle. Nor can poor morale be linked to cultural changes; 60 percent support homosexuals to serve openly in uniform, and a similar percentage of veterans and active duty solders supported opening up ground units to women. But that still leaves a powerful 40 percent who may not welcome these service members.

Cohen found dissatisfaction with outcomes to be more important. A 2013 study found active duty troops about evenly divided over whether the Iraq War was worth fighting. However, 80 percent of veterans feel proud of what they did in Iraq and Afghanistan, at least "often" or "sometimes." But 24 percent said that they committed actions that "often" or "sometimes" made them question their mission. So despite their pride in their service, few called the mission a success.[5]

This might be termed an existential crisis, a crisis of confidence within the military itself. Cohen concluded that this crisis cannot be resolved by motivational speeches or added benefits. Instead, the morale problem requires hard critical thinking about what went wrong with those wars, with the hope that future military campaigns—to be engaged only if all other conflict-solving means have been tried and have failed—produce better results than past ones did.

Takeaway Points

- Suicides in the military have not decreased, despite much money and effort invested in resilience programs.
- Low military morale has many causes, but its existential roots—questions of meaning—may be critical.

Notes

1. Forbes, S., & Fikretoglu, D. (2014). Building resilience: The conceptual basis and research evidence for resilience training programs. *Review of General Psychology, 22*, 452–468.

2. Seligman, M. E., & Fowler, R. D. (2011). Comprehensive Soldier Fitness and the future of psychology. *American Psychologist, 66*, 80–86.

3. Eidelson, R., Pilisuk, M., & Soldz, S. (2011). The dark side of "Comprehensive Soldier Fitness." *Psychology Today, 66*, 643–644.

4. Brown, N. J. L. (2014, July). A critical examination of the U.S. Army's Comprehensive Soldier Fitness program. *Winnower*, pp. 1–24.

5. Cohen, R. S. (2015, June 29). Understanding the U.S. military's morale "crisis." *Lawfare* (online).

CHAPTER FORTY-ONE

Skills for Self-Regulation

Self-regulation is the ability to bounce back from disappointments, to contain unwise enthusiasms, and generally to be actively in charge of oneself. There are many ways of doing this: breathing deeply, confiding in a friend, turning to art or music, reading a self-help book, or attending a support group. In this book, we have shown you additional ways to self-regulate, such as engaging in exercise, disputing irrational beliefs, learning spiritual practices, using critical thinking, considering medications or psychoactive plants, and exploring the many forms of treatment available for anxiety, depression, and hopelessness. Most of the commonly used self-regulation strategies share many elements and have comparable efficacy.

Implicit, unstated cognitive and emotional regulation involves perception, comprehension, and memory processes that occur with a person's direct awareness.[1] The Implicit Association Test is a clever measure of a person's implicit processes and has been used to study at-risk people's unconscious intentions and to predict with a fairly high degree of accuracy which people who self-harm will later make suicide attempts.[2]

Mindfulness

The American Psychological Association defines *mindfulness* as the full awareness of one's internal states and surroundings. Meditation as profound and extended contemplation was traditionally associated with spiritual and religious exercises. Today, it is increasingly used to provide relaxation and relief from stress. Mindfulness is a type of meditation in which thoughts, feelings, and sensations are experienced fully, but without judgment, as they arise and subside.[3] It is intended to enable individuals to become highly attentive to sensory information, focusing on each moment. In most forms, there is a strong element of compassionate acceptance, especially self-acceptance. It can be practiced on one's own, and many mental health professionals have used mindfulness meditation (MM) to treat symptoms of PTSD and several other disorders. MM seems to be beneficial to most of those who practice it.[4]

Similar practices are transcendental meditation, prayer, imagery, visualization, and body-centered procedures such as progressive relaxation, autogenic training, and yoga; mindfulness-based stress reduction; and mindfulness-based cognitive therapy. All of these are associated with a reduction in symptoms of anxiety and depression, can be mastered in relatively brief time frames, and are relatively cost-effective. Functional magnetic resonance imaging (fRMI) studies suggest that MM, like other mind-body techniques, can influence brain centers that regulate stress—for example, eliciting increased activity in cerebral areas related to attention and emotion.[5]

Mindfulness and meditation have many similarities, but they are not exactly the same. Meditation is an intentional practice, and the forms range from breathing meditation to mantra meditation (focusing on a sound such as "aum" or one given by a guru, as in Transcendental Meditation). Meditation is usually practiced in a particular place or "setting." Mindfulness is simply being aware, and it can be practiced apart from any structured procedure. It is the act of paying attention, noticing, and being present.[6] One could be mindfully washing the dishes or listening to a friend rather than inwardly fretting about the future or regretting the past.

In progressive relaxation, one learns to relax the entire body by becoming aware of tension in various muscle groups and then relaxing them. In autogenic training, one self-regulates functions of the autonomic nervous system through mental imagery, breath control, and bodily sensations. There are many types of yoga; the practice was originally designed to achieve union with the Supreme Being through self-regulated breathing, body postures, and other practices. Currently, many people bypass the spiritual aspect of yoga and use it to reduce stress and enhance mind-body functioning.

Mindfulness-Based Stress Reduction (MBSR) is an eight-week course developed by Jon Kabat-Zinn, a psychologist who has specialized in mindfulness meditation. The course combines this type of meditation with yoga and other self-regulation practices. MBSR is used in treating PTSD at several locations. The overall results strongly support the use of MBSR for this condition, noting overall improvement and a reduction of particular symptoms of PTSD.[7]

Meditation is not for everyone. Some people can go too far into the recesses of their minds and become overwhelmed with unfamiliar material. Suppressed emotions and memories of trauma may surface. Paula Watkins, a clinical psychologist and meditation teacher, observes that intensive meditation retreats are the most common places for this to occur, especially for those people who have been suppressing their negative emotions for decades.[8]

Meditation may trigger other negative reactions. When relaxation increases anxiety, it is referred to as "relaxation-induced anxiety," which is characterized by unexpected anxiety, muscle tension, and anxious thoughts and images while one is attempting to relax. Those people reporting this condition are those who need it the most, people with anxiety disorders. Practitioners who utilize relaxation training should be aware of the risks so as not to offer to their clients what one team of researchers has called a "poisoned chalice"[9]; they should perhaps offer one of the other methods described here instead.

Biofeedback, Neurofeedback, and Hypnosis

Biofeedback uses an external monitoring device to provide information about individuals' physiological status so they can use voluntary control to make changes. This type of self-regulation is used to treat stress disorders, migraine headaches, and hyperactivity. Neurofeedback is the type of biofeedback that monitors brain activity; other types of biofeedback monitor muscle tension, heart rate, and other autonomic nervous system functions. Biofeedback shares many similarities with other self-regulation approaches and can be used in combination with them or as part of a program fostering healthy lifestyle changes.[10]

With hypnosis, a health practitioner or researcher suggests that a client, patient, or research participant experience changes in sensations, perceptions, thoughts, or behavior. The style of hypnotic induction depends on the context; the goal is to increase concentration and decrease attention to peripheral distractions. Indirect, informal hypnosis can be just as effective as direct, ritualized hypnotic induction. Hypnosis is not a therapy itself; it is used to facilitate other therapies, as in hypnotically facilitated cognitive behavioral therapy." Hypnosis has been found to help clients work through traumatic memories, increasing coping skills and promoting a sense of competency. It has also been useful in treating dissociation, pain, insomnia, and other symptoms of PTSD.[11]

Some practitioners believe that all hypnosis is basically self-hypnosis because the practitioner's suggestions are directed toward a mutually agreed upon goal. In clinical practice, the client is often taught self-hypnosis to reinforce the suggestions made during intervention.[12] Like other self-regulation programs, self-hypnosis is especially compatible with the cognitive behavioral perspectives that we have described in this book.

To conclude, we encourage readers, whether or not they are stressed or suicidal, to investigate this wonderful cornucopia of self-regulation techniques that have been developed in many times and places.

Takeaway Points

- Self-regulation involves a person's voluntary control of internal states and can foster clients' collaboration with their health care providers.
- Biofeedback, neurofeedback, hypnosis, and self-hypnosis can be useful adjuncts in a program for people vulnerable to the allure of suicide.

Notes

1. Howes, M. B. (2007). *Human memory: Structures and images*. Los Angeles: Sage.

2. Nock, M. R., Park, J. M., Finn, C. T., et al. (2010). Measuring the suicidal mind: Implicit cognition predicts suicide. *Psychological Science, 21*, 511–517.

3. VandenBos, G. R. (2007). *APA Dictionary of Psychology*. Washington, DC: American Psychological Association.

4. Kabat-Zinn, J. (1991). *Full catastrophe living*. New York: Delta Trade.

5. Peper, E., Harvey, R., & Lin, I-M. (2019). Mindfulness training has elements common to other techniques. *Biofeedback, 47*, 50–57.

6. Eisler, M. (2018, June 29). What's the difference between meditation and mindfulness? *Chopra Newsletter* (online).

7. Davis, L. L., Whetsell, C., & Hamner, M. B. (2018). A multisite randomized controlled trial of mindfulness-based stress reduction in the treatment of posttraumatic stress disorder. *Psychiatric Research and Clinical Practice, 1*(2), 39–48.

8. House, L. (2015, June 28). Revealed: Meditation can trigger depression and anxiety. Daily Mail.com (online).

9. Kim, H., & Newman, M. G. (2019). The paradox of relaxation training: Relaxation induced anxiety and mediation effects of negative contrast sensitivity in generalized anxiety disorder and major depressive disorder. *Journal of Affective Disorders, 259*, 271–278.

10. Moss, D. (2019). Special issue: Integrating mindfulness training with clinical biofeedback: Practical applications. *Biofeedback, 47*, 49.

11. Cardeña, E., Maldonaldo, J. R., Van der Hart, O., & Spiegel, D. (2008). Hypnosis. In E. B. Foa, T. M. Keane, M. J. Friedman, & J. A. Cohen (Eds.), *Effective treatments for PTSD* (pp. 427–457). New York: Guilford Press.

12. Fromm, E., Brown, D. P., Hurt, S. W., et al. (1981). The phenomena and characteristics of self-hypnosis. *International Journal of Clinical and Experimental Hypnosis, 29*, 189–254.

CHAPTER FORTY-TWO

Building a Better Teenage Brain

In the teen years, the brain is not fully formed. Impulsive acts and poor judgments can be fatal. We believe that one of the best ways to prevent suicide among teenagers is to facilitate their neurological development—to build a better teenage brain.

It was long assumed that brain development was completed by the age of ten, as human brains most rapidly develop during the first two years of life. Researchers at the National Institute of Mental Health studied adolescents' neurology at the turn of the millennium and found, much to their surprise, that brains continue to develop throughout the teenage years and into the early twenties, especially in the prefrontal cortex. The prefrontal cortex plays a critical part in shifting attention, organizing behavior, and strategic decision-making.[1]

This was important news. Many parents had assumed that the bizarre and unpredictable behavior of their teenagers was "just a phase" that they would eventually outgrow. But some adolescents get stuck and become addicted to nicotine, drugs, alcohol, video games, social networks, or thrill-seeking behaviors such as drag racing, shoplifting, or petty crime. Alcohol and drugs, both legal and illegal, pose serious hazards to the developing brain.

On the other hand, many teenagers exert considerable discipline to do well in sports or to develop physical strength and a sculpted body. Furthermore, it has been found that exercise physically strengthens the brain by delivering more oxygen-rich blood to it. Exercise is also a well-known antidote to depression, so we should respect the desire of children and teens to participate in sports.

Most young people pass through these growing pains and emerge safely into adulthood, but others do not. Sometimes an overreaction to a perceived insult or a dip into despondency can lead to a rash decision that ends a life. But it is possible for them to learn and practice life-affirming thinking skills, intentionally rewiring their prefrontal cortex. Like physical exercise, using thinking skills develops brain circuits and neurological connections.

Foundational Thinking Skills

Teenagers need to take advantage of the spurt in neurological growth that begins at around the age of fourteen (at least in Western cultures, which have been the most studied). This is the time to learn to discriminate functional from dysfunctional personal myths and rational from irrational beliefs. Girls and boys mature at different rates, but both need to develop foundational thinking skills.[2]

Foreseeing Consequences

Children begin to comprehend cause and effect: actions have consequences, and certain behaviors usually lead to predictable outcomes. Adolescents need to set goals, make plans, and begin to manage their lives. They can delay gratification if it will lead to greater rewards at a later time. They can foresee the advantages and disadvantages of taking a course of action or make step-by-step plans to initiate a complex project. Young people can be asked to think about something they really want (a piece of sports equipment, entering college, or a road trip) and to foresee how their first step will help them reach the goal.[3]

Learning from Experience

Teens can learn to consider what happened, why it happened, and the results of what happened. They can reflect on the costs and benefits and on whether the end result could have been achieved another way. As with other foundational skills, the more proactive teenagers are, and the more they reflect at the time of the experience, the greater the growth in the prefrontal cortex will be. A teen could be asked why a certain project ended in failure. What would be done differently if another try were made?

Evaluation

Evaluation is an important foundational skill. Children are told when something is good, bad, right, or wrong. Teenagers build on these judgments or develop their own standards. Either way, we believe it is important for them to think through the evaluation process rather than to automatically accept the judgments of family, friends, or celebrities. Rigid parenting styles and black-and-white religious beliefs can delay this important development. Adolescents need to ask how much an object is worth, how well it was made, whether it contained flaws, how nutritious a food choice may be, how safe a game might be, and how important it is to eat that food or play that game. They also need to make moral and ethical judgments. Does partaking in an activity violate the moral code of one's family or friends? A child is more likely to adopt parental values, while a teenager is more likely to be swayed by peers. But learning how to establish standards is a foundational skill because it will help provide needed consistency in a world of options, disagreements, and risks. Teenagers also need to be aware of the consequences of committing an illegal act.

Reasoning

Chapters 35, 39, and 45 on rational emotive behavior therapy demonstrated the importance of careful reasoning. Sometimes an intuitive hunch may provide a useful insight, but it still should be evaluated. Reasoning skills include ways to detect fallacies (conclusions based on improper reasoning) and to determine whether a conclusion makes sense, whether it violates other principles, and whether it is consistent with other conclusions. A group of teens could be asked to watch a candidate for political office speak on television and to remember key statements. Afterward, they evaluate the truth or falsity of these statements.

Problem-Solving

Children often turn to a parent or other adult when they cannot solve a problem. Both children and adolescents tend to take a hit-or-miss approach to solving a problem, whether it is a malfunctioning toy or game, a missing object, the best route to a destination, or a problematic relationship. Adolescents need to learn basic problem-solving skills. First, identify the problem. Next, speculate on various ways to solve the problem. Is this similar to a problem that was solved in the past? How have other people solved it? Who can provide useful advice? If there are several approaches, which yields fewer costs and greater benefits?

Creative Thinking

Sometimes logic and reasoning reach a dead end, and other ways of knowing are needed. Several parts of the brain and body are nonverbal and do not employ logical thinking skills. Creative thinking can access them. Sometimes a solution will come in a dream, a reverie, or an intuitive flash. Most programs that teach creative thinking consist of following a process of identifying a problem, immersing oneself in the parameters of the problem, allowing the information to consolidate (usually unconsciously), having an insight (an answer to the problem), applying the insight, and evaluating how well the application worked.[4]

Decision-Making

Whether a problem is resolved by logical thinking or creative thinking, the results are put into action. Teenagers need to learn how to choose between alternatives and foresee the consequences. What are the risks, rewards, costs, and benefits? Besides critical and creative thinking, there are visceral sensations that many scientists are beginning to refer to as the "second brain." Intuitions and gut reactions, while often useful, need to be considered carefully. Teenagers can pay attention to intuitive insights and also develop ways of evaluating them.

Planning and Organizing

Many adolescents do not know how to plan for the future. This requires the activation of the prefrontal cortex to make mental maps that can be used to chart one's way through life. Without these maps, young people can flounder. Ironically, poor organization saved the lives of many young people who attempted suicide; they had not thought through their suicide: they didn't take enough medication, cut their wrists in the wrong way, or tried to use a firearm that had been equipped with safety locks.

Attention and Focus

Humans do not have the capacity to attend to everything, having evolved to focus on those stimuli that would ensure their survival. Young people can be thrown off track by competing stimuli, shifting their attention to social networking, snacking, or other distractions. Adolescents need to learn to set priorities and to use those skills in implementing their decisions: how to turn down a surprise invitation and how to resist tantalizing online links that can lead down an endless rabbit hole.

Self-Regulation and Impulse Control

These skills are especially important because many suicide attempts are impulsive. Recall Tex, who realized he had made a mistake as soon as he saw the blood spurt from his slit wrists. Teenagers can be overwhelmed by strong, powerful feelings that may dictate risky courses of action. Learning impulse control does not mean blocking feelings or bottling them up. It means *reflecting* on a strong feeling, *determining the origin* of that feeling, and *postponing* immediate action. Developing self-regulation prevents teenagers from making hasty decisions. Once they feel a strong reaction, such as rage or fear, young people can learn to calm themselves, breathe deeply, and attain a sense of stability. Self-regulation does not entail repressing feelings but, rather, being mindful and making a considered response.

Independent Thinking

Teenagers are keenly aware of the norms and expectations of their peers, often to the dismay of adults. One of the strongest social pressures urges them to obey strict gender roles. We have seen how this pressure can be disastrous for those who do not fit neatly into binary male-or-female stereotypes—but it can also harm those who do. We refer here to "traditional masculinity," which is not the same as "toxic masculinity" mentioned in an earlier chapter.

A suicide researcher theorized that traditional masculinity, defined as "a set of social norms that includes an emphasis on competition, strength, avoiding emotions and perceived femininity, an action-orientation, and the acceptability of anger and violence,"[5] could actually put men at risk for suicide. A study confirmed the link, finding that the only other risk factor of equal peril was depression.[6] And having several risk factors multiplies the hazard. The researchers found that "high traditional masculinity was associated with a host of other significant risk factors for suicide death. So not only does high traditional masculinity add to the risk of suicide death, it also may have indirect effects through other variables."[7]

We also want to call out hazardous racial entitlement. In the United States, the worst injustices of racism fall on black and brown citizens, requiring concerted, powerful social and legal actions to end them. Whites may be interested to learn that believing in racial entitlement is not so good for them either. The pressure of living up to social expectations—even unjust ones—can contribute to depression and death. A 2019 study found that even *thinking* one is losing status can contribute to mortality (not just suicide) among whites. "Short-term rising white mortality seems to be driven principally by anxiety among whites about losing social status, even in the absence of evidence that they are, in fact, ceding status to blacks."[8]

Learning to rise above restrictive gender roles and racial expectations is something every teenager should strive to do and every adult should support.

Being Mindful

Throughout this chapter, we have advocated what is often called "being mindful." The term *mindfulness* refers to being aware in the moment rather than getting caught up in upsetting memories, regrets, fears, or fantasies of the future. Instead, one learns to fully experience the present moment's sensations, thoughts, and feelings without judgment as they arise and dissolve. Taking this skill into everyday life enables one to become highly attentive to internal and external stimulation.[9]

Mindfulness is especially important given the blossoming of neural growth during adolescence. The neurological blossoming includes the manufacture of additional dendrites, the brain's connection fibers. Until enough dendrites are available for decision-making, adolescents may fall back on the amygdala and other parts of the brain that do not apply reflective judgment. If an adolescent does not develop and exercise foundational skills, the stock of dendrites gets pruned away and the best age for learning them ends.

The Default Mode Network

In addition to the prefrontal cortex, other parts of the brain develop during adolescence. One of these is the default mode network (DMN), which seems to shut down during focused activity and attention but is active during mind wandering, mental imagery, imagination, and daydreaming. Its development during the teenage years is important because among the DMN functions are those that establish a person's "future self," autobiographical memories, social functioning, and a "theory of mind" that helps explain the actions of other people, though not always accurately.[10]

A 2016 neuroimaging study of teenagers who ruminated about suicide and teens who did not discovered major differences in their DMN functioning. Suicidal teens demonstrated different abnormalities than those who were depressed but nonsuicidal. Healthy teenagers showed no DMN malfunctioning, indicating another diagnostic clue that could be used in suicide prevention.[11]

Neuroplasticity

Over the years, feral children have been found in various places around the world, boys and girls lost or cast aside by their parents to fend for themselves in isolated places, such as rainforests. Remarkably, these children survived, having befriended animals and learning which plants could be eaten. However, despite later help, they never developed the speaking and social skills needed for them to adapt to civilization. Help came too late—after age-specific windows of neurological blossoming, when the language areas of the brain best develop.

Still, even an adult can make improvements. *Neuroplasticity* refers to the brain's ability to develop new circuits. Meditation, psychotherapy, and other activities have been shown to facilitate brain functioning; this is due to neuroplasticity, and it refutes the discredited notion that one's brain is set in childhood and cannot thereafter be altered.

Meditation, which can enhance brain functioning, involves the self-regulation of attention, and there are dozens of meditative practices. Some teenagers prefer movement meditations such as Qigong, Tai Chi, and yoga. Like other forms of meditation, they require focus and repetition to become effective and play a role in building a better teenage brain.

Young people who ask questions, who are curious, who exercise and meditate, and who reflect on their behavior are improving their brains and conferring lifelong advantages, including the ability to resist the allure of suicide.

Takeaway Points

- Adolescents have a limited time window to take best advantage of their neurological blossoming and brain plasticity to learn foundation skills.
- Critical thinking, self-regulation, impulse control, and other foundational thinking skills are valuable assets for suicide prevention.

Notes

1. Coates, D. E. (2018). *How your teen can grow a smarter brain.* Washington, DC: First Summit Publishing.

2. Gurion, M., & Stevens, K. (2010). *How boys and girls learn differently.* San Francisco: Jossey-Bass.

3. Yensen, F. E., & Nutt, A. E. (2015). *The teenage brain: A neuroscientist's survival guide to raising adolescents and young adults.* New York: HarperCollins.

4. Richards, R. (2018). *Everyday creativity and the healthy mind.* New York: Palgrave/Macmillan.

5. Coleman, D. (2015). Traditional masculinity as a risk factor for suicidal ideation: Cross-sectional and prospective evidence from a study of young adults. *Archives of Suicide Research, 19*(3), 366–384.

6. Coleman, D., Feigelman, W., & Rosen, Z. (2020). Association of high traditional masculinity and risk of suicide death: Secondary analysis of the ADD health study. *JAMA Psychiatry.* Published online February 12.

7. Vlessides, M. (2020). Excessive masculinity linked to high suicide risk. *Medscape Medical News* (online).

8. Siddiqi, A., Sod-Erdene, O., Hamilton, D., McMillan-Cottom, T., & Darity, W. (2019, December). Growing sense of social status threat and concomitant deaths of despair among whites. *Population Health, 9,* 1–20.

9. Kabat-Zinn, J. (2013). *Full catastrophe living: Using the wisdom of your body to face stress, pain and illness.* New York: Bantam Dell.

10. Domhoff, G. W. (2018). *The emergence of dreaming.* New York: Oxford University Press.

11. Zhang, S., Chen, J., Kuan, L., et al. (2016). Association between abnormal DMN activity and suicidality in depressed adolescents. *BMC Psychiatry, 16.* https://bmcpsychiatry.biomedcentral.com/articles/10.1186/s12888-016-1047-7.

CHAPTER FORTY-THREE

Preventing Suicide behind Bars

Suicide is a common cause of death in prisons. A notable one was the 2019 apparent suicide of financier and child sex trafficker Jeffrey Epstein. Factors involved in inmates' self-harm include medical and mental health challenges, family issues, the stress of incarceration, and a lack of meaningful activity. Hopelessness and helplessness, characteristic of many settings for suicide, are pervasive. Most suicides occur during the first few months after a convict arrives in prison. Juvenile offenders are at the highest risk, probably because they lack the skills to cope with the prison environment, understand their emotional reactions, or control their impulses because their brains are still developing. More female than male prisoners attempt to kill themselves. They are also more likely to inflict other forms of self-harm.[1]

The most common method of inmate suicide is strangulation using ropes fashioned of bedsheets, clothes, or shoelaces. The second most common method is blood loss from cutting or stabbing. Unlike suicides on the "outside," most prison suicides do not occur when convicts are under the influence of drugs or alcohol. Social support from family and friends is a factor in the prevention of prison suicides, but being married does not seem to make a difference. Some institutions have implemented suicide prevention programs: these involve careful supervision, monitoring shower activity and telephone calls, and suicide-resistant housing and clothing. In addition, staff training sessions emphasize developing communication skills and observing clues that a prisoner is at risk.[2]

Unnecessary Roughness

When attorney José Baez first met Aaron Hernandez in 2016, the former National Football League star was already serving a life term in prison. After three seasons with the New England Patriots, Hernandez had been convicted for the murder of an acquaintance and hanged himself in his cell. A brain scan revealed that Hernandez had suffered several brain injuries due to repeated head blows while playing football. This type of brain damage, chronic traumatic encephalopathy, is now a recognized hazard of football, but it had been covered up by league officials for years.

Baez recounts his interaction with Hernandez in his book *Unnecessary Roughness: Inside the Trials and Final Days of Aaron Hernandez*, mentioning letters Hernandez wrote to loved ones. Baez commented, "I don't believe he was in sound mind in doing this. I have mixed emotions when I read these notes. In one context, I'm reading them as his lawyer while investigating his case, but in another context he's a young man I knew, liked, and cared about. He had a serious brain disease. We need more awareness of it or we're going to miss something." Two other books and a documentary describe Hernandez's childhood traumas, conflicted sexuality, drug addiction, many injuries, and his trial for murder. He was acquitted just before he killed himself.

"I Was Not Born for That"

Sometimes the mere *threat* of imprisonment can lead to suicide. In 2019, Peru's former president, Alan García, shot himself when police arrived to arrest him for a massive corruption scandal. Previously, when asked about possible arrest, García had said, "I was not born for that." He added that he would never submit to the humiliating spectacle of an arrest and imprisonment and often showed friends a pistol that he carried. In a letter he left for friends and family, he wrote, "I've seen others paraded around in handcuffs holding on to their miserable existence, but Alan García has no reason to suffer such indignities."

García insisted he was innocent and had faith in his historic legacy. "I am a Christian. I believe in life after death. I think I have earned a small place in the history of Peru." A former classmate's reminiscences suggested that there might have been a predisposing cause of García's demise. "There was something missing, replaced, as it were, by ambition. García didn't seem to be completely *there*. And those who are not *there* tend to make stupendous candidates because others can project onto them whatever they wish."[3]

In Durkheim's categories, García's death may have been an instance of fatalistic suicide, as, in oppressive situations, a person would rather die than continue enduring suffocating conditions. He lists imprisonment as one example; although García was not in prison at the time, he made no secret of his determination to avoid incarceration.

Human Kindness

The Human Kindness Foundation's mission is to encourage incarcerated people to use their time for spiritual growth. The foundation sends free books about interfaith spirituality to people in jails, including *We're All Doing*

Time, written by Bo Lozoff, the organization's founder. Lozoff points out that people who are incarcerated can devote themselves to their inward journeys without the distractions of ordinary life. They can turn their jail cell, and perhaps other cells as well, into ashrams—places where people live for a while to strengthen their spiritual practice and self-discipline.[4]

Catherine Dumas, the executive director of the foundation, notes that letters arrive every week from inmates who had contemplated suicide but decided against it after reading the foundation's literature. She shared some of these letters with us. One letter from June 2019 was from a man named Charlie:

> You guys recently sent me a copy of *We're All Doing Time*. I was in a funk when I got it and just set it on the table beside my bed. Things just seemed to keep getting worse that week. Solitary and 24/7 lockdown take their toll, no matter who you are. I've never been as low as I was the other night. I was through contemplating and 100% decided it was time to move on. I was deep in thought and working up the courage to make that final step. I was sitting on the edge of my bed and staring at my table. I was looking at Bo's book, without really seeing it, just kind of staring blankly, when suddenly the title's words registered because I had just heard them spoken by some guy on the television show "The Redemption Project." He had just said the title and the author's name, and the hope it gave him.
>
> Curiously, I picked it up again, and when I opened the book a little paper fell out and on it was printed, "Faith. No fear," and on the back were a few handwritten words from you. I'm not sure what the moral is, but it could be "Don't put off helping yourself when others are willing to help you do it," or maybe "Despite the reservoir of wisdom and knowledge right in front of you, it's up to you to want to apply it." But personally, I think everything happens just when it's supposed to, just when you need it the most. Something comes along, makes itself known, and reinstates that flicker of hope. That doesn't fix anything. It doesn't suddenly turn the world right side up, but instead allows us to make peace with everything that's broken because we know that we are loved, and, as everyone knows, "All you need is love."

The end of Charlie's letter demonstrated that he had begun to accept his situation. You might recall that rational emotive behavior therapy (REBT) emphasizes self-acceptance, other acceptance, and life acceptance—the foundations for growth and development.

We're All Doing Time contains a wealth of insights and ideas, many of which have dissuaded at-risk prisoners from suicide. Here are a few of these insights:

The cause of all of our personal problems and nearly all the problems of the world can be summed up in a single sentence: human life is very deep, and our modern dominant lifestyle is not.

Simple kindness may be the most vital key to the riddle of how human beings can live with each other in peace and care properly for this planet we all share.

In some respects, if I had to choose just one virtue on the spiritual path, I'd feel safest with a sense of humor. We pick ourselves up, dust ourselves off, have a good laugh about human nature, and get on with our journeys.

We're all doing time. As soon as we get born, we find ourselves assigned to one little body, one set of desires and fears, one family, city, state, country, and planet. Who can ever understand exactly why or how it comes down as it does? The bottom line is, here we are. Whatever, wherever we are, this is what we've got. It's up to us whether we do it as easy time or hard time.

Takeaway Points

- Hopelessness and helplessness characterize many of the suicides behind bars.
- Human kindness can prevent suicides and transform people's lives in positive ways.

Notes

1. Fazel, S., Ramesh, T., & Hawton, K. (2017). Suicide in prisons: An international study of prevalence and contributory factors. *Lancet Psychiatry, 4*, 946–952.

2. Fazel, S., Cartwright, J., Norman-Nott, A., & Hawton, K. (2008). Suicide in prisoners: A systematic review of risk factors. *Journal of Clinical Psychiatry, 69*, 1721–1731.

3. Alacon, D. (2019, July 8–15). Executive decision: What led Peru's former president to take his own life? *The New Yorker*, pp. 26–31.

4. Lozoff, B. (1985). *We're all doing time*. Durham, NC: Human Kindness Foundation.

CHAPTER FORTY-FOUR

Spirituality as a Path away from Suicide

Spirituality differs from religion in several ways. A spiritual person is devoted to human betterment, behaving ethically, transcending the earthly plane, preserving nature, or all of these. Many secular activists share these concerns, but a spiritual perspective also assumes that there is an underlying unity to life and a transcendent reality beyond what is tangible and visible. Religion, on the other hand, is a system of beliefs and practices organized around the veneration and worship of a powerful deity (or deities) and a set of principles and practices that define the boundaries of the religion—whether one is in or out.

Over the centuries, religion has often been badly misused. Some believers feel justified in carrying out or condoning atrocities or causing harm in the name of their religion. Some religious persons also obey or enforce the letter of their ethics but entirely miss the spirit. These deviations from the heart of a faith may have contributed to a tendency among young Americans to declare themselves "spiritual but not religious," indicating that they do not identify with any organized faith system. Of course, it is possible to be both religious and spiritual—belonging to an established religion and also adhering to high moral standards and a sense of participating in the mystery of life. It's also possible to be neither religious nor spiritual, finding life's meaning in secular beliefs and pursuits.

How Religion Impacts Daily Life

One's Religious Orienting System (ROS) is one aspect of the General Orientation System (GOS) that defines a person's typical ways of viewing the world and dealing with its challenges. (This resembles what we call "personal mythology.") Both systems have cognitive, behavioral, social, and emotional aspects. A strong ROS helps people adapt and even thrive in stressful situations. By contrast, a weak ROS leaves people vulnerable to decline in psychological and spiritual functioning.[1] Those people with a strong ROS believed that they could collaborate with God to reach solutions, reframing suffering to find its beneficial aspects and finding meaning in their struggles. They felt God as loving and adapted successfully to a stressful situation. Those with a weak ROS exhibited an anxious attachment to God, viewed God as cruel or distant, and often felt alienated from life.

Many psychotherapists use the term *religious/spiritual struggles* (R/S struggles), noting that these conflicts may have positive or negative outcomes. R/S struggles are not reducible to other forms of distress, such as anxiety or depression, and should not be ignored or dismissed. Indeed, they may represent the most important part of a person's inner life.

One of the R/S struggles that therapists encounter is the "moral injury" that some war veterans experience. These struggles can lead to suicide. When associated with trauma, they may manifest as one of the following:

- Perceived conflicts with deities or demons
- Conflicts with individuals or institutions
- Existential conflicts regarding one's beliefs, morality, or meaning in life

Religious/Spiritual Struggles

In 2019, Joshua Witt, Kenneth Pargament, and others published results of their attempt to identify patterns of spiritual growth or decline that could serve as predictors of ongoing distress. They obtained an ethnically and religiously heterogeneous group of 248 men and 30 women through a Veterans Administration hospital and its associated clinics, all of them participants in the country's four most recent wars. Participants completed several questionnaires, including one that focused on their ROS and another that identified R/S struggles. Both positive and negative outcomes of their wartime experiences were monitored.[2]

The results indicated that the "typical veteran" reported a moderate to strong ROS with low levels of R/S struggle and social support during the struggle. On average, veterans showed relatively positive spiritual change related to the R/S struggle but noted both positive and negative effects on their lives resulting from it. Spiritual decline was related to high levels of R/S struggle and to difficult religious coping.

The authors noted that these results mirror those found previously in civilian samples. For both groups, finding meaning in a struggle may restore one's belief that the world is coherent, which could be associated with more positive perceptions of the R/S struggle. Positive religious coping includes several strategies: reconceptualizing the stressor as positive, working together with a higher power, and seeking greater connection with "Spirit." High levels of R/S struggle are not always negative; there were instance in which they were associated with spiritual growth.[3] As may be remembered, even great spiritual leaders such as Mother Teresa and St. John of the Cross suffered profound spiritual crises but survived them to offer great wisdom to others. These are also examples of what Stanislav Grof called a shift from spiritual emergency into spiritual emergence.

Whether or not there is a God, either loving or cruel or distant, is not the crucial issue for our purposes. Of greater importance is the meaning attributed to the R/S struggle and its support for a person's survival. Both veterans and nonveterans reported discussing existential issues with friends and loved ones, and these discussions may well have refined and reinforced the positive coping, reconceptualization, and reframing that appeared to have been crucial to their resilience.

Clinical Implications

Some veterans seeking mental health support may be more highly motivated by faith-related and meaning-related issues than by the hope of relieving depression or anxiety. Moral injuries are often overlooked by a system that focuses on symptoms. Far too few therapists are familiar with the R/S struggle concept or the category of "religious or spiritual conflict" that appears in the DSM. But there is evidence that therapeutic interventions that address R/S struggles among veterans may *improve* treatment efficacy, especially for those with suicidal ideation.[4] In this book, we have constantly argued for the inclusion of existential issues in psychotherapy for trauma survivors.

Mental health care providers need to be aware of their clients' ROS strengths, their religious concepts and coping strategies, and their ability to find meaning. This need not be done directly, but it would not be out of place in an intake interview or in group-based interventions. Therapists, counselors, and chaplains who work with veterans need to be aware of these factors and perhaps include them in intervention. A 2015 study revealed that almost half of the chaplains and assistant chaplains queried thought that they needed additional instruction in suicide prevention.[5]

Of course, these issues are far from simple. What would happen if a veteran discloses to a health care provider a God concept that is cruel and justifies the elimination of nonbelievers? What if the client earnestly attempted to convert the therapist to ensure his or her eternal life? What if a client confessed considering suicide following a terrorist act—or considered committing one?

All professional organizations have their codes of ethics, and mental health care providers should review them before engaging in important but sensitive areas. For example, the American Psychological Association forbids badgering clients in regard to their religious beliefs by disparaging their faith or trying to convert them to another one. Similar positions can be found in ethical codes of other organizations.

Sandra Rogers's Suicide Attempt and Near-Death Experience

Sandra Rogers's case is unusual because she has revealed her identity, hoping that her experience will be useful to suicidologists and people at risk for suicide. Sandra grew up believing that God is unfair. She was taught that only those who publicly profess their faith in Christ will go to heaven.[6]

Life did not go well for Sandra; she endured destructive relationships, pregnancies, miscarriages, broken marriages, drug overdoses, and suicide attempts. She could not understand how a loving God could allow these events to happen. Sandra hated her existence. It was an extreme case of "psychestress." In 1976, following an unsuccessful suicide attempt via drug overdose, she placed a .38-caliber pistol to her chest, aimed it at her heart, and pulled the trigger. She expected to die. Instead, she found herself in the presence of a brilliant light. This light gave Sandra the choice of remaining in the light or returning to live out the rest of her life. She chose to return so that she could communicate what she had learned to other people. She lived another twenty-four years and wrote and lectured about her near-death experience (NDE).

Like many people who have had NDEs, Sandra experienced a life review; she saw her decades of poor choices and the pain she had caused herself and others. However, the light never judged her; instead, it "understood and loved me." She also learned that "forgiveness is the capacity to give Love in the most difficult circumstances. Forgiveness sows God's Love in action. It is as close as we get to God's nature in this physical world."

NDEs have been reported for millennia, under one name or another, but did not enter the medical literature until 1892, when a German author published a collection of accounts from mountain climbers, wounded soldiers, survivors of construction accidents, and people who had nearly drowned. All had been pronounced dead but revived, relating various experiences from the "afterlife." The nature of NDEs is to some a matter of controversy, but there is general agreement that they can permanently alter the survivor's ROS and personal mythology. The strong objections to suicide expressed by the survivors, based on their new or enhanced understanding, are especially notable.

Takeaway Points

- Religious/spiritual struggles are overlooked by many mental health care providers, despite their importance in suicide prevention and treatment.
- A strong Religious Orienting System can provide positive meaning to a person's religious/spiritual struggles and help prevent or mitigate suicidal despair.

Notes

1. Pargament, K. I., Wong, S., & Exline, J. J. (2016). Wholeness and holiness: The spiritual dimension of eudaimonics. In J. Viterso (Ed.), *Handbook of eudaimonic well-being* (pp. 379–394). Cham, Switzerland: Springer International.

2. Wilt, J. A., Pargament, K. I., Exline, J. J., et al. (2019). Spiritual transformation among veterans in response to religious/spiritual struggle. *Psychology of Religion and Spirituality, 11*, 266–277.

3. Kopacz, M. S. (2014). The spiritual health of veterans with suicidal ideation. *Health Psychology and Behavioral Medicine, 2*, 349–358.

4. Ramchand, R., Ayer, L., Geyer, L., & Kofner, A. (2015). Army chaplains' perceptions about identifying, intervening, and referring soldiers at risk of suicide. *Spirituality in Clinical Practice, 2*, 36–47.

5. Rogers, S. (2019). Sandra Rogers' suicide near-death experience. https://www.near-death.com/experiences/suicide/sandra-rogers.html.

6. Greyson, B. (1992–1993). Near-death experiences and anti-suicidal attitudes. *Omega, 26*, 81–89.

THOSE WHO SURVIVED: THE SISTER WHO LIVED

Edwin Shneidman related an incident in which he used an approach similar to that employed in rational emotive behavior therapy (REBT):

A young woman in her 20s, a nurse at the hospital where I worked, pleaded with me to see her sister who she believed to be highly suicidal. The younger woman was agitated and tearful, [a] bit incoherent. She told me that she was single, pregnant, and was going to kill herself. She showed me a small automatic pistol she kept in her purse. Her pregnancy was such a mortal shame to her, laced with feelings of rage and guilt, that [she] simply could not bear to live (or live to bear the child). Suicide was the only answer, and shooting herself was the only way to do it. Either she had to be the way she was before the pregnancy or she had to be dead.

I did several things. For one, I took out a sheet of paper and began to widen her blinders. I said, "You could have an abortion here locally." She replied, "I couldn't do that." It is the "can'ts" and "won'ts" and "have to's" and "nevers" and "always" and "onlys" that have to be negotiated in psychotherapy. I continued.

"You could go away and have an abortion."
"I couldn't do that."
"You could bring the baby to term and keep the baby."
"I couldn't do that."
"You could have the baby and adopt it out."
"I couldn't do that."
"You could get in touch with the young man involved."
"I couldn't do that."
"We could invite the help of your parents."
"I couldn't do that."
"You could always commit suicide, but there is no need to do that today."

No response.

"Now first let me take the gun and then let's look at this list and rank them in order and see what their advantages and disadvantages might be and what their implications are, remembering that none of them will be perfect."

The very making of the list had a calming effect on her. Within fifteen minutes, her lability [mood swings] had begun to de-escalate. She actually rank ordered the list, commenting negatively on each item. But what was of critical importance was that suicide was now ranked third, no longer first or even second. She decided that she reluctantly would talk to the father of her child. Not only had they never discussed the issue, he did not even know about it. But there was another issue. He lived in another city, almost across the country. And that involved a long-distance phone call.

It only took a few seconds to obtain the area code from the long-distance operator and the phone number from information. And then, with some trepidation, and ambivalence for her to dial the number, even though it was at the university's expense, she finally made the call. The ensuing conversation only began to resolve the issue, but the point is that it was possible to lower her lethality.[1]

Our Comment on This Vignette

This excerpt from a therapist/client interaction demonstrates Shneidman's calm and reasoned approach to his client's dilemma. Some readers may feel that he was being overly intellectual and did not plumb the deeper recesses of his client's psyche. Others may argue that Shneidman did not address his client's feelings, making the interaction overly ordered and logical. Yet other critics would have liked Shneidman to become even *more* logical. However, we take the position that reason and emotion work together, and an adroit therapist will recognize this interaction. The notion that thought and emotion are two separate processes is obsolete, yet it often stands in the way of effective psychotherapy as well as progress in medicine and neuropsychology.

Note

1. Leenaars, A. A. (2010). Edwin A. Shneidman on suicide. *Suicidology 1*, 4–18 (online).

SECTION IX

Healing

CHAPTER FORTY-FIVE

Achieving Self-Empowerment

Earlier chapters presented the basics of the REBT approach and how it can help prevent suicide. This chapter describes more ways to change suicidal thoughts and activities by replacing them with ones promoting self-empowerment.

Human beings can act in cruel ways. Groups of people may be treated inhumanely, mocked, and bullied. Others experience ugly discrimination. Viktor Frankl, the creator of logotherapy, was imprisoned in concentration camps during World War II amid indescribable cruelty, but he chose to maintain purpose in life by focusing on things that gave him respite.[1] He observed his fellow prisoners, noticing who survived and who did not, and began to formulate his philosophy of meaning.

Frankl's admirable resilience shows that external forces are not the last word. There are many racial, societal, and relationship rules and roles that deprive people of their liberties and humane living conditions. This is deplorable, but a cognitively able person who is determined to vigorously adopt realistically positive and rational beliefs can still live an empowered and fulfilling life.

When working with clients who had contemplated or attempted suicide, one of the authors of this book (Joffe Ellis) observed that most of them felt disempowered. They made similar statements to the following:

No matter how hard I work, I will never get ahead.

I belong to a racial minority in a majority-white town. No one likes or accepts me, and I will always have to work harder than white people to achieve things—and maybe not even then.

I have tried everything. Nothing helps.

My wife left and took the kids. I will never get to see them. The courts are always on the woman's side.

Some believed that ending their lives would demonstrate their power to other people, who would feel guilty forever. Others succumbed to utter hopelessness, shame, and guilt and could not find the means for restoring some hope. Prior to REBT therapy, none of these clients had learned about the power of their thoughts or techniques for replacing irrational ones with realistically positive ones.

You may recall that disempowering thoughts go like this:

1. This situation is terrible, the worst, and will never change.
2. I am worthless and hopeless.
3. I fail at everything. I am a complete failure.
4. I can never right the wrongs I have done and will always be miserable as a result.
5. Life should be fair.
6. My life should have turned out differently. I have wrecked it.
7. No one will ever understand me.
8. People will never treat me the way they should.
9. I will never be as successful/pretty/handsome/rich as others. I am not and will never be good enough.
10. I hate myself.
11. No one will ever love or accept me the way I am.
12. Life is not worth living.

We ask our readers whether they feel the weight of these beliefs as they read them. If so, perhaps they can better understand why people who are burdened by such thoughts can feel like giving up.

Here are some of the disputes that can be applied to the above destructive beliefs:

1. Where is the evidence that this situation is the worst ever and cannot change?
2. Where is solid evidence that there is no hope and that I am worthless?
3. Have I truly failed at everything I have done? And even if I failed at some things, how does that make me a complete failure?
4. Is there any proof that I cannot right some of the wrongs I have done?
5. Where is the evidence that life should be, or can be, fair all the time?
6. Where is the evidence that my life should have turned out differently and that it is wrecked?
7. Where is the evidence that no one understands me or ever will? And even if no one does, does that mean I cannot have a meaningful life?

8. Where is it written that people must always treat me the way I think they should?

9. Where is the evidence that if I do not have certain qualities or material goods that others have, I am not good enough?

10. Where is it getting me to hate myself? Is it reasonable to do so?

11. Where is the evidence that no one will ever love or accept me the way I am?

12. Where is the evidence that life is not worth living?

Although reading all these disputes at once may seem confrontational, the therapist asks such questions one at a time in a supportive tone. Effective REBT therapists listen well, are empathic, and demonstrate unconditional acceptance of the client. Using sensitivity in choosing the most beneficial time, the therapist teaches the principles of REBT and assigns homework activities to be done between sessions that put the principles into action. Once the irrational beliefs have been confronted and disputed, new beliefs can emerge. These are not feel-good statements such as, "Everything always works out for the best." They are thought-out evaluations that are believable. They are based on evidence, often from the person's own life. They are "realistic optimism."

REBT reminds us that lasting change requires ongoing effort and offers many practices and techniques. Readers are encouraged to read more about REBT and practice it.[2]

One quite different approach is helpful for some people. Medication can help shift clients to a more biologically healthy state that enables them to engage in therapy. REBT discourages medication that is unnecessary or prolonged, but appropriate medication is like one wing of a bird that wants to fly. In itself, medication is not empowering, but medication may serve as a temporary wing. The second wing, which allows elevation and flight, is putting relevant techniques into daily practice.

Here are a few suggestions related to the ABCDE tool (described in chapter 35) and some additional practices:

- Get into the habit of thinking about your thinking, catching the irrational thoughts, and nipping them in the bud through the ABCDE framework.
- After doing the ABCDE self-help practice, make a list of the E's (Effective new beliefs) and read them regularly throughout the day for at least thirty days.
- Make a vigorous effort to practice unconditional self-acceptance.
- Find absorbing activities to practice regularly.
- Find ways of helping other people. This can include the simple action of smiling at strangers and offering kind and encouraging words to others.
- Be vigorously alert to tendencies of catastrophizing or awfulizing, and immediately take a healthier perspective.

- Seek the humorous side of things, and have a daily intention of not taking life, others, or yourself too seriously.
- Remind yourself not to take it personally if others act in bullying or obnoxious ways.
- Practice daily gratitude, even during the most challenging times.

Takeaway Points

- The earlier in life that one can learn and practice REBT, the better. Nonetheless, for most people, it is not too late to start at any age.
- The more that REBT is practiced during less challenging times, the easier it will be to apply it during urgent moments or times of crisis.

Notes

1. Frankl, V. (1963). *Man's search for meaning.* New York: Pocket Books.
2. Ellis, A. (2001). *Overcoming destructive beliefs, feelings and behaviors.* Amherst, NY: Prometheus Books.

CHAPTER FORTY-SIX

Deal with PTSD Nightmares First

By now, you know that the word *trauma* refers to an assault on the human mind or body that disrupts ordinary functioning. Psychological trauma can lead to disorders that do not seem to mend, such as persistent anxiety and depression, which are often reflected in recurring nightmares.[1] Because nightmares reflect the disrupted brain functioning of clients with a post-traumatic stress disorder (PTSD) diagnosis, we recommend that therapists work with nightmares directly instead of hoping that they will disappear when other interventions begin to work. This approach can also prevent suicides of people who kill themselves because they can no longer abide constant nightmarish stress.

Nightmares Are Frightening Dreams

Nightmares are frightening dreams that awaken the dreamer, who typically has a clear memory of the terrifying images. These dreams most frequently occur during rapid eye movement (REM) sleep and are characterized by terror, grief, or rage. We have discussed how normal dreams seem to help the dreamer download and process emotions. But when the emotion is too overwhelming to be effectively downloaded and processed, dangerous nightmares can recur.

A key adaptive function of normal dreaming is the extinction of fearful memories, which is accomplished by activating and downloading emotions that had been connected to unpleasant memories.[2] The pioneer dream researcher Rosalind Cartwright concluded that, during sleep, dreamers review emotional experiences from the day, defuse their emotional impact with similar experiences from memory, update an organized sense of self, and rehearse new coping behaviors.[3] PTSD nightmares are an exception; they fail to perform these functions.

According to neuropsychologists Ross Levin and Tore Nielsen, the first process, *memory element activation*, refers to the increased availability of a wide range of memory elements during dreaming. Most dreams do not represent specific memories but rather a variety of memories from multiple times and places. The second process, *memory element recombination*, continuously assembles the isolated memory units into a coherent flow of imagery and narrative, often providing new contexts for highly arousing (positive and negative) memory elements. Emotional processing is one of the major functions of dreaming. However, PTSD nightmares do not follow this sequence. New contexts do not replace the existing context; therefore, nightmares are ineffective at maintaining the extinction of the fear memories.[4]

The third process in normal dreaming, *emotional expression*, maximizes the involvement of neurological structures, primarily limited by limbic system activity, to further downregulate negative emotional arousal. The PTSD nightmare is incapable of regulating emotions; in fact, it may reflect an increase of emotion that prevents the extinction of fear memories. PTSD nightmares tend to repeat themselves on successive nights; this may represent failed attempts at extinction. The continuing accumulation of stressful negative experiences hinders an individual's capacity to effectively regulate emotion. Indeed, emotional distress may result, bringing the negative emotionality of the dreamers' nighttime dreams into their waking activities.

In brief, PTSD nightmares resist being extinguished. Instead, they reproduce past fearful experiences such as the accidental shooting of an innocent villager thought to have been carrying a weapon, witnessing a friend's body being shattered by an improvised explosive device, or engaging in face-to-face combat with an enemy who spurted blood when bayoneted and killed. Civilian examples include being raped by a trusted family friend, becoming engulfed in a tsunami and swept into the ocean, or being constantly taunted, bullied, and physically abused by members of one's high school peer group.

For the PTSD dreamer, this self-regulation process has broken down. Fear memories are directly expressed in PTSD nightmares rather than transformed in a way that would reduce daytime distress. As long as the PTSD nightmare recurs, the dreamer is blocked from resolving basic existential conflicts, which prevents him or her from moving ahead. The PTSD nightmare could be considered a "chaotic attractor" that is at the core of the entire disorder, as it represents both the neurological and the cognitive dimensions of PTSD.[5] Therefore, we recommend that treatment directly focus on nightmare modification as early as possible. If repetitive nightmares begin to shift, this could initiate a cascade of positive changes in work and relationships.

Treatment for PTSD Nightmares

How can PTSD-related nightmares be treated? One of the most encouraging medications is prazosin, an alpha-1 adrenergic, and its effect may be partly due to the placebo effect (expectation of success). When it is discontinued, the nightmares often return. Ernest Hartmann observed that although medication may reduce anxiety and the immediate intensity of the nightmares, it may do so at a price. Many medications reduce REM sleep and delay the resumption of normal dreaming. In some cases, traumatic nightmares become chronic and even more difficult to treat.[6]

For some reason, there is less verbal content in nightmares of patients with PTSD than those without. Psychotherapy for PTSD nightmares, which often recognizes this lack of verbal content, may supplement cognitive interventions with breathing, relaxation, artistic expression, bodily movement, mindfulness meditation, biofeedback, neurofeedback, and other nonverbal self-regulatory activities.[7] Several interventions deal directly with nightmares, and we will describe them here and in the next chapter.

Exposure Therapy

Exposure therapy (ET) is a frequently used intervention for nightmares, and it is one of the most successful treatments for PTSD. A psychotherapist guides clients to recall memories in a controlled situation until they have mastered their thoughts and feelings surrounding their traumatic experiences.[8]

An examination of the effects of ET on the brains of PTSD clients revealed decreased amygdala activation during fear processing and increased prefrontal cortex activity.[9] In other words, ET can enhance the inhibition of fear responses. The eight participants in this small study had developed PTSD as a result of assault or car accidents. Other studies support the use of ET for treating the nightmares of clients with different histories of trauma.

Imagery Rehearsal Therapy

Sleep disorders specialist Barry Krakow has observed that nightmares will not always necessarily fade away with time, and so he developed imagery rehearsal therapy (IRT) to tackle the nightmare directly. IRT involves some degree of exposure to nightmare content followed by rewriting or rescripting components of the nightmare. Controlled and uncontrolled case studies found promising results for the efficacy of IRT for chronic nightmares, both in people who were exposed to trauma and those who were not.[10]

Because ordinary dreaming serves the adaptive functions of extinguishing fearful memories and regulating emotions, dreams desensitize the disturbing experience through repeated exposure in a less frightening setting. The IRT practitioner asks dreamers to write down a disturbing dream and then rewrite it in any way they wish. The dreamers spend time each day mentally rehearsing the revised dream. Eventually, the nightmare itself begins to shift, completing the desensitization.

Some studies have compared ET and IRT. In one such study, two hundred participants received an eight-week self-help intervention and completed questionnaires at three intervals after the treatment ended. Initial progress was almost completely sustained after forty-two weeks; no differences were found between the two therapies.[11]

Exposure, Relaxation, and Rescripting Therapy (ERRT)

J. L. Davis developed exposure, relaxation, and rescripting therapy (ERRT) after she discovered patients' attempts to engage in pleasant imagery before sleep had little effect on their nightmares. Borrowing techniques from IRT, Davis targeted three systems in which anxiety was manifested: physiological (increased arousal at bedtime), behavioral (using legal and illegal substances to fall asleep), and cognitive (the belief that sleep is inevitably accompanied by nightmares). She directly engaged the fear network using both written and oral exposure to nightmare content.[12]

The four basic treatment components were educational (providing accurate information about PTSD nightmares), exposure (directly engaging the fear network), relaxation (progressive muscle relaxation), and rescripting (altering the nightmare's emotion, such as shifting from insecurity to security). Davis emphasized the difference between the nightmare and the trauma itself. An event may or may not be traumatizing, but only the *experience* of it can be described as traumatic.[13]

This perspective is introduced in the educational component of ERRT. Clients are informed that people respond to potentially traumatizing events in different ways. Indeed, some experience few difficulties at all, while others are distressed months or years after the event. Clients are told about the various forms a traumatic experience may take, including nightmares. Depending on the group being studied, 50–90 percent report PTSD nightmares, and the nature and frequency of these reports may change over time. A nightmare set in Iraq may change to one in which a terrorist invades the client's home. A nightmare reflecting an assault on a dark street may shift to one in which the setting is the dreamer's workplace.

In ERRT, clients are informed of the benefits of the exposure procedure. One client commented, "I used to be afraid of harmless snakes, but the more contact I had with them, the more comfortable I was with them. It might work the same way with my wartime trauma."

The second component, relaxation, does not come easily to PTSD clients and usually must be taught. Progressive muscle relaxation (PMR) involves alternatively tensing and relaxing different muscle groups of the body. This procedure can be utilized whenever a client notices a buildup of tension and anxiety. Diaphragmatic breathing is also taught. The client places one hand on his or her chest and the other on the belly and then tries to shift his or her breathing to the abdominal area.

When clients rescript their nightmares, they sometimes use humor. This is so incongruous with the traumatizing event that it often becomes incorporated into the nightmare itself. One veteran in the study changed the female terrorist who blew herself up into a Playboy bunny who jumped out of a huge party cake. Similar to PMR, where relaxation replaces tension, with this technique, humor replaces fear, which allows the brain to associate a new emotion with the respective memory. As the Boggart, a fear-inducing creature from the Harry Potter series, is dispelled by a Riddikulus spell (replacing its horrifying appearance with a hilarious one) and ensuing laughter, so may a nightmare dissolve back into a dream when juxtaposed with that very dreamlike element of bizarreness.

The behavioral component involves diminishing the use of legal and illegal substances, including alcohol; increasing social engagement; or exploring employment opportunities. All of these components interact; for example, proper sleep hygiene consists of behavioral choices (such as not watching the nightly news, taking the television out of the bedroom, or getting out of bed instead of tossing and turning for hours), and rescripting reflects one's education about PTSD.

In one study, more PTSD clients found education about sleep hygiene to be more helpful than education about PTSD.[14] Research on ERRT has ranged from case studies to randomized control trials. An example of the latter involved forty-nine participants (82% female), of whom 84 percent reported positive "end-state functioning" (in other words, an absence of nightmares in the week before the report); this was even higher than the 79 percent who reported positive "end-state functioning" for PTSD symptoms as a whole.

Having ERRT clients write their own account of the traumatizing event was surprisingly beneficial, possibly because it combined both cognitive and emotional elements of the trauma, helping them to develop a more coherent narrative of the traumatizing event.[15] The thematic exploration of nightmares is one of the components that differentiates ERRT from other nightmare treatments, possibly because it leads to resolution, control, and mastery.

Conclusion

David Jenkins sees the nightmare as a narrative that "needs improvement," which is what the interventions we have cited attempt to do.[16] PTSD nightmares reveal what we might call an "existential shattering"; treatment needs to help clients put those pieces together again, perhaps in a manner that is wiser, deeper, and more resilient.

Another psychologist, Daniel Pitchford, applied this perspective to PTSD and called for more research on informed activism in trauma treatment.[17] More support systems for and community outreach to families are needed as well as more holistic and less stigmatizing models of treatment and intervention. PTSD is a consequence of modern life, and the nightmares that accompany it both reflect contemporary violence and present a challenge for those valiant practitioners who attempt to treat those who have been devastated by it.

Two more points should be mentioned. A 2019 study found that experiencing a trauma influences a person to *feel fear*, which leads to *avoiding* certain things or places, which leads to the person feeling *continued fear*. Thus, fear and avoidance intensify each other. The treatment should therefore be prompt.[18] A second factor is the power of hope. We have known for a long time that expecting a treatment to work actually helps it to work—the famous placebo effect. Researchers who studied combat veterans with PTSD found that when clinicians worked to enhance their clients' expectation of improvement, it helped.[19]

Takeaway Points

- Addressing a person's PTSD nightmares should probably be initiated as soon as the client is agreeable.
- There are various methods to extinguish fear responses through working with clients' dreams and nightmares.
- Expecting treatment to help actually improves its effectiveness.

Notes

1. Barrett, D. (2001). *Trauma and dreams*. Cambridge, MA: Harvard University Press.

2. Levin, R., & Nielsen, T. (2009). Nightmares, bad dreams, and emotion dysregulation: A review and new neurocognitive model of dreaming. *Current Directions in Psychological Science, 18*(2), 84–88.

3. Cartwright, R. D. (2012). *The twenty-four hour mind: The role of sleep and dreaming in our emotional lives*. New York: Oxford University Press.

4. Levin, R., & Nielsen, T. A. (2007). Disturbed dreaming, posttraumatic stress disorder, and affect distress: A review and neurocognitive model. *Psychological Bulletin, 133*, 482–528.

5. Krippner, S., & Combs, A. (2007). Chaos, complexity, and self-organization in the dreaming brain. In R. Kay & K. A. Richardson (Eds.), *Building and sustaining resilience in complex organizations* (pp. 129–147). Mansfield, MA: ISCE Publishing.

6. Hartmann, E. (1984). *The nightmare: The psychology and biology of terrifying dreams.* New York: Basic Books.

7. Davis, J. L. (2008). *Treating post-trauma nightmares: A cognitive behavioral approach.* New York: Springer.

8. Foa, E. R., Molnar, C., & Cashman, L. (1995). Change in rape narratives during exposure therapy for posttraumatic stress disorder. *Journal of Traumatic Stress, 8,* 675–699.

9. Felmingham, K. I., Kemp, A. H., Williams, A. M., Das, P., et al. (2007). Changes in anterior cingulate and amygdala after cognitive behavior therapy of posttraumatic stress disorder. *Journal of Psychological Science, 18,* 127–129.

10. Krakow, B., & Zadra, M. (2006). Clinical management of chronic nightmares: Imagery rehearsal therapy. *Behavioral Sleep Medicine, 4,* 45–70.

11. Lancee, J., Van Den Bout, J., & Spoormaker, V. I. (2010). Expanding self-help imagery rehearsal therapy for nightmares with sleep hygiene and lucid dreaming: A waiting-list controlled trial. *International Journal of Dream Research, 3*(2), 111–120.

12. Davis, J. L. (2008). *Treating post-trauma nightmares: A cognitive behavioral approach.* New York: Springer.

13. Krippner, S., Pitchford, D. B., & Davies, J. (2012). *Post-traumatic stress disorder: Biographies of disease.* Santa Barbara, CA: Greenwood.

14. Davis, J. L., & Wright, D. C. (2007). Randomized clinical trial for treatment of chronic nightmares in trauma-exposed adults. *Journal of Traumatic Stress, 20,* 223–233.

15. Davis, J. L., Rhudy, J. L., Byrd, P. M., & Wright, D. C. (2009). Efficacy of exposure, relaxation, and rescripting therapy. In J. L. Davis (Ed.), *Treating post-traumatic nightmares* (pp. 187–213). New York: Springer.

16. Jenkins, D. (2012). The nightmare and the narrative. *Dreaming, 20,* 101–114.

17. Pitchford, D. B. (2009). The neuropsychology of nightmares reported by Iraq War veterans. In S. Krippner & D. J. Ellis (Eds.), *Perchance to dream: The frontiers of dream psychology* (pp. 113–130). New York: Nova Science.

18. Price, M., Legrand, A. C., Brier, Z. M. F., Gratton, J., & Skalka, C. (2020). The short-term dynamics of posttraumatic stress disorder symptoms during the acute posttrauma period. *Depression and Anxiety, 37*(4), 313–320. https://doi.org /10.1002/da.22976.

19. Price, M., Maples, J. L., Jovanovic, T., Norrholm, S. D., Heekin, M., & Rothbaum, B. O. (2015). An investigation of outcome expectancies as a predictor of treatment response for combat veterans with PTSD: Comparison of clinician, self-report, and biological measures. *Depression and Anxiety, 32*(6), 392–399.

CHAPTER FORTY-SEVEN

Nightmare Dream Revision and Lucid Dreaming

In the previous chapter, we discussed several methods of working with PTSD nightmares. In this chapter, we discuss two additional methods that are not as well known. Just as there are many ways of working with other PTSD symptoms,[1] there are several ways of alleviating PTSD nightmares, and all of them seem to work with some people.[2]

Dream Revision Therapy

Bruce Dow, neuroscientist and psychiatrist, has developed a comprehensive method to treat nightmares, flashbacks, anxiety, depression, and other debilitating effects of PTSD.[3] Like some methods discussed in the previous chapter, Dow's approach involves "rescripting" the nightmare and rehearsing the revision, but in a group context. He was inspired by the group dream-working method developed by the psychoanalyst Montague Ullman.[4] In the Ullman method, a group member presents a dream, members of the group ask basic questions about the dream content, and then the members project their own meaning into the dream. They accomplish this by saying, "If this were my dream, this is what it would mean to me." No interpretation is forced on the dreamer because Ullman believes that dreamers are the best interpreters of their own dreams. However, they can learn a great deal by listening to group members' projections, attending to the subsequent discussions, and eventually reaching their own interpretation. If the dream insights yield positive results in daily life, this lends support to the conjecture that the dreamer's interpretation was valid and useful.

Dow minimizes his clients' reexposure to their traumatizing events, making his treatment more benign than some other methods. His step-by-step group procedure can be followed by the therapist or, in some cases, by the PTSD survivors themselves. Dow developed his method, dream revision therapy, when he was working with groups of Vietnam War veterans. A patient volunteered a nightmare, which a staff member wrote on a white-board. Other members of the group then asked questions, including frequency and variations of the nightmare and daytime triggers that often preceded the nightmare. Next, the dreamer described accompanying emotions. Dow observed that this helped avoid *alexithymia*, the inability to name an emotion that one is feeling. Group members then brainstormed the possible overt and covert meanings of the nightmare without forcing an interpretation on the dreamer.

The next step was for the dreamer's fellow group members to propose changes to the dream that would make it less terrifying and more optimistic. A staff member wrote these alterations on a whiteboard, and the dreamer was able to select his own revision or perhaps combine elements of several suggestions. The dreamer was instructed to rehearse the revised dream during the day and look for possible changes the next time he dreamed. The dreamer gave a report to the group at its next meeting, usually one week later. Dow observed that peer support and encouragement became an important part of the process. Although dream revision therapy can be used in one-on-one counseling, Dow found many advantages to group dreamwork.

One veteran reported a repetitive nightmare in which he relived, with great agony, the death of his friend, Paul. "The helicopters are there. The helicopter is up, but my buddy Paul is still holding on to my hand. They're saying, 'He's dead; he's dead.' I feel like I'm flying, but I worry about landing on my feet. I go up with him until they say, 'He's dead.' Then I'm floating. The feeling of floating, the sound of the helicopter, and him holding my hand all stay after I'm awake until I stand up." Following group input, the dreamer revised the nightmare: "My guardian angel, Paul, is protecting me. He keeps me safe by holding my hand. Holding my hand makes me feel stronger, like a survivor." Eventually, the negative emotions disappeared, and the scenario became an ordinary dream, not a nightmare.

Dow has used this method as the core of psychotherapy with veterans, other trauma survivors, and even teenagers. In contrast to exposure therapy, the goal of dream revision therapy is not just to recall the trauma but to change its impact and weaken its negativity, eventually eliminating the fear associated with the original nightmare. Dream revision therapy may turn out to be a robust method to extinguish fear.

Allyson's Story

Allyson worked late, and it was dusk when she began her walk home. Suddenly, a husky man grabbed her and tried to push her into a patch of bushes. Allyson, although badly bruised, escaped being sexually assaulted, but she was terrified whenever she went near the site of the attack and had night-mares virtually every time she went to sleep. In group therapy, the therapist used dream revision therapy. Allyson received several suggestions on how her nightmare could be revised, ranging from shooting her assailant to per-suading him to adopt a more peaceful way of life. Allyson opted for a sce-nario in which she persuades a friend to join her for the walk home, both of them carrying powerful flashlights, and she arrives home safely.

Dream revision therapy also encourages creativity, both on the part of the dreamer and from other members of the group. When used in individual therapy sessions, the therapist makes suggestions, taking care that no inter-pretation is forced upon the dreamer. Allyson drew upon her creativity to reduce both the frequency of her nightmares and their intensity.

Lucid Dreaming Interventions

Lucid dreaming therapy (LDT) is a rising approach that combines ele-ments of imagery rehearsal, exposure therapy, and cognitive behavioral ther-apy. Lucid dreaming (LD) is defined as knowing one is dreaming without waking up.[5] Research has indicated that LD is associated with an increased activation in a part of the prefrontal cortex that is normally quiet while dreaming.[6] During wakefulness, this brain area is associated with metacog-nition, being aware that one is aware. It is also active during decision-making, particularly in ambiguous situations where complexity demands a thought-ful response. Activation of this part of the brain appears to produce the para-doxical feeling that one is awake and dreaming at the same time.

When LD occurs naturally, it seems to protect the dreamer from psychologi-cal distress.[7] Many of these insights were first put into practice by Ernest Hart-mann and Frank Galvin in 1990.[8] LD can be learned through various methods, such as asking oneself, "Am I dreaming?" This may be why some therapists have put LD to practical use, reducing the frequency and intensity of nightmares after their clients have learned to increase the time spent dreaming lucidly.[9]

Positive sleep habits have been well established by a field known as sleep medicine, which teaches sleep hygiene: finding a comfortable bed, using it for sleep and sex only, and maintaining a regular sleeping and waking sched-ule. Separately, practitioners have observed that people reporting PTSD nightmares may have sleep apnea (interruptions of breathing that compro-mise sleep quality).

Roger's Story

Roger was thirty-nine years of age when he arrived at the emergency unit of an Australian hospital after having tried to kill himself five times during the previous week. He had been admitted to three previous psychiatric wards, receiving diagnoses of depression, alcohol abuse, and PTSD. He was admitted a few weeks before Christmas, which was the anniversary of the murder of his fiancée by an unknown assailant. He averaged sixteen drinks per day, convinced he could not fall asleep without alcoholic intake. While in the psychiatric ward, standard medication did not provide Roger sufficient sleep. When he did fall asleep, he awakened after about two hours and reported nightmares so frightening that he could not fall asleep again for the rest of the night. His nightmares were replays of various traumas, including witnessing his father holding a shotgun to his mother's head, finding a dead baby in a bathtub while doing construction work, and being first at the scene of an automobile accident in which two people had been decapitated.

Roger was put on an alcohol withdrawal program and prescribed several medications. He was given reading material about LD and was asked to write down his dreams upon awakening and then altering the narrative before falling back to sleep. Within a few days, Roger was able to become aware that he was dreaming during the nightmare and could change the dream so it was not as alarming. Within two weeks, Roger's sleep had improved, his dreams were no longer as troublesome, and he was able to sleep for about six hours without medication. Roger insisted that this psychoeducational program was the primary factor in his improvement, and he was discharged after sixteen days of inpatient stay. Roger's story was published in a psychiatric journal in 2010, and there had been no apparent relapse at that time.[10]

Takeaway Points

- Lucid dreaming, when occurring naturally, could have evolved to serve as a buffer against intense nightmare imagery and to engage in solving problems regarding trauma and similar challenges.

- There are several innovative dreamwork interventions that can assist at-risk people whose issues are reflected in their nightmares.

- If you intend to work with any type of dream, we suggest you join the International Association for the Study of Dreams (www.IASDreams .com), attend its conferences, and read its authoritative publications. IASD does not advocate any specific dreamworking method, but it urges its members to explore a variety of approaches.

Notes

1. Benish, S., Imel, Z., & Wampold, Z. (2008). The relative efficacy of bona fide psychotherapies for treating post-traumatic stress disorder: A meta-analysis of direct comparisons. *Clinical Psychiatry Review, 28,* 746–758.

2. Krippner, S. (2016). Working with posttraumatic stress disorder night-mares. In J. E. Lewis & S. Krippner (Eds.), *Working with dreams and PTSD night-mares: 14 approaches for psychotherapists and counselors* (pp. 251–268). Santa Barbara, CA: Praeger.

3. Dow, B. M. (2015). *Dream therapy for PTSD.* Santa Barbara, CA: ABC-CLIO.

4. Ullman, M. (1996). *Dream appreciation: A group approach.* Santa Barbara, CA: ABC-CLIO.

5. LeBerge, S. (1985). *Lucid dreaming.* New York: Ballantine.

6. Voss, U., Holzmann, R., Tuin, I., & Hobson, J. A. (2009). Lucid dreaming: A state of consciousness with features of both waking and non-lucid dreaming. *Sleep, 32,* 1191–1200.

7. McGaugh, J. L. (2004). The amygdala modulates the consolidation of memories of emotionally arousing experiences. *Annual Review of Neuroscience, 27,* 1–28.

8. Galvin, F., & Hartmann, E. (1990). Nightmares: Terror in the night. In S. Krippner (Ed.), *Dreamtime and dreamwork: Decoding the language of the night* (pp. 233–243). Los Angeles: Jeremy P. Tarcher/Perigee.

9. Holzinger, B., Klösch, G., & Saletu, B. (2015). Studies with lucid dream-ing as add-on therapy to Gestalt therapy. *Acta Neurologica Scandinavica, 131*(6), 355–363.

10. Been, G., & Garg, V. (2010). Nightmares in the context of PTSD treated with psychoeducation regarding lucid dreaming. *Royal Australian and New Zealand College of Psychiatry, 44,* 583.

Eye Movement Desensitization and Reprocessing

Eye movement desensitization and reprocessing (EMDR),[1] combined with the existential orientation that we have emphasized throughout this book, saved the life of a suicidal client. The existential perspective can add depth to virtually any intervention.

Marcia's Story

Marcia (pseudonym) was thirty years old when she was released from a hospital following a suicide attempt. Her family told Dr. Glenn Graves that conventional therapy and medication had not stopped Marcia from fantasizing about killing herself and that her recent attempt had been the latest of several. Dr. Graves discussed Marcia's case with one of us (Krippner) and gave permission to use it.

Marcia told Graves that she had a firm commitment to die and spoke of it very comfortably, admitting she had spent a considerable amount of time fantasizing about how to do it. She could not express a clear motivation for her behavior and thoughts, only speaking vaguely about "transcendence."

Using EMDR, Graves opened the second session with bilateral eye movement reprocessing. Their interaction spontaneously uncovered a trauma Marcia had experienced when she was twelve years old. Marcia was a passenger in a car with other family members. The car was hit by another automobile, and Marcia lost consciousness. During the EMDR session, she recalled walking down a road, drawn toward a beautiful white light. Suddenly, Marcia heard her name being called. She turned and saw the car accident and her cousin's dead body lying on the ground.

At the hospital, her grandmother cried out, "Oh, why did it have to be her?" Marcia thought this meant that her grandmother wished that she, the surviving granddaughter, had been the one to die. This appalling comment gave Marcia tremendous, persistent survivor's guilt. Through EMDR, Marcia was able to confront what this comment had meant for her, realizing that the survivor's guilt could have motivated her suicidal thoughts.

Although the EMDR process uncovered the reason for Marcia's suicidal ideation, it did not resolve her attraction to the white light and "transcendence." Graves was concerned that more processing might actually enhance her death wish. In his experience, EMDR is effective unless the client has secondary gain, a reason for retaining the negative thoughts and behaviors. He felt that Marcia needed more time to work through her survivor's guilt and to grieve the loss of her cousin and the end of her own childhood.

After another hospitalization, Marcia returned to therapy. Subsequent sessions utilized an existential framework, allowing Marcia to explore the meaning that emerged from her grandmother's unfortunate comment. In Marcia's culture, children and adolescents can rarely confide in adults, much less confront them. In one EMDR session, Marcia imagined telling her grandmother about the aftereffects of her statement. Surprisingly, she received an apology from her grandmother, who had long since passed away. Marcia took this imagined apology as a message from the spirit world.

In another session, Marcia's grandmother was joined by the deceased cousin. Both were living in the white light, and they told Marcia that her time to join them was years away. Her guilty feelings about surviving the automobile accident were resolved and did not return. Marcia began to make concrete plans to continue a life that had been put on hold for years.

Graves adopted an agnostic attitude regarding these reports. Marcia's family members verified the accident. This verification was important because false memories are all too common when a client is asked to recall a past trauma during EMDR sessions, those involving hypnosis, or certain other interventions that attempt to retrieve experiences only dimly remembered or long since forgotten. Indeed, there is scant evidence that material deliberately evoked is reliable or accurate.[2] In Marcia's case, the information came spontaneously, not through any attempt by Graves to retrieve information.

The bottom line is that Graves's skillful use of EMDR and its integration with existential perspectives probably saved the life of a client who had been in love with the light.

EMDR Is Not Simple

Some well-meaning practitioners add eye movement tracking into their treatments without sufficient training. EMDR is not an easy gimmick; it is part of a detailed treatment plan. Experienced practitioners first take a client's history, prepare the client for the intervention, and assess the trauma memories. The client describes the distressing images and associated negative thoughts, proposes positive thoughts (which will be used later), identifies the emotions associated with the memories, describes and locates the accompanying physical sensations, and rates the degree of disturbance associated with the trauma memories. These qualitative responses are supplemented by reports that quantify the client's distress.[3]

At this point, the client is asked to hold the distressing image in mind, along with the negative thoughts and the bodily sensations. All of this is done while the client is tracking the therapist's fingers across the client's entire field of vision in rhythmic sweeps of one full back-and-forth sweep per second. Following twenty sweeps, the client is asked to "blank it out," to let go of the memory, and to take a deep breath. The client is requested to provide feedback of any changes in the images, thoughts, sensations, or emotions.

The therapist then initiates the next set of bilateral eye movements, adapting the procedure to reflect any reported changes during feedback. Once the client has reported a lower score on the Subjective Units of Distress Scale, the client is asked to hold the previously identified positive thoughts in mind while tracking the therapist's fingers. This time, the client is not asked to report changes in symptoms but to evaluate the validity of the positive thoughts.

The client is then asked to report any continuing body sensations. If these are negative in character, each one of them is attended to while the client is tracking the therapist's fingers. Finally, the client is taught coping skills, including relaxation exercises and positive visualizations. Keeping a journal is often recommended so that the client can keep track of pertinent thoughts, feelings, and dreams. The therapist determines whether treatment goals are being met and maintained from session to session. Extra sessions may be scheduled if needed, and the client takes an active role in evaluating and planning the program.

How Does EMDR Work?

The American Psychological Association's guidelines included EMDR on its short list of suggested treatments for PTSD. Many research studies were evaluated, some of which suggested that EMDR is effective even without bilateral eye tracking. Other studies have indicated that modified EMDR intervention is helpful for both children and adolescents. Additional investigations have found that EMDR has long-term results that compare favorably with more conventional treatments. The accumulation of supporting evidence for EMDR's effectiveness has quickened the search for the underlying mechanisms with the hope that understanding them may help alleviate trauma's distressing aftereffects.[4]

One model has been proposed by Canadian psychologist Don Kuiken and his associates, who have observed an analogy between EMDR and the naturally occurring rapid eye movements (REMs) that are a concomitant of nighttime sleeping.[5] Kuiken and his team focused on two orienting systems, one involving the processing of threat and fear and the other involving attempts to cope with threat and pain, sometimes in unsatisfactory ways. Both are relevant to trauma and to the possibility of self-harm.

The orienting response occurs when a person experiences an altered, novel, or unexpected stimulus, for example, turning one's head toward a sudden noise. The orienting response is accompanied by physiological changes, including dilation of blood vessels and eye pupils and changes in skin resistance and heart rate. Experimentally induced eye movements can modify these changes, all of which occur naturally during traumatic experiences, especially those including the threat of loss or separation. They also resemble the bilateral tracing movements that characterize EMDR.

The Canadian team reviewed experimental literature in which eye movements induced by researchers persist even following their induction. In other research studies, startle has been connected to perceived threats, both during wakefulness and REM sleep. Other brain centers are activated, especially the amygdala, which you may recall from our previous discussions of flight, fight, and freeze responses. The amygdala and the hippocampus usually work together, but in startle reactions, their regulation of working memory is hampered. As a result, startle reactions are poorly handled in both sleep and wakefulness; the parts of the cortex that usually regulate the threat of pain and separation cannot operate well, so the trauma persists.

Some traumatic experiences overwhelm the brain's ability to process the emotion and recollection that are ordinarily downloaded by the amygdala and hippocampus during sleep. Ordinarily, the cortex continues this downloading, often recasting emotion-laden events into symbols and metaphors that connect old and new experiences, but PTSD prevents this function. In an ingenious series of experiments, Kuiken and his colleagues induced rapid eye movements in various participants, some of whom had ongoing issues with trauma and some who were relatively free of trauma. The participants who had unresolved trauma exhibited longer reaction times than those who did not. That is, they took longer to recover from the startles induced by the researchers, and their orientation responses were longer as well.

EMDR for Survivors of Sexual Assault and Domestic Violence

EMDR has also been tested to heal the aftereffects of rape and domestic violence. Eight sessions were offered to forty-one participants, and levels of anxiety, depression, and PTSD fell dramatically.[6] Jill Schwarz, the lead author of the study, told a reporter,

One of the most powerful moments of the study for me was talking to a woman who, for 22 years, was not able to shower on her own because she had been assaulted in the shower," Schwarz says. "She had to have a family member sit right outside the door." Like most of the women, she had already been in counseling; in her case, on and off, for two decades. Yet after three sessions of EMDR, she was showering independently. "I sat face to face with her as she sobbed, telling me this. This is something [that] numbers on the assessments can't tell you."[7]

Takeaway Points

- Although its mechanisms are not well understood, eye movement desensitization and reprocessing (EMDR) is a valuable intervention for many traumatized people, including those at risk for self-harm.
- EMDR should only be used for at-risk individuals by a clinician well trained in the technique.

Notes

1. Shapiro, F. (2018). *Eye movement desensitization and reprocessing (EMDR): Basic principles, protocols, and procedures* (3rd ed.). New York: Guilford Press.

2. Spanos, N. P. (1996). *Multiple identities and false memories: A sociocognitive perspective* (p. 103). Washington, DC: American Psychological Association.

3. Spates, C. R., Koch, E., Cusak, K., et al. (2009). Eye movement desensitizing and reprocessing. In E. B. Foa, T. M. Keane, M. J. Friedman, et al. (Eds.), *Effective treatments for PTSD: Practice guidelines from the International Society for Traumatic Stress Studies* (2nd ed., pp. 279–305). New York: Guilford Press.

4. Courtois, C. A., Sonis, J., Brown, L. S. et al. (2019). *Clinical practice guidelines for the treatment of posttraumatic stress disorder (PTSD) in adults.* Washington, DC: American Psychological Association.

5. Kuiken, D., Chudleigh, M., & Racher, D. (2010). Bilateral eye movements, attentional flexibility and metaphor comprehension: The substrate of REM dreaming? *Dreaming, 20,* 227–217.

6. Schwartz, J. E., Baber, D., Barter, A., & Dorfman, K. (2019). A mixed methods evaluation of EMDR for treating female survivors of sexual and domestic violence. *Counseling Outcome Research and Evaluation, 11*(1), 4–18.

7. Conway, C. (2019, December 3). Pioneers in bringing a promising PTSD treatment to survivors of domestic violence, Jill Schwarz and her grad students hope to spread it statewide. *College of New Jersey Magazine.*

CHAPTER FORTY-NINE

Narrative Exposure Therapy

Narrative exposure therapy (NET) is a treatment for trauma-related disorders in which a therapist helps the client to establish a narrative of his or her life, weaving both the negative and positive memories into a coherent, meaningful story. One of several types of exposure therapies, NET asks the client to retell traumatic experiences over and over again.[1] Because oral narratives are an integral part of every human culture, and because imagined exposure is a basic part of most successful trauma therapies, NET promotes healing through these components.[2]

The client is asked to talk about the traumatizing events that triggered the traumatic experience within the context of the previously created life narrative. The client is asked to relive or imagine as many emotions associated with the trauma (or traumas) as possible. This process is repeated several times in as much detail as possible. It is hoped that fear reactions will be processed in much the same way that some dreams download emotions. Many therapists encourage their clients to bring their notable dream reports to the therapy sessions.

Some NET therapists ask their clients to draw or construct a "lifeline," a horizontal line that represents their chronological age, and to make drawings or use photos, flowers, or colorful objects to represent pleasant experiences and stones to represent unhappy, traumatic experiences. NET has been utilized with children, adolescents, and small groups with purported success, according its proponents, including Maggie Shauer, who has coauthored training manuals for NET.[3] Homework assignments often involve clients exposing themselves to something that they ordinarily fear in the hope that they become desensitized (less reactive) to that trigger. Homework can also involve writing assignments and role-playing. Group therapy sessions can include psychodrama techniques, such as role-playing, rewriting the ending, and so on. During all these activities, clients are urged to engage in activities that will bring enjoyment into their lives. This is especially important for suicide-prone clients; as we have noted before, this group is often characterized by anhedonia, the inability to experience pleasure.

NET combines creative arts such as drawing, music, and drama with cognitive behavioral therapies. Many of the early psychoanalysts, Freud and Jung among them, wrote extensively on creativity, mythology, and the arts. Many concepts in the creative arts therapies draw upon psychoanalytic concepts such as projection (the attribution of one's own characteristics to another person or group), externalization (the attribution of one's thoughts, feelings, and perceptions to the external world), and abreaction (bringing unconscious material into awareness with emotional release and the discharge of tension and anxiety). The use of imagination is found in many other interventions. Its powerful effects have been observed in such diverse fields as athletics and theatrical training.[4]

Narrative Exposure Therapy in Action

For maximum effectiveness, the narrative needs to have a developmental aspect. Clients identify their first trauma and use exposure techniques to desensitize themselves to it. This corresponds to the myth, legend, or fairy tale they have chosen. They can progress through the various stages of the creative process: immersing oneself in the problem, assimilating relevant information about the problem and letting it incubate, illuminating possible solutions to the problem, and then expressing that solution by putting it to work. Later, evaluation can occur, which provides clues for future problem-solving.[5]

In 2017, the Montreal Museum of Fine Arts presented an exhibit called *Seeds of Hope: An Arts-Based Approach to Suicide and Resilience*. This exhibit presented the works of many individuals whose lives had been affected by suicide; facial masks represented the stigma, and other media were used, including sculpture, music, and dance. The director of the exhibit, Yehudit Silverman, had written, produced, and directed an award-winning film, *The Hidden Face of Suicide*,[6] that focuses on suicide survivors and those who have lost loved ones to suicide and how they had to break the silence they encountered with other family members. Silverman also helped design an arts-based suicide prevention project.[7] These projects have reached out to diverse groups, including seniors and adolescents, Jews and Christians, Canadian First Peoples, and ethnic and sexual minorities.

NET is one of several creative art therapies that involve a trained therapist's intentional use of storytelling, drama, poetry, art, dance, movement, or music in psychotherapy, counseling, special education, and rehabilitation. All forms of these therapies involve imaginative exposure, in that the trauma is represented by the artwork, dramatic role-play, or verse. There are also similarities between NET and cognitive restructuring, role-playing, and role modeling. Reenacting and replaying health-promoting options allows the client to confront a dysfunctional personal myth, an irrational set of beliefs, or a distorted view of a situation. This reframing and reprocessing is implemented through journaling, writing and rewriting, and telling one's story. Anxiety and stress are managed through progressive relaxation, deep breathing, and the use of humor and spontaneity.

NET can be used with nonverbal clients, as art often allows them to access implicit memory systems as well as visual and kinesthetic schemas, and it allows expression by clients who have difficulty describing their trauma verbally. NET also has cross-cultural advantages in that traumatizing events can be portrayed by clients who do not share the therapist's language.[8]

The 2019 New York production of Christopher Shinn's play *Dying City* struck a responsive chord with many trauma survivors in its depiction of twin brothers, one of whom had PTSD after returning from Baghdad, Iraq, the "dying city" of the title. Because both brothers were played by the same actor, the audience had the opportunity to see each brother's development, one of which ended in suicide. This is one of several dramatic productions that focus on the topic. Others from various decades include a daughter's carefully planned suicide in Marsha Norman's *'night Mother*, the double suicides in Henrik Ibsen's *Hedda Gabler*, and Ntozake Shange's play *For Colored Girls Who Have Considered Suicide/When the Rainbow Is Enuf*. These powerful dramatic works can be mentioned to help motivate clients who are engaged in NET, perhaps inspiring some of them to create a dramatization that could be performed for other vulnerable groups.

Takeaway Points

- Arts-based therapy can be especially effective with suicidal people, especially those who find verbal dialogue difficult.

- For maximum effectiveness, narrative exposure therapy makes extensive use of the imagination, both on the part of the client and that of the therapist.

Notes

1. Courtois, C. A., Sonis, J., Brown, L. S., et al. (2019). *Clinical practice guidelines for the treatment of posttraumatic stress disorder (PTSD) in adults*. Washington, DC: American Psychological Association.

2. Zandberg, L. J., Porter, E., & Foa, E. B. (2017). Exposure therapy. In S. N. Gold (Ed.), *APA handbook of trauma psychology: Trauma practice* (Vol. 2, pp. 169–192). Washington, DC. American Psychological Association.

3. Schauer, M. (2015). Narrative exposure therapy. In J. D. Wright (Ed.). *International encyclopedia of the social and behavioral sciences* (2nd ed., Vol. 16, pp. 198–203). Oxford, UK: Elsevier.

4. Johnson, D. R., Lahad, M., & Gray, A. (2009). Creative therapies for adults. In E. B. Foa, T. M., Leame, M. J. Friedman, & J. A. Cohen (Eds.), *Effective treatments for PTSD* (2nd ed., pp. 270–490). New York: Guilford.

5. Murphy, G. (1958). *Human possibilities* (pp. 129–131). New York: Basic Books.

6. Silverman, Y. (2004). The story within: Myth and fairy tale in therapy. *The Arts and Psychotherapy, 31*(3), 127–135.

7. Silverman, Y., Smith, F., & Burns, M. (2013). Coming together in pain and joy: A multicultural and arts-based suicide awareness project. *The Arts in Psychotherapy, 40*, 216–223.

8. Foa, E. B., Keane, T. M., Friedman, M. J., & Cohen, J. A. (2008). Creative therapies for adults. In E. B. Foa, T. M. Keane, M. J. Friedman, & J. A. Cohen (Eds.), *Effective treatments for PTSD* (pp. 600–603). New York: Guilford.

CHAPTER FIFTY

Time Perspective Therapy

A traumatized person who seeks help will discover that dozens of treatments are available. One encouraging study revealed that all bona fide treatments improved the mental health of traumatized patients.[1] This chapter focuses on time perspective therapy (TPT) because of its success in preventing suicide. TPT is based on the ways that people describe time (past, present, and future) and how they assign positive and negative descriptions to each time segment.[2] This model of time was first described by psychologist Philip Zimbardo in his book *The Time Paradox*.[3]

Instead of replaying the trauma repeatedly, TPT asks the trauma survivor to remember the *positive* experiences of one's past rather than only the *negative*. The survivor is asked to stay in the present while working to create a brighter tomorrow. TPT does not ignore traumatic memories but keeps survivors from getting stuck in their negative past. In TPT, survivors move forward rather than continually looking back. They learn from the past and recall their happy experiences, especially those that took place around the time of their traumatic experiences.[4]

TPT uses these time-related terms instead of negative labels that can be discouraging. TPT therapists reframe their clients' "illness" as a *mental injury*, or even a *moral injury*, recasting their depression and anxiety as a "negative past" experience that they can replace with a "positive present" and a "brighter future." To PTSD survivors, the idea of having a forward-leaning framework often comes as an enormous relief.

Six Time Perspectives in TPT

TPT employs six basic perspectives on time:

1. *Past positive* is a focus on the positive experiences.
2. *Past negative* is a focus on what went wrong in the past.

3. *Present hedonistic* lives in the moment, seeking pleasure and avoiding pain.
4. *Present fatalistic* ignores planning, as bad luck or "fate" will decide.
5. *Future positive* plans and trusts that decisions will usually work out.
6. *Future negative* feels that the future is certain to be doomed.

Some people are *transcendental positive future oriented*, believing that by leading a moral, compassionate, and spiritual life on earth, they will be rewarded in the afterlife. But if such people killed children or civilians in the line of duty, or if they believe they have engaged in an unjust war, they may suffer from a moral injury that may increase their thoughts of suicide. Some are also future oriented, but, for them, punishment awaits them in a *transcendental negative future*. Some have no future orientation at all. Thoughts of suicide are very common in this group of survivors, many of whom succumb to suicide's allure.

The typical time perspective profile of a survivor with PTSD is one who is low past positive, high past negative; low (or high) present hedonism, high present fatalism; and low on negative future orientation. The goal in TPT is to balance negative time perspectives with positive time perspectives. In other words, with PTSD survivors, the goal is to boost past positive memories to help curb past negatives, to introduce and practice moderate (instead of extreme) present hedonism to offset present fatalism, and to focus on building a brighter future to enhance hope, as opposed to thoughts of a negative future, especially a transcendent negative future.

There is nothing wrong with *moderate* present hedonism, which includes mindfulness of the present moment, sensory awareness, and enjoyable relationships. We have recommended this attitude throughout this book.

TPT is a humanistic, client-centered, and collaborative style of therapy that promotes the healing of the PTSD survivor through greater self-awareness, self-care, and social integration. TPT begins by respecting the trauma for what it can *teach* survivors rather than dwelling on how it *harmed* them.

No matter what their experiences have been, it is essential for survivors to realize that they can change the way they view themselves and their lives. While participating in TPT, survivors move away from their traumatizing past, pessimistic present, or negative thoughts of the future. Instead, they work their way toward a balanced time perspective in which it seems possible to live a full and promising life in the present. They learn to make time for what matters most to them, such as family, friends, nature, hobbies, or constructive work.

Putting TPT to Work

Richard Sword, the founder of TPT (and a former student of Krippner), was fond of saying, "We are going to take TPT out of the ivory tower and place it squarely in the hands of the people." Following through with

Richard's idea, his wife, Rose, and the eminent psychologist Philip Zimbardo determined that individuals with an undergraduate degree in psychology could practice TPT. Although TPT was developed as a treatment for PTSD, aspects of TPT, such as refocusing from past negatives to past positives and making plans for a positive future, are practical for medical practitioners, physical and massage therapists, practitioners of complementary medicine, and high school and university counselors. The twenty-minute *The River of Time* video on YouTube was created to assist clients in the TPT process.[5]

Evidence-Based Research on TPT

Richard and Rose Sword kept a detailed account of their clients' progress—or lack of it. They analyzed the tests their clients had taken to determine whether any improvement was due to the treatment or the placebo effect, positive results that are produced from the expectation that the treatment will work. In the six-month period of January–June 2009, their clients' levels of depression decreased 89 percent, their levels of anxiety decreased 70 percent, and their levels of trauma decreased 39 percent. Clearly, TPT helped these veterans attain better scores on clinical assessments in comparison to their pretherapy test levels. The scores also matched the self-reports of the veterans themselves.

All thirty-two veterans were retested in 2010. The improvements had endured, and there was some further progress. This is an important finding. The significant improvement in symptoms demonstrated in the first phase of the study was maintained, and nearly two-thirds of the cases improved still further over a one-year period. The improvement persisted in a second retest in 2011.

With each retest, the reduction in symptoms endured. Overall, 87 percent of the veterans reported decreased trauma and PTSD symptoms, with an astonishing 100 percent of them reporting a decrease in their depression rating. This indicates that TPT is not a temporary fix; improvements can be sustained. In addition, during this four-year period, not a single veteran attempted suicide—in dramatic contrast to the high percentage of untreated veterans who attempted or committed suicide during that same time frame. It was apparent that TPT had diminished suicide's allure for this group of veterans. TPT can also be applied to the challenges and opportunities of everyday life.[6]

Takeaway Points

- Time perspective therapy has been successful in reducing suicides, in part because it regards therapists and clients as partners.
- Though TPT is helpful for various healing professionals, it does not require a professionally trained guide.

Notes

1. Benish, S., Imel, Z., & Wampold, B. (2008). The relative efficacy of bona fide psychotherapies for treating post-traumatic stress disorder: A meta-analysis of direct comparisons. *Clinical Psychology Review, 28,* 746–758.

2. Sword, R. M., Sword, R. K. M., & Brunskill, S. R. (2015). Time perspective therapy: Transforming Zimbardo's temporal theory into clinical practice. In M. Stolarski, N. Fieulaine, & W. van Beek (Eds.), *Time perspective theory; Review, research and application* (pp. 481–98). New York: Springer.

3. Zimbardo, P. G., & Boyd, J. (2010). *The time paradox: The new psychology of time that will change your life.* New York: Rider. Visit www.timeparadox.com to view the ZTPI long form, which can be taken online and scored automatically.

4. Zimbardo, P. G., Sword, R., & Sword, R. (2012). *The time cure: Overcoming PTSD with the new psychology of time perspective therapy.* San Francisco: John Wiley & Sons.

5. Twin Peaks Creative. (2012, July 27). *The River of Time* (Video). https://www.youtube.com/watch?v=r4ZX0XVAa2A.

6. Zimbardo, P. G., & Sword, R. K. M. (2017). *Living & loving better with time perspective therapy: Healing from the past, embracing the present, creating an ideal future.* Jefferson, NC: Exposit.

CHAPTER FIFTY-ONE

How TPT Saved Jamie from PTSD

Jamie (not his real name) joined the U.S. Army after graduating from high school, where he had received excellent grades. Although Jamie wanted to continue his education and had received an academic scholarship to a nearby college, his parents could not afford the additional tuition and expenses. Jamie enlisted so that he could attend university on the G.I. Bill once he had completed his service. Four years later, after two tours in Iraq and several close quarters firefights in which some of his friends were killed or maimed, he returned home and finally enrolled in college.

Jamie had been a bright and enthusiastic student in high school, but now he had difficulty focusing. At the end of the first semester, he dropped out of school due to failing grades. Jamie knew that his time in the military had changed him, and not for the better. Further, he realized that he missed two vital elements in civilian life: the unique camaraderie he had with his brothers-in-arms and the adrenaline rush of living amid danger. Jamie thought about civilian service-oriented organizations, such as the fire or police departments; perhaps they might offer the camaraderie and excitement that he was missing. The local fire department was not accepting recruits, but the police department had some openings.

While at the Police Academy, Marisa (pseudonym), a fellow candidate, taken by Jamie's pensive mood and good looks, pursued him, and they commenced a romantic relationship. Upon graduation, they married and before long had a baby.

The Triggering Incident

One day, while Marisa was on maternity leave, Jamie was called as backup for a dangerous situation involving an active shooter in a low-income neighborhood. During the ensuing incident, Jamie underwent an on-the-job psychological breakdown. In his mind, the present had evaporated and been replaced with a firefight Jamie had experienced in Iraq. His fellow law enforcement officers suddenly became his platoon buddies. The active shooter turned into an Iraqi insurgent. One of the police officers noted that while crouched behind a wall, Jamie was shaking uncontrollably and sweating profusely, and he had called him by a different name. He told Jamie to stay put while he called headquarters.

Jamie was admitted to the psychiatric ward at the local hospital and put on paid leave. During his time there, he told the psychiatrist he was suffering suicidal thoughts. After a few weeks of intensive therapy, he was released under the condition that he would continue seeing a psychiatrist for medication and a psychologist for psychotherapy. Jamie was to remain on leave until he was either cleared by both practitioners or was deemed unfit to serve in the police department.

Jamie's Time Perspective

Richard Sword was contacted by the chief of police and asked to take Jamie as a client. Not knowing much about Jamie's background as a veteran, they felt TPT[1] might help this young officer. Rosemary Sword was the cotherapist for Jamie and gave us permission to use his story.

Session One. During his first session, Jamie mentioned he had served two tours in Iraq before becoming a police officer. The Swords suspected he had some form of post-traumatic stress and gave him psychological tests that diagnosed him with depression, anxiety, and PTSD.

Session Two. The test results were explained. Jamie's stress was so severe that he definitely had PTSD. The therapist told him that the recent incident as a police officer had triggered it. Jamie described the triggering incident and realized that he had been experiencing PTSD since he returned home. The symptoms had worsened since he had joined the police force, married, and had a child.

Session Three. The third session was devoted to Jamie's military service, especially the life-threatening firefights—past negatives. Jamie had an excellent memory and was prompted to relive these experiences in as much detail as he could manage. At the end of these exhausting sessions, the therapist encouraged self-care, such as listening to soothing music, engaging in meditation, and recalling positive memories, such as experiences with family and friends, playing sports, riding horses in the countryside, hiking his favorite trails, and swimming in the ocean. When past negative thoughts arose, Jamie was told to immediately replace them with these past positive memories.

Session Four. During the fourth session, while sharing how he was doing at the present time, Jamie admitted to having suicidal thoughts. In TPT, this is called *extreme present fatalism.*

Jamie volunteered that he owned a gun and thought that if he were to kill himself, it would probably be with that weapon. He was not sure that he really loved Marisa and felt that she had pressured him into marriage and having a child. He did not know whether he could keep up with their house payments. In addition to feeling overwhelmed with responsibility, he now realized that his time in Iraq had left him with extreme post-traumatic stress.

Deeply concerned about Jamie's suicidal thoughts and the handgun in his home, the therapist suggested he turn over the firearm to the police department. Jamie eventually agreed, muttering that although he had not thought about it previously, there were other ways he could take his life if he wanted to do so. The therapist called Jamie's wife and asked her to remove the gun from the premises before Jamie returned home. She took the gun directly to the police department.

The therapist then asked Jamie to once more focus on his past positives in the outdoors: surfing, diving, fishing, hunting, hiking, and farming. Jamie still enjoyed some of these (present hedonistic), but with a wife on maternity leave and a baby at home that he helped care for, most of these activities were out of reach. The therapist suggested that he clear some of his land and plant his favorite vegetables. Jamie agreed to give it a try.

Then the therapist turned the conversation and asked Jamie to consider all the positives in his life. Together they made a list: a loving partner and caring parents, loyal friends, a roof over his head, and a baby he was getting to know and love. When Jamie found himself feeling depressed, he was to recount his many blessings and do some farm work on his land. The therapist also taught Jamie self-soothing breathing techniques and simple guided meditations, which Jamie practiced between sessions, especially when he felt anxious or depressed.

Subsequent Sessions. Although Jaime's suicidal thoughts had decreased, he continued to have them on occasion. He frequently shared one of his main concerns about the future: that he would be unable to provide for his family if he lost his job on the police force (future negative). As a veteran, Jamie had taken advantage of the G.I. Bill, but he had not considered other VA benefits. At the suggestion of the therapist, Jamie agreed they would work together applying to the VA for a disability claim due to service-connected PTSD. In earlier sessions, they had reviewed his past negative experiences in the military. Adding additional details and placing them into the format required by the VA would be fairly straightforward. The thought of receiving well-deserved compensation gave Jamie hope (future positive).

As Jamie improved, his sessions were reduced to once a week. He had taken the therapist's suggestion seriously and had cleared a portion of his land. A counseling session was conducted on Jamie's property, and the therapist marveled at the large vegetable garden Jamie had planted. Jamie shared that he had plans to clear another tract of land to plant fruit trees.

Within four months of his first session, Jamie no longer suffered from suicidal thoughts. Within six months, he was cleared by both his psychiatrist and therapist to return to work. Simultaneously, he received a 100 percent service-connected PTSD rating from the VA.

Jaime had also received a job offer from a former high school friend to work on a ranch a few hundred miles away. After discussions and two couples therapy sessions, Jamie and his wife decided they wanted to start over. The thought of working outdoors on a ranch excited Jamie, and Marisa, reluctant to return to work, wanted to spend more time with their baby. They sold their house and purchased a modest home near the friend's cattle ranch. At his last contact with the therapist, Jamie and Marisa were living the "brighter future" they had created together. Combining TPT with many of the other techniques mentioned in this book worked for Jamie.

Jamie's story reminds us of a sobering statistic. While firearms are used in less than 6 percent of suicide attempts, over 50 percent of suicide deaths occur with firearms. In other words, guns are eight times as lethal as other means and cause over half the suicide deaths. Of the most commonly used methods of self-harm, firearms are by far the most lethal, with a fatality rate of approximately 85 percent. Conversely, fewer than 5 percent of people who attempt suicide using other methods will die, and the vast majority of all those who survive do *not* go on to die by suicide.[2] This suggests that a reduction in suicide attempts by firearm would result in an overall decline in the suicide rate.

Takeaway Points

- Time perspective therapy can make the difference between life and death for veterans at risk for suicide.
- As is the case with all therapies, TPT therapists need to be well trained, attentive, and capable of forming a healing relationship with their clients.

Notes

1. Zimbardo, P., Sword, R., & Sword, R. (2012). *The time cure: Overcoming PTSD with the new psychology of time perspective therapy.* San Francisco: John Wiley & Sons.

2. EverytownResearch.org. (2018, September 10). "Firearm Suicide in the United States." https://everytownresearch.org/wp-content/uploads/2018/08/Firearm-Suicide-CDC-Update-022020D.pdf.

CHAPTER FIFTY-TWO

Nature's Gift

Turning to nature is one of the quickest and least expensive activities a person can do for his or her mental and spiritual health, costing only a pair of sturdy shoes and a bus ticket or gallon of gas—or no cost at all outside one's back door. Bringing nature indoors can be done with house plants, opened curtains for natural light, and a furry dog or cat. This is not wishful thinking: decades of research show that nature heals, and even exposure as limited as access to a view can hasten recovery in hospitalized patients and reduce violence in prison inmates. More generally, regular contact with natural settings is linked to better health, and a feeling of connectedness with nature is linked to well-being.[1]

When Nature Heals

Nature can heal through a gentle walk in the woods. According to the Association of Nature and Forest Therapy Guides and Programs, "The forest itself is the therapist. We don't train therapists; we train guides. By slowing people down and facilitating sensory experiencing, guides open the doorways through which the forest can accomplish its healing work."[2] One participant in a small Irish study commented, "Peace, I love the peace. . . . Just being out in nature is very healing. I think it's the calmness, quietness, lack of noise, just the beauty of the birds, you know the wind, just the natural elements, I think. I do find it helps my sleeping. I am not tossing around and turning."[3]

On the other hand, Outward Bound and other adventure education programs devise challenging, even strenuous activities. This focus is particularly helpful for returning service members, who face a stigma often associated in the military with admitting problems and seeking help. As one participant explained,

How can I go from jumping out of airplanes and sitting in trenches in foreign countries to being afraid to getting out of my basement. . . . Self-stigma, it's probably the worst now that you mention it, because there's this sense of bravado as you know, we just joke around that we're bulletproof type thing—I always said this, I wish I could have broken a leg, my back, an arm amputation instead of breaking my mental health, or more or less breaking my soul.[4]

Adventure groups composed solely of veterans help by offering comradeship, teamwork, trust, and belonging. "Being in a group of other military personnel within a unique adventure setting often allows the participants to feel connected with other soldiers again, and this connection can be clearly beneficial in their recovery."[5] The authors of a Canadian study noted the metaphorical value of "anchor building and finding sources of personal support and connection during rock- and ice-climbing courses, or navigating rapids and getting through stressful and rough patches in life during white-water canoe courses."[6]

Gardening and animal care programs help many people, including prison inmates, to find meaning in their lives, learn useful skills, and form healthy relationships. Nature has such a powerful healing effect that even *looking* at images of natural landscapes (photos, 3D images, virtual reality, and videos) is reliably shown to produce relaxation,[7] and taking outdoor "micro-breaks" as brief as one to five minutes made a positive difference for college students.[8]

Animal-assisted therapy (AAT) is a well-established discipline, with applications for disabled children, elders with dementia, victims of sexual abuse, substance abusers in recovery, and more. K9s for Warriors is one of many programs that match veterans with companion animals. According to their website, "K9s for Warriors is ending veteran suicide and returning our warriors to a life of dignity and independence. We rescue and train shelter dogs to be paired as Service Dogs for warriors with service-connected Post-Traumatic Stress, Traumatic Brain Injury and/or Military Sexual Trauma." K9s for Warriors saves lives in more ways than one. They acquire the dogs from high-kill shelters and rescue groups and train them at no cost to the veterans. In praise of the program, one man wrote, "Suicide doesn't take away the pain; it gives it to someone else. I chose the program to get my life back."

Juliet's Story

A friendly therapy dog helped another suicidal patient. Bullying, mental illness, and abusive family dynamics led a girl we will call Juliet to become suicidal in childhood. Suzanne Engelman's therapy dog, CJ, became instrumental in Juliet's recovery. Dr. Engelman has given us permission to share Juliet's story.

Sitting atop her family's refrigerator, six-year-old Juliet finally felt safe. Her rapid breathing slowed, and the tension in her stomach finally lessened. Her latest asthma attack also subsided. She gazed at her schizophrenic mother from her perch of safety. As Juliet recalled, "She was trying to eat me and absorb me like I was being sucked into quicksand." In her psychotic state, the mother would never have realized she was bullying Juliet. But she was, and her daughter was coming closer to the brink of suicide.

Juliet had developed intense anxiety, panic, and depression. In addition, after all the horrible things her mother had told her about what "outsiders" would do to her, social interactions were too risky and frightening. The house was always darkened, shades drawn, so that "they" could not peek in, and she was isolated, even at school, where classmates ridiculed the outgrown clothes her mother made her wear. The teasing verified her mom's rants that other people are dangerous and to be avoided. Juliet's anxiety turned into agoraphobia—fear of being outdoors in public places—and she became terrified of leaving home, though she was desperate to get away from her mother.

Juliet began overdosing on pills at age eleven, after her mother temporarily abandoned her. And then the cutting started. There was another pill overdose at age fifteen and more cutting. Juliet recalled, "Each cut was like a mouth screaming, and it made me feel better, because I dared not scream myself." By the time local social services referred Juliet to Dr. Engelman at age twenty, she was covered with tattoos, cuts, and scars hidden under long-sleeved shirts. Although not actively suicidal, Juliet had suicidal ideation. She kept cutting herself, and she sometimes needed hospitalization to get stitches to stop the bleeding. A social worker received permission from Juliet's mother to transport her to Dr. Engelman's office and back.

Juliet felt like a "wounded animal" and yet she also identified a "spark in me that doesn't want to die." Animals felt safer to her than people. This dynamic allowed her to bond with CJ, Dr. Engelman's therapy dog. CJ greeted Juliet in the waiting room with a wagging tail and friskiness that instantly helped Juliet feel accepted.

To begin safely exploring the various chapters of her life, Juliet began petting CJ, which helped evoke feelings of calmness. Dr. Engelman taught Juliet how to use slow-paced diaphragmatic breathing to counter anxiety and hyperarousal. Then, after Juliet signaled with her finger that she was ready, Dr. Engelman utilized guided, relaxing imagery to arrive at a painful life episode, symbolized by colorful rooms. In her imagination, Juliet carefully picked which room to go into for a safe confrontation with her mother.

Eventually, she could visualize going outside the therapy room with CJ leading her through fields of flowers. At other times, in her imagination, CJ reunited her with the few positive figures she had encountered during her daily life, including Dr. Engelman. Upon returning to awareness back in the therapy room, Juliet would be aglow with her discoveries that she had made with CJ's help.

As their work proceeded, Juliet's cutting diminished. When Juliet felt like cutting herself, she remembered CJ's loving gaze and the protection that she had bestowed upon Juliet in her imaginal world. Juliet became convinced that Dr. Engelman's intent was benevolent, and this sense of safety was transferred to other people.

With the help of Dr. Engelman and CJ, Juliet's negative beliefs about herself began to change. "I am a worthless person" changed to "Just the fact that I am human makes me worthwhile." The belief "The outside world is filled with danger" changed to "The outside world can be dangerous, but there are more positive than negative aspects to it; I have the intelligence to know the difference." The personal myth "I can never separate from my mother" shifted to "I am an adult capable of living my own life and making my own decisions." Perhaps most important, "There is no joy and love in my dismal life" altered to "The warmth and happiness I have discovered with Dr. Engelman and CJ exists elsewhere, and I am capable of discovering it."

Juliet then developed the courage to explore the external world. As the length of the walks in public increased from one minute to five minutes, Juliet was able to soothe her social anxiety more readily. At home, Juliet's agoraphobia diminished; she now felt comfortable enough to open her front door and gaze outside. This activity evolved into actually leaving the house. Juliet was able to walk down the sidewalk of her house to the street without feeling overwhelming tension.

Gradually, over several months of weekly psychotherapy and with the assistance of CJ, Juliet's incapacitating migraines ceased, and she was able to enroll in a class at the local community college. Her asthma attacks lessened in intensity, and she applied for a part-time job doing bookkeeping.

CJ, like other therapy dogs, had come to the rescue. Just as the legendary St. Bernard dogs were said to bring lifesaving food and water to stranded hikers in the Swiss Alps, CJ brought hope and help to Juliet. Could Dr. Engelman have done this without CJ's help? One never knows. But Juliet's recovery probably moved more quickly and went far deeper than work with a human psychotherapist alone.

One does not need a formal therapy animal organization to find and adopt a companion animal, as hundreds of shelters and private groups rescue and rehome cats, dogs, horses, and other animals. Of course, companion animals require ongoing expenditures of food, supplies, and veterinary visits. The authors of this book think it is money well spent.

Takeaway Points

- Immersion in nature is an overlooked resource for traumatized individuals.
- Animal-assisted intervention and companion animals can play an important role in both suicide prevention and recovery.

Notes

1. University of Plymouth. (2020, February 13). Reconnecting with nature key for the health of people and the planet. *ScienceDaily* (online).

2. Hart, J. (2016). Prescribing nature therapy for improved mental health. *Alternative and Complementary Therapies, 22*(4), 161–163.

3. Iwata, Y., Dhubhain, A. N., Brophy, J., et al. (2016). Benefits of group walking in forests for people with significant mental ill-health. *Ecopsychology, 8*(1), 16–26.

4. Forsyth, A., Lysaght, R., Aiken, A., & Cramm, H. (2020, February). Wilderness adventure program may help combat perceptions of stigma among veterans. *Ecopsychology, 12*(1), 8–18 (online).

5. Ewert, A. (2014). Military veterans and the use of adventure education experiences in natural environments for therapeutic outcomes. *Ecopsychology, 6*(3), 155–164 (online).

6. Harper, N. J., Norris, J., & D'astous, M. (2014, September). Veterans and the Outward Bound experience: An evaluation of impact and meaning. *Ecopsychology, 6*(3), 165–173 (online).

7. Jo, H., Song, C., & Miyazaki, Y. (2019, November 27). Physiological benefits of viewing nature: A systematic review of indoor experiments. *International Journal of Environmental Research and Public Health, 16*(23), 4739. https://doi.org/10.3390/ijerph16234739.

8. Ibes, D., Hirama, I., & Schuyler, C. (2018, September). Greenspace ecotherapy interventions: The stress-reduction potential of green micro-breaks integrating nature connection and mind-body skills. *Ecopsychology, 10*(3), 137–150 (online).

CHAPTER FIFTY-THREE

Psychedelics Old and New

In 1974, one of us (Krippner) published an essay predicting the eventual legalization of marijuana in the United States.[1] This prediction was based on research showing that marijuana had been used for medicinal purposes for centuries. Sure enough, by the third decade of the twenty-first century, many U.S. states had decriminalized marijuana and permitted the birth of the medicinal and recreational marijuana industries. With proper precautions, it can be helpful in many ways.[2]

There are two major stains of cannabis: *Cannabis sativa* and *Cannabis indica*. Both have two main psychoactive components:

- Delta 9 tetrahydrocannabinol (THC) can produce mind-altering sensations, both pleasant (the "psychedelic effects") and unpleasant (such as paranoia and anxiety).
- Cannabidiol (CBD) has distinctly different effects, suggesting it may have therapeutic potential.

In one study with cannabis in which a control group took a placebo, eighty-eight patients with symptoms of schizophrenia were given either CBD or a placebo for six weeks, alongside any other antipsychotic drug they were taking. After six weeks, those treated with CBD had fewer symptoms of schizophrenia (hearing voices, paranoid thoughts, visual hallucinations, etc.) than those taking the placebo. They also found it easier to work with others and to carry out daily functions, and they received higher improvement ratings from their psychiatrists. Their cognitive functioning improved, they were able to think more clearly, and they manifested no serious side effects, such as thoughts about committing suicide.[3]

These favorable results could be attributed to marijuana's psychedelic or "mind-manifesting" properties. A 1968 study of artists and musicians found that marijuana was cited by the artists and musicians along with LSD-type drugs as having positive effects on their cognition and perception, "making manifest" their creative potential.[4]

The Psychedelic Resurgence

Advances in psychopharmacology have benefited people around the world, most notably those with schizophrenia and bipolar disorders. Antipsychotic, antidepressant, and mood-stabilizing drugs have helped millions of patients. However, these drugs do not correct existential issues, and their side effects are often problematic.

By contrast, most forms of psychotherapy focus on processes underlying a client's problems. Evidence-based psychotherapy often yields better results than medication, especially for clients experiencing depression, post-traumatic stress disorder (PTSD), or existential distress due to life-threatening illnesses.[5] Furthermore, clients' preference for psychotherapy is three times greater than for medication.[6] However, many people with PTSD do not make adequate progress or drop out because they cannot tolerate emotionally challenging aspects of treatment, such as prolonged exposure. These factors led Michael Mithoefer, Charles Grob, and Timothy Brewerton to explore psychedelic drugs to augment psychotherapy.[7] They do not offer psychedelics regularly, only on one or a few occasions to overcome obstacles to psychotherapy or to catalyze a healing experience.

After decades of the War on Drugs, when psychedelics were banned, even for research, the first aboveground project in the United States involved twelve patients with advanced cancer and concomitant anxiety who were given psilocybin on one occasion and an inert placebo on another. They received extensive preparation, including discussions of what to expect and experiences they might encounter. When patients were retested and reinterviewed one month later, they reported significant reductions in anxiety and depression, which remained three months later.[8] A study conducted in Switzerland with LSD produced similar results.[9]

Most participants in these and similar investigations reported profound psychospiritual experiences. Mithoefer and his colleagues ascribed this to the drugs' abilities to evoke innate inner mechanisms for spiritual healing, especially on the part of those with life-threatening conditions. Some writers use the term *entheogenic*, implying that psychedelics can awaken the "God within." Mithoefer's participants' experiences included transcending space and time, a profound sense of unity, a deeply felt positive mood, and a renewed sense of purpose. This existential shift remained a year later when participants were retested. Moreover, anxiety and depression, two conditions reported by people who attempt suicide, were reduced.

MDMA-Assisted Psychotherapy

Ecstasy (methylenedioxymethamphetamine or MDMA) is often associated with rave clubs, disco dancing, and recreational use, but it also has legitimate healing potential. Called an *empathogen* because of its capacity to increase participants' empathy, MDMA was used by many psychotherapists worldwide before the U.S. Food and Drug administration (FDA) classified it as a Schedule 1 drug in the 1980s, meaning it had no recognized medical use. Like LSD-type drugs, MDMA has staged a dramatic comeback, as it can be legally used for "investigative" purposes in government-approved trials, but it is not without risks. Like psychedelics, MDMA should be administered as part of an overall treatment plan by psychotherapists who have had special training. Special training is necessary for many reasons, including being prepared to treat episodes of nostalgia and sadness after the session ends.

MDMA-assisted psychotherapy has been successful in treating intractable PTSD. Mithoefer and a team of psychotherapists worked with twenty patients whose PTSD had not responded to treatment. Following MDMA-assisted psychotherapy, 83 percent of them no longer met the criteria for PTSD. Remarkably, 25 percent of the placebo group made similar changes, demonstrating the power of expectation and the necessity of including a placebo group when evaluating any type of medication. Later, seven members of the placebo group were given MDMA-assisted psychotherapy and experienced similar reductions in PTSD symptoms.[10] Follow-up indicated that most patients had retained their gains, even without further administration of MDMA.[11]

Ketamine, with and without Psychotherapy

Originally used as an anesthetic, ketamine is frequently used for severe depression, which is extremely relevant in preventing suicide. However, its occasional psychedelic effects worried conventional psychiatrists, who sought to minimize the visions that patients often reported.[12] They did not consider that these visions may have played an important role in ketamine's positive results.

A 2016 review discovered seventy-seven publications on the therapeutic uses of ketamine.[13] Over six hundred people received ketamine, most only once, usually for depression that had not responded to psychotherapy, antidepressant medication, or electroconvulsive (shock) treatment. Only two of the seventy-seven were randomized control trials, and many of the rest were collections of case studies. There were a few adverse reactions, but some members receiving placebos also reported negative side effects. There were few long-term follow-ups, and some patients showed positive responses only after a second or third administration of ketamine.

Despite the many limitations of these studies, the reviewers concluded that ketamine appears to have had "remarkably robust efficacy in short-term relief of severe and treatment resistant depression, with onset in hours, and duration of at least a few days." It was observed that "ketamine's effectiveness in relief of acute suicidal ideation is also a highly valuable finding."

Unlike conventional pharmacological treatments for depression, ketamine induces "an altered state of self that can lead to a new state of contentment."[14] Better-known psychedelics often induce dissociation as well, with frequent reductions in depression. All these drugs alter ordinary brain functioning, a condition that can be used positively by skilled psychotherapists. In unsupervised sessions, the results may be euphoric but are sometimes disastrous.

Psychedelics and Human Evolution

Did psychedelics play a role in human evolution? Anthropologist Michael Winkelman used neurophenomenological findings to explain how psychedelics and similar mind-altering substances may have done so.[15] The neurotransmitters serotonin and dopamine (which help nerve cells communicate) are affected by varieties of mushrooms (later synthesized as psilocybin), cacti (later synthesized as mescaline), and fungi (containing lysergic acid, related to LSD). The use of these plants was ritualized with dancing, drumming, chanting, and controlled dreaming, giving rise to what is now called *shamanism*, the core of a community's social life and central to healing, hunting, social bonding, and protection from enemies and wild animals. Sources of information that were usually unconscious were brought to awareness by psychedelic rituals. Perhaps the genes that supported these functions were useful enough to pass on to subsequent generations.

Conclusion

Controversial though they may be, natural and synthesized mind-altering substances are finding a place in modern society and its healing practices. They should be used with caution but can be helpful in preventing suicide.

Takeaway Points

- Marijuana, psilocybin, LSD, MDMA, and ketamine appear to have important psychotherapeutic uses if administered properly by qualified psychotherapists.
- Psychedelics may have played an important role in human evolution. In contemporary times, their proper usage can both enhance life and prevent suicides.

Notes

1. Krippner, S. (1974). Marijuana and Viet Nam: Twin dilemmas for American youth. In R. S. Parker (Ed.), *The emotional threat of war, violence, and peace* (pp. 176–221). Pittsburgh, PA: Stanwix House.

2. Englund, A., Freeman, T., Murray, R., et al. (2017). Can we make cannabis safer? *Lancet Psychiatry, 4,* 643–648.

3. McGuire, P., Robson, P., Cubala, W. J., Vasile, D., et al. (2017). Cannabidiol (CBD) as an adjunctive therapy in schizophrenia: A multicenter randomized control trial. *American Journal of Psychiatry, 175,* 225–231.

4. Krippner, S. (1968). The psychedelic artist. In R. E. L. Masters & J. Houston, *Psychedelic art* (pp. 163–182). New York: Grove Press.

5. Watts, B. V., Schnurr, P. P., Mayo, L., et al. (2004). Meta-analysis of the efficacy of treatments for posttraumatic stress disorder. *Journal of Clinical Psychiatry, 74,* 541–550.

6. LeMay, K., & Wilson, K. G. (2008). Treatment of existential distress in life-threatening illness: A review of manualized interventions. *Clinical Psychology Review, 28,* 472–493.

7. Mithoefer, M. L., Grob, C. S., & Brewerton, T. D. (2016). Novel psychopharmacological therapies for psychiatric disorders: Psilocybin and MDMA. *Lancet Psychiatry, 3,* 481–488.

8. Grob, C. S., Danforth, A. I., & Chopra, C. S., et al. (2011). Pilot study of psilocybin treatment for anxiety in patients with advanced stage cancer. *Archives of General Psychiatry, 68,* 71–78.

9. Gasser, P., Holstein, D., Michel, Y., et al. (2014). Safety and efficacy of lysergic acid diethylamide-assisted psychotherapy for anxiety associated with life-threatening diseases. *Journal of Nervous and Mental Disease, 202,* 513–520.

10. Mithoefer, M. L., Wagner, M. T., Mithoefer, M. T., et al. (2011). The safety and efficacy of 4/-3 4-methylenedioxymethamphetamine-assisted psychotherapy in subjects with chronic treatment-resistant posttraumatic stress disorder: The first randomized control pilot study. *Journal of Psychopharmacology, 25,* 439–452.

11. Mithoefer, M. L., Wagner, M. T., Mithoefer, M. T., et al. (2013). Durability of improvement in post-traumatic symptoms and absence of harmful effects or drug dependence after 3, 4 methylenedioxymethamphetamine-assisted psychotherapy: A prospective long-term follow-up study. *Journal of Psychopharmacology, 27,* 28–39.

12. Wolfson, P. (2016). Introduction. In P. Wolfson & G. Hartelius (Eds.), *The Ketamine Papers: Science, therapy, and transformation* (pp. 1–23). Santa Cruz, CA: Multidisciplinary Association for Psychedelic Studies.

13. Ryan, W. C., Marta, C. J., & Koek, R. J. (2016). Ketamine, depression, and current research: A review of the literature. In P. Wolfson & G. Hartelius (Eds.), *The Ketamine Papers: Science, therapy, and transformation* (pp. 199–273). Santa

Cruz, CA: Multidisciplinary Association for Psychedelic Studies. Quotations on pages 214–215, 221–222.

14. Ryan, Marta, & Koek, Ketamine, depression, and current research, 214–215, 221–222.

15. Winkelman, M. J. (2017). The mechanisms of psychedelic visionary experiences: Hypotheses from evolutionary psychology. *Frontiers in Neuroscience, 11*, 539.

CHAPTER FIFTY-FOUR

Vine of the Spirits

Ayahuasca, a psychedelic brew that originated in the Amazon, has spread to distant lands, including Estonia. Two psychologists, eager to learn more, conducted a questionnaire study and received many intriguing surprises. One of them was from a woman who had been contemplating suicide for some time, but she heard about an ayahuasca session in her vicinity and promptly registered. The experience was life changing. She told the psychologists, "Thanks to ayahuasca, I am still alive." Years later, she is still alive and coping.[1]

The Concoction

Serious Western research into the nature of ayahuasca and similar preparations began with Richard Spruce, an ethnobotanist who explored the Amazon and the Andes between 1849 and 1864. Among other species, he discovered the *Banisteriopsis caapi* jungle vine. He observed that concoctions containing elements of this vine were ingested ritually by locals to "travel" to "other worlds" to visit their tribal divinities but also for the healing of tribal members who had become ill.[2] In addition to the term *ayahuasca*, the brew is called *yage*, *caapi*, *kahpi*, *cadana*, *pinde*, *natem*, *natema*, and other names, depending on the tribe, its location, and the exact combination of substances and method of preparation.[3]

In the Tukano tribe of Colombia, ingestion is preceded by a period of fasting and, at the time of the ceremony, recitation of creation myths and genealogies accompanied by the sounds of instruments such as drums, rattles, flutes, whistles, and even singing and dancing. The participant's report usually begins with a description of circles, triangles, spirals, and later such culturally meaningful images as jaguars, snakes, and mythical landscapes. The experience is considered superior to one's ordinary state of consciousness and is reflected in artistic decorations, architectural designs, and the pottery decorations found on Tukano pottery and musical instruments. Richard Rudgley observed that this imagery reinforces key cultural concepts and values.[4]

You may recall from our previous discussions that serotonin is a neurotransmitter, a molecular messenger that helps nerve cells in the brain communicate with each other. Neurotransmitters are the foundations of most medical psychiatric treatments such as Prozac and other selective serotonin reuptake inhibitors (SSRIs). Some serotonin receptors are also targets of psychedelics such as LSD and psilocybin. SSRI antidepressants and psychedelics are biochemically related, and this underlies their ability to manage certain mental health problems, though their mechanisms of action are quite different.

Effects of Ayahuasca on Suicidality

In 2019, researchers from Brazil and England published the first study on the effect of ayahuasca on suicidality that used a comparison group, whose members took a placebo.[5] Their twenty-nine participants, all Brazilians, were deeply depressed people for whom treatment had been ineffective, even with antidepressant medications. All participants underwent psychiatric interviews and took a psychological test to ensure that they met the criteria of major depressive disorder but were not at imminent suicidal risk. Participants were told to discontinue their medication an average of two weeks prior to the experiment and for at least a week following the experiment. Daily use of benzodiazepines (tranquilizing medicines) was permitted, except during the acute phases of the intervention. The mean age of the participants was forty-two, three out of four were female, and half of the group was unemployed. Half of the group members had made a suicide attempt, and three out of four had a serious problem in addition to suicidality. There were fourteen members in the ayahuasca group and fifteen members in the placebo group.

On the morning of the intervention, participants were reminded of how to deal with their experiences and of strategies for coping with those that seemed to be difficult. They were told to pay special attention to their bodily sensations, their thoughts, and their emotions. A previously determined playlist of musical performances was used during the entire intervention. In individual settings, participants were administered a single dose of ayahuasca or a placebo that had been designed to mimic the color, taste, and bodily feelings that characterize ayahuasca. A staff member, who did not know which participants had been administered ayahuasca, was available to provide support if needed. The sessions lasted about eight hours.

Suicidality was assessed before the intervention began, a day after the intervention, two days after, and seven days after. The scores at the end of the first day following intervention showed a greater decrease in suicidality on the part of the ayahuasca group than that of the placebo group, a difference that held up during the second- and seventh-day follow-ups. The investigators concluded that ayahuasca leads to decreases in suicidality that are sustained from one to seven days after administration.

From our perspective, the results may have been stronger if there had been more interaction between staff members and the participants. Also, there were no integration sessions in which participants could have discussed how they brought the lessons from the session into their daily lives. In addition, a longer period of follow-up would have been useful to determine the long-lasting effects of the treatment. So this study offers only mild support for the use of ayahuasca for suicidality.

Russ's Story

Let's look at one individual's experience. Russ (not his real name) spent his early years at his family's home in rural Colorado. As soon as he was able, he joined the military and was sent to Vietnam, where he was assigned to an air ambulance crew that evacuated soldiers who were severely wounded or dying. Ross was wounded several times and was constantly immersed in the horror of war.

After Vietnam, he returned to Colorado, where he worked on a ranch and enrolled in college, earning a master's degree in counseling psychology and another in social work. Ross worked in the health care industry, human resources, and administration. But when the Persian Gulf War commenced, Russ began experiencing symptoms of PTSD. He had never taken the term seriously until he began experiencing it himself. He had outbursts of anger, disturbing thoughts, and chronic stress. His health deteriorated, and he had bypass surgery and was diagnosed as a diabetic.

Russ was also diagnosed as suffering from PTSD and underwent treatment at a VA hospital, where he was placed on antidepressants. For five months, he received individual and group therapy at the VA hospital. These treatments helped Russ control his symptoms, but he felt that he was not healing. He recalled that his grandmother had been an herbalist, and he became interested in traditional healing procedures. He discovered a center in Peru where plant medicines and shamanic methods were employed and arranged for treatment with ayahuasca. Russ weaned himself off the antidepressant medication before his first psychedelic session, which was preceded by interviews with a physician and a shaman.

After ingesting ayahuasca, Russ reported seeing black leeches emerging from his body. When the shaman began to sing, the leeches seemed to fly from Russ's stomach and intestines. Russ began to vomit, which the shaman interpreted as another indication of purification; the "dark energies" were leaving his body. Russ retreated to the washroom, and when he did not return, the physician went after him, only to be told by Russ that he was enjoying the colorful snakes that were surrounding his body. Later, the shaman mentioned that snakes are frequently seen during ceremonies because they represent the spirit of ayahuasca.

Between sessions, Russ was placed on a plant-based diet and given herbs to reinforce what he had learned. During subsequent sessions, he talked with his deceased parents, reviewing critical life incidents with apologies on both sides. He also visualized visiting his sleeping children and apologizing for how harshly he had treated them. Russ reported feeling as if "every synapse in my brain was firing. . . . I think it helped reroute some of my patterns, my neuropatterns." Later, he added, "I think forgiving myself for a lot of things I've done" was his greatest accomplishment.

Once he returned from Peru, Russ began to counsel young veterans returning from the Middle East who were struggling with PTSD. He enrolled in an integrative PTSD program at the VA hospital in Tucson, Arizona. He later commented, "That integrative program was very helpful for me. I never would have gone if I had not done that work in Peru." A few years later, he returned to Peru for a three-week program. This time, he took smaller doses of ayahuasca and focused on his physical healing. When he left Peru, he had lost weight, his hypertension and diabetes had improved, and his blood pressure and diabetes medications had been reduced. He had no further need for antidepressants.[6]

Conclusion

We have summarized the promising effects of psychedelics and similar substances in treating conditions associated with suicide. In 2019, the U.S. Food and Drug Administration (FDA) approved the use of another novel psychopharmacological agent, ketamine, to treat depression.[7] The FDA also recently granted "breakthrough therapy" status to study MDMA (or ecstasy) as a treatment for PTSD and psilocybin as a treatment for major depression. This designation hastens research because of the success of early results. FDA approval means that psychiatrists could also prescribe these substances for other purposes, such as to improve the quality of close relationships. MDMA, for example, often enhances emotional empathy, feelings of closeness, and thoughtfulness. Psilocybin has a track record of enhancing life satisfaction and a sense of well-being. Hence, one need not be suffering from an emotional disorder to benefit from these preparations. However, many psychiatrists hesitate to meet a patient's request because the Controlled Substances Act bars medical practitioners from writing prescriptions without a "legitimate medical purpose."[8]

Participants in the 2019 ayahuasca study displayed beta and theta brain waves resembling those characteristic of dreaming sleep. In addition, many of the verbal reports resembled those already on file from people reporting "near-death experiences." One member of the team remarked that participants seemed to be "dreaming while awake," a description often given to lucid dreaming. It seems likely that ayahuasca, under carefully prepared and monitored conditions, has potential for psychotherapy, even though its precise use has yet to be determined.[9]

We believe that preventing suicide is a legitimate medical purpose and look forward to responsible understanding and use of mind-altering plants and related preparations. Their use has been limited, but the results are so positive that psychedelic research should be accelerated and current prohibitive legislation should be modified.

Takeaway Points

- Ayahuasca, a brew used for centuries by indigenous healers, shows promise in preventing suicides and treating suicidal people, although solid research on this topic has recently been initiated.

- Psychedelics and similar mind-altering substances show promise in treating at-risk people, but the legal provisions have not kept pace with developments along these lines.

Notes

1. Kaasik, H., & Kreegipuu, K. (2020). Ayahuasca users in Estonia: Ceremonial practices, subjective long-term effects, mental health and quality of life. *Journal of Psychoactive Drugs.* https://doi.org/10.1080/02791072.2020.1748773.

2. Krippner, S., & Sulla, J. (2011). Spiritual content in experiential reports from ayahuasca sessions. *NeuroQuantology, 9*, 333–350.

3. Labate, B. C., & MacRae E. (Ed.). (2010). *Ayahuasca: Ritual and religion in Brazil.* London: Equinox.

4. Rudgley, R. (1994). *Essential substances: A cultural history of intoxicants in society.* New York: Kodansha International.

5. Zeifman, R. J., Palhano-Fontes, F., Hallak, J., et al. (2019, November 19). The impact of ayahuasca on suicidality: Results from a randomized controlled trial. *Frontiers in Pharmacology, 10,* 1325.

6. Tafur, J. (2017). *The fellowship of the river: A medical doctor's exploration of traditional Amazonian plant medicine.* Santa Cruz, CA: MAPS.

7. Meisner, R. C. (2019, May 22). Ketamine for major depression: New tool, new questions. *Harvard Health Blog.* https://www.health.harvard.edu/blog/ketamine-for-major-depression-new-tool-new-questions-2019052216673.

8. Lamkin, M. (2019, July 31). Psychedelic medicine is coming. The law isn't ready. *Scientific American.*

9. Timmermann, C., Roseman, L., Schartner, M., et al. (2019). Neural correlates of the DMT experience assessed with multivariate EEG. *Scientific Reports, 9,* 16324.

Those Who Survived: Saved by the Vine

This story was told to us by Emily Sinclair, who adds that the protagonist "would be happy to know his story is being shared. He always encouraged me to share it!"

A young man from Australia attended a retreat in the Iquitos region of Peru, an event that consisted of five ceremonies that included ingestion of the mind-altering brew ayahuasca. He did not reveal he was suicidal or even depressed until a crisis occurred during the third ceremony, when he shouted to the rest of the group that they were all crazy. He seemed to enter a manic state and ran down the local community street shouting obscenities. As the group leader, I managed to bring him inside to his lodging. Two of his friends were with me, and we engaged him in conversation. He said he had been depressed and suicidal for a long time and had actually written a suicide note following the second ceremony. He felt trapped in his job and life, seeing no purpose in them, and thought that most people lived pointless and stupid existences.

Clearly, he felt isolated and alone. Through our conversations and the realization that we empathized with him, an incredible change occurred. He emerged relaxed and much happier. The next morning, he seemed like a different person, calmer and with brightness in his eyes. He expressed his feelings more openly and had long conversations with others in the retreat. Simply finding the ability to express his feelings honestly and openly and finding that others empathized with him may have really been his cure.

In a follow-up interview six months later, he looked back on this ceremony as the turning point in his life and expressed huge gratitude to ayahuasca and those who had been involved in his experience. He had become open to the spiritual element of existence and had begun practicing meditation and yoga. He had quit his job and begun happily working on a cannabis farm in the United States with a young woman he had met at the same ayahuasca retreat. He did say that his depression had returned a few months following the retreat, but he had felt able to deal with it and was helped by his new girlfriend, with whom he spoke about his feelings.

Was ayahuasca the cure? Or did it just create a psychological opening that allowed him to reclaim parts of himself, as could happen in many kinds of psychotherapy or friendship? Perhaps it does not matter. He is one who survived.

SECTION X

Turning the Tide

CHAPTER FIFTY-FIVE

Turning the Tide

The four of us began this odyssey out of curiosity. We wondered why, after millions of years of evolution and the development of adaptive traits to produce human beings, some people end their lives prematurely. In this chapter, we summarize what we discovered and present some innovations that could turn the tide on this woeful epidemic.

First, we learned that suicide can be explained from an evolutionary perspective. Strangely enough, suicide is not necessarily at odds with Darwin's ideas. We concluded that suicidal thoughts and behavior in some people can be expected for the foreseeable future. In line with this evolutionary perspective, we have highlighted pertinent findings by neuroscientists about suicidal thoughts and behaviors.

Second, we discovered that the field of suicidology covers a vast number of issues. We gave special attention to military service, sexual assault, and bullying. These topics demonstrate how suicide can be a fatal outcome to events that perpetrators and participants did not expect. We then expanded our lens to look at suicide among children, the elderly, farmers, teenagers, minorities, and many others.

Third, the four of us are psychologists; hence, we gravitated to the psychological literature. We were gratified that the American Psychological Association (APA) has devoted considerable attention and resources to suicidal behavior and have used many of its guidelines and definitions.

Fourth, we were relieved to find so many psychotherapeutic inventions that alleviate factors associated with suicide, such as depression, anxiety, and trauma. We gave our readers overviews of evidence-based practices, such as exposure therapies, eye movement desensitization and reintegration (EMDR), and cognitive behavioral therapies (CBT), notably their original source, rational emotive behavior therapy (REBT). We also mentioned interventions that have not yet been sufficiently researched to be considered evidence-based:

time perspective therapy (TPT), deconstructing anxiety, and some transpersonal therapies, especially those of Carl Jung and Stanislav Grof.

Fifth, we expressed concern about the possible misuse of psychiatric medication. Antidepressants and other medicines have saved lives and deserve to be considered in treating suicidal thoughts and behavior. But we also provided instances where these medications failed to prevent suicide and may have even been a factor in provoking suicide attempts.

Sixth, we emphasized the importance of active learning and practice. Vulnerable people can respond positively to the homework assignments provided by TPT, REBT, and others. People can learn self-hypnosis, biofeedback and neurofeedback, and mindfulness and meditation as procedures to decrease suicidal thoughts, to handle negative emotional feelings, and to enjoy ordinary daily activities. They can decrease the frequency and intensity of trauma nightmares through image rehearsal therapy, lucid dreaming, and similar practices.

Seventh, we learned the basic sociological categories of suicide, including a few cases that are difficult to categorize. We reviewed the important roles played by such pioneers as Edwin Shneidman, the first suicidologist, and acknowledged the contributions of Kazimierz Dabrowski, Émile Durkheim, and Karen Mason, whose work on suicide prevention is both practical and theoretically sound.

Eighth, we included case histories and stories of those who survived. All these stories are authentic, but names and some details have been changed to protect personal identities. Some accounts were written by the people who attempted suicide, whose poignant narratives provide a first-person depth to the discussion.

Ninth, we paid homage to indigenous healers and their traditions, especially psychedelic and psychedelic-like preparations. Some of these plant medicines are finding their way into mainstream psychotherapy, and we regret that these contributions were not accepted in Western health care earlier. Spirituality and religion also play an important role for many people, in both helpful and destructive ways. We frankly discussed the possibility of life after death and how this affects many vulnerable people.

Tenth, we emphasized existential perspectives, which hold that people are responsible for making their own decisions. For some people, the decision to end one's life is haphazard, almost frivolous. For others, it is a well-planned, deliberate act, and if their first attempt is aborted, the second or third attempt may be completed. Existential psychotherapists grant that people have the right to terminate their lives, but they do this within a context that often informs clients of other possibilities. Existential psychotherapists also focus on their clients' search for meaning, a life dimension often woefully underdeveloped among suiciders and neglected in many healing approaches.

Eleventh, we concluded that suicide is a public health issue that sometimes reaches epidemic proportions. One person's suicide usually affects dozens of other people, almost always in negative ways. Those left behind may require counseling or psychotherapy. In addition, suicide has economic consequences, not only for families but also for workplaces and neighborhoods. We have stressed the link between poverty and suicide; community development can address both in transformative ways. Instead of viewing suicide as a sin or a crime, we view it as a community problem, just as AIDS, opiate addiction, the coronavirus, and vaping challenge the health of countless people. Suicide can be prevented by telephone and internet hotlines, nets installed on bridges, reasonable restrictions on access to firearms, and monitoring of medication prescriptions.

Finally, we have emphasized the role of social support and positive relationships in preventing suicides and treating vulnerable people. Friendships can counter anhedonia, the inability to experience pleasure. Intimate relationships can provide the romance, humor, and joy that serve as healthy buffers against harmful thoughts and impulses. Family ties can be both preventive and therapeutic if handled properly. Health care providers play a vital role, especially if they display wise acceptance. Just one benevolent act by a kind person can change an irrational belief or dysfunctional personal myth from "Nobody cares about me" to "Perhaps people are not as malevolent as I thought." Most suicidal people need more than love, but it is a promising start.

An Example of Success: Suicide Prevention in Hong Kong

There are many promising suicide prevention programs around the world, but the one in Hong Kong deserves special attention. Hong Kong has about seven million residents, and its gross domestic product per person is one of the highest in Asia. However, the cost of living is high, and its inhabitants work long hours, often twelve hours a day. Many residents bring unfinished work home, even though most apartments are small and cramped. Young people often feel little obligation to care for their aging parents, which adds to the elders' stress. In 2003, Hong Kong's suicide rate reached an all-time high, 18.6 per 100,000 persons. That same year, there was an increase in unemployment, divorce, and illness and death due to an epidemic of severe acute respiratory syndrome (SARS). Inability to manage debt, often caused by gambling and overspending, was a recurring finding. Hanging was the most common means of suicide, followed by burning charcoal, which creates carbon monoxide poisoning.

The increase in suicides was especially apparent among the elderly and young people, stimulating a massive governmental and community response. Innovative services included outreach programs (such as the government's

Suicide Prevention Services), programs for the elderly (Outreach Befriending Service for the Suicidal Elderly), crisis intervention (the Samaritan Befrienders Hong Kong), family crisis support (Family Crisis Support Center), and debt counseling (Debt and Financial Capability Project of the Caritas Family Crisis Support Center), various community education activities, and the establishment of the Hong Kong Centre for Suicide Research and Prevention at the University of Hong Kong.

In addition to Hong Kong's governmental efforts, several nongovernmental organizations were set up, including three twenty-four-hour-a-day hotline services. One of them, the Samaritan Befrienders Hong Kong, created a Suicide Crisis Intervention Center that targeted people at risk and provided assessments, outreach, and crisis interventions for up to eight weeks, with follow-up services for up to twelve weeks. The center also provided services for family members affected by a suicidal crisis and training for family and friends, especially alerting them to warning signs. Because the suicide of a celebrity often stoked other suicide attempts, the media were instructed to use responsible reporting methods that did not sensationalize the prominent person's death.

These programs took a public health approach to suicide, employing evidence-based programs that had been effective in other settings. The scope of this approach extended from vulnerable individuals to the community at large. Access to charcoal was reduced, barriers were installed on railways, and a school program named "The Little Prince Is Depressed" helped children recognize and manage negative emotions. Web-based role-playing games were developed to counter cyberbullying and other challenges posed by social media.

The 2003 suicide rate of 18.6 per 100,000 dropped to 13.1 in 2007 and to 10.6 in 2011. Faculty members of the University of Hong Kong's suicide research center concluded that the public health approach appeared successful in reducing suicide. They noted that hard work and commitment by all stakeholders in the community were important because there is no "quick fix" to suicide prevention.[1]

In 2018, the Hong Kong Centre for Suicide Research and Prevention reported an all-time low of 10.2 suicides per 100,000. Unfortunately, this success was interrupted by the dispute in 2019 over a controversial extradition bill that would have made it easier to send accused individuals to China. Some observers estimated that one out of every three residents of Hong Kong had developed post-traumatic stress disorder (PTSD). The suicide rate went back up, as did calls to the Samaritan Befrienders Hong Kong and other hotlines. People making the calls reported depression concerning the bill (which fortunately was rescinded) and over the long-term future of Hong Kong.[2]

Despite the setback, we are impressed by the comprehensive efforts undertaken in this region. It shows that broad-based prevention can succeed in reducing the rate at which individuals take their lives.

Military Veterans

We have explored the high suicide rate among veterans; surprisingly, those who never saw combat kill themselves at about the same rate as those who did experience combat. In its 2019 report, the Department of Veterans Affairs noted that suicide among the military continues to rise, and there is no simple explanation. Some experts blame demographics; 85 percent of the military is male, and men die by suicide more often than women. However, the 2019 report noted that the suicide rate for women veterans was 2.2 times greater than the suicide rate for nonveteran women.

Other specialists have cited such factors as insomnia, anxiety, depression, sexual assault, gun ownership, and substance misuse. Older veterans are especially vulnerable because of age-related problems and stress and lingering effects of their military service that had never been resolved. But younger veterans are vulnerable as well, especially in readjusting to civilian life, finding and retaining employment, and in coping with relationships in a nonmilitary setting.

In August 2019, the VA and the Department of Defense released revised Clinical Guidelines for the Assessment and Management of Patients at Risk for Suicide.[3] The guidelines were developed by an interdisciplinary team composed of psychologists, psychiatrists, pharmacists, nurses, social workers, and primary care physicians. A major recommendation from this team was to integrate screening for suicide risk into all military clinical settings using the Patient Health Questionnaire-9. If the questionnaire yields a positive score, the Columbia Suicide Severity Rating Scale is administered. If this also provides a worrisome score, the primary care provider or a colleague administers a comprehensive evaluation for suicide risk.

An alternative form of evaluation is REACH-VET, a computer-based program that identifies at-risk veterans based on their health records. The aim of the program is prevention, in some cases even before the veteran is aware of suicidal thoughts. These men and women are referred to their primary care physician or VA mental health specialist to determine whether enhanced care is needed. This program was implemented at all VA facilities in 2017; a year later, more veterans were making appointments with specialists, few appointments were cancelled or broken, there were fewer mental health admissions to VA hospitals, and there were fewer deaths from any causes.

The guidelines recommended evidence-based interventions, as a decade of research had identified cognitive behavioral and other therapies as able to reduce veterans' suicidal thoughts and behaviors. But these interventions required several sessions to be effective, and they could not be implemented in acute and emergency settings. This dilemma led to the development of the twenty- to forty-minute Safety Planning Intervention, which was designed to help veterans develop coping strategies, reduce their access to firearms and lethal medications, and help them establish follow-up treatments. A pilot study reported that the Safety Planning Intervention cut suicide attempts in half, as compared to veterans who were merely referred for follow-up care. The emphasis on inquiring about firearm access was especially important because 70 percent of military suicides involve guns and rifles compared to 50 percent of suicides among the general population.

The guidelines also identified technology that appeared to reduce suicidal risk. A specially designed smartphone increased veterans' ability to cope with unpleasant thoughts and emotions. Another development, the Virtual Hope Box, contains items that remind veterans of positive life experiences, people who care about them, resources in the area, and reasons to go on living. This latter goal, of course, is a cornerstone of existential psychotherapy. The Virtual Hope Box can include personalized photos, recorded songs, quotations, puzzles, videos, guided meditations, relaxation exercises, and a phone contact list.

The guidelines also offer suggestions for smoother transitions points between health care providers, hospitals, and residences because these are times when suicide-prone people are especially vulnerable. VA services are uneven and have been frequently criticized; only one out of three veterans requests health care services from the VA. However, the 2019 National Veteran Suicide Prevention Annual Report noted that the suicide rate of veterans receiving recent VA care increased by 1.3 percent, and the rate for veterans who were not receiving VA care increased by 11.8 percent. This difference held up even after age and gender differences between the two groups were accounted for.

The VA guidelines did not mention the Comprehensive Soldier and Family Fitness program, which we reviewed and critiqued in an earlier chapter. However, the implementation of the guidelines has already yielded positive results due, at least in part, to their reliance on evidence-based interventions and the collaboration of members of several disciplines.

Sexual Assault

The second issue that received our special focus was the role that sexual assault plays in suicidal behavior. The most notorious recent case centered on the Hollywood producer Harvey Weinstein, about whom rumors had been circulating for years. In 2017, *New York Times* reporters Jodi Kantor and Megan Twohey interviewed several people with whom Weinstein had worked—female actors, employees, and business associates. Hearing about this effort, Weinstein employed a cadre of lawyers and investigators to stop the investigation, but Kantor and Twohey had already convinced some of their key sources to go on the record.

Their first story was published in October 2017. Within days, numerous women, some from abroad, came forward with their own traumatic stories. The searchlight widened. Hundreds of men in positions of power were subjects of allegations of wrongdoing. This sterling example of investigative journalism, *She Said*, is a remarkable account that not only describes the consequences of their reporting for the #MeToo movement but also the inspiring and affecting journeys of the women who spoke up.

Over and over again, respondents condemned a system that protected Weinstein and other predators by compensating their victims for remaining silent, offering them money in exchange for signing nondisclosure agreements. Many women with no connection to the film industry reported similar experiences in other industries where men held inordinate amounts of power. Their testimony has already initiated major changes in some U.S. businesses and has put new generations of workers, both female and male, on guard against improper statements and actions. Weinstein was convicted in 2020, a jury finding that vindicated those who testified. The testimony of Kantor and Twohey's respondents was helpful not only for themselves but also for their contemporaries and for future generations. Numerous lives have been saved by these investigative reporters and their courageous collaborators.[4]

Being Bullied

Bullying has reached epidemic proportions in the United States, and no attempt to change the bullying culture has been a resounding success. So in our final discussion of bullying, we will provide the results of a statewide survey on the topic and discuss what was learned from it.

The Arizona Youth Survey of 2016 queried fifty thousand students from the eighth, tenth, and twelfth grades. Questions were adapted from the Risk and Protector Feeder model and the Youth Risk Behavior Surveillance System Behavioral Risk Factor. The results demonstrated the magnitude of the problem. One out of five girls and boys admitted that they had bullied someone else during the previous twelve months. One out of three stated that they had been bullied, and most of these young people claimed that they had been cyberbullied. Social networking and similar technologies have become dangerous vehicles for bullying.

Only one out of four young people reported never having been bullied, and the same number claimed that they had been bullied once during the past year. An astonishing 16 percent of youth stated that they had been bullied four or more times, either at school, at home, or elsewhere in the community. When ethnic and racial background were recorded, 80 percent of white students reported having been bullied as compared to 41 percent of Hispanics, 8 percent of Native Americans, 6 percent of African Americans, 4 percent of Asian Americans, about 1 percent of Hawaiians and Pacific Islanders, and 11 percent of those reporting "multi" ethnicity.

But bullying was only one of several "adverse childhood experiences" studied. One out of two youth reported one or more such experiences within the past year: physical abuse, emotional abuse, and sexual abuse, either in the home or outside the home setting. We have emphasized the importance of attachment in previous chapters; the large number of adverse experiences demonstrates how fortunate those children are who have formed a deep relationship with one or both parents or with other significant adults. This permits them to become resilient so that a potentially traumatizing event need not become a traumatic experience with severe consequences.[5]

In Retrospect

Social critic Christopher Ryan has vividly portrayed the contemporary milieu that, in too many ways, facilitates suicide rather than preventing it. Citing authoritative sources, Ryan observes that only 30 percent of Americans are enthusiastic about their jobs, which occupy at least forty hours of their time each week. Since 1990, the use of antidepressants has increased 400 percent; one out of four women between the ages of forty and fifty-nine is taking at least one. When asked if they had at least one friend with whom they could confide, in 1985, 10 percent said "nobody," and in 2004, that number had risen to 25 percent. Regarding suicide, Ryan cites the Centers for Disease Control and Prevention's findings that the number of Americans who take their lives now surpasses, for the first time, the number killed in car accidents.

Ryan believes that our society has two major shortcomings: lives that lack meaning and activities that bypass other people.[6] These themes run through our book as well. There are multiple predisposing factors for suicide; a systems approach is needed to chart them all.

Suicide is complicated, and we do not claim to have fully explained its many forms, reasons, and variations. We have offered information on prevention and treatment and hope that our readers will find something of value in our search that they can apply to the present and future adversities that may be faced by their families, their loved ones, and themselves.

In this book, you have read about many ways to heal from suicidality. You may have wondered, "Why are there so many treatments?" It is because no two people's situations and personalities are exactly alike. What works for person X is not helpful or even relevant for person Y. You, or your loved one, or your clients must be carefully interviewed and assessed to find which factors contribute to the despair and which treatments are best suited to each individual.

We also make this recommendation: to counter the appalling negativity of media reporting, find some publications, organizations, or websites that showcase good news, kindness, and heroism. You will get a more balanced view of your fellow humans! For instance, GoodNewsNetwork.org, MyPositiveOutlooks.com, and Kindspring.org specifically exist to share the best in human nature. You can also watch videos (easily found online) of rescuers caring enough and even taking risks to interrupt suicides. People do care—even people the at-risk person does not know.

Remembering that "Those Who Survived" are many in number, and that many individuals, groups, and governments are working with intelligence and dedication to reduce the rates of suicide, we are hopeful that the peak of this epidemic will soon pass and that more people will find ways to overcome obstacles and find meaning and satisfaction in life.

Takeaway Points

- There are evidence-based programs that have been effective in curbing suicide rates, but they require the collaboration of all public health stakeholders.
- People whose lives lack meaning and social connections are vulnerable to suicide, and the same can be said of societies with similar deficits.

Notes

1. Yip, P., Yik, W. L., & Chan, M. (2013). Suicide prevention in Hong Kong. In D. Lester & J. L. Rogers (Eds.), *Suicide: A global issue, Vol. 2, Prevention* (pp. 219–247). Santa Barbara, CA: Praeger.

2. Chui, A. (2019, July 4). Protest suicides spark concern in Hong Kong. *Asia Times* (online).

3. Novotney, A. (2020, January–February). Stopping suicide in the military. *Monitor on Psychology*, pp. 32–34.

4. Kantor, J., & Twohey, M. (2019). *She said: Breaking the sexual harassment story that helped ignite a movement*. New York: Penguin/Random House.

5. Arizona Criminal Justice Commission. (2016). *Arizona youth survey state report 2016*. Phoenix: Arizona Criminal Justice Commission.

6. Ryan, C. (2019). *Civilized to death: The price of progress* (p. 259). New York: Avid Reader Press.

Index

ABCDE self-help formula, 209–210, 273–274

Active euthanasia, 53

Adios, 192

Adventure education programs, 305–306

Afghanistan, 19, 69

African Americans and suicide, 21–22

After-death communications (ADCs), 55

Agricultural, farmers and suicide, 161–165

Alaskan Natives and suicide, 23

"Alchemist" technique, 146, 148

Alcohol, 169

Algorithm, 219–221

Alienation dream, 40

Allen, Woody, 6

Allure, 5

Altruistic suicide, 16, 17

American Counseling Association, 230–231

Analytical psychology, 213–214

Angry rapist, 104

Anhedonia, 203–204

Animal-assisted therapy (AAT), 306–308

Anna Karenina (Tolstoy), 15

Anomic suicide, 16, 17, 167

Antidepressants, 141

Anxiety, 135, 143–148

Apollonia, 192

Applewhite, Marshall, 199

Archetypal field theory, 193

Archila, Ana Maria, 94

Arizona Youth Survey (2016), 331–332

Asian Americans and suicide, 24–25

Assagioli, Roberto, 140, 214–215

Attractor sites, 193

Autonomic nervous system (ANS), 80

Ayahuasca, 316–320, 322

Azibo, Daudi Ajani ya, 22

Baez, José, 258–259

Bauer, Henry, 81

Beck, Aaron, 134, 151

Benga, Ota, 21

Bering, Jesse, 81, 188

Bertini, Kristine, 32, 232

Best, Katherine, 191

Billings, Bart, 77–78, 79–80, 81

Billy the Kid, 14

Binswanger, Ludwig, 12

Biofeedback, 248

Bogzaran, Fariba, 39–40

Borderline personality disorder, 44–46

Boring, E. B., 17

Bourdain, Anthony, 8, 13

Breggin, Peter, 81, 141

Brewerton, Timothy, 311

Brief eclectic psychotherapy (BEP), 150
Bullying, 7–8, 111–114; Arizona Youth Survey (2016), 331–332; cyberbullying, 117–118; prevention of, 126–129; sexual violence, 117; system, 121–124; victims and bystanders, 120–124; and the vulnerable, 115–118
Bullying rapist, 104
Burke, Tarana, 6, 95
Bystander, 127–128

Cajete, Gregory, 167
Campbell, Joseph, 197
Camus, Albert, 43
Cannabidiol (CBD), 310
Cannabis, 310–311
Carter, Michelle, 75–76
Cartwright, Rosalind, 275
Casey, George W., 241
Catanzarite, Zachary, 183
Chapman, Allen, 40, 75
Child abuse and suicide, 31–32
Child maltreatment, 31
Child neglect, 32
Children and suicide, 176, 203–204
Chronic traumatic encephalopathy, 259
Churches, sexual assault in, 98–102
Cleopatra VII of Egypt, 196
Cliques, 126
Cobain, Kurt, 196
Cocaine, 169
Cognitive behavioral therapy (CBT), 136, 140–141, 150, 151, 229
Cognitive processing therapy (CPT), 150, 151
Cognitive therapy (CT), 150, 151
Cohen, Raphael, 244
Colectivismo, 23–24
Collective suicide, 192
Community Supported Agriculture (CSA), 164
Core fear, 144–146
Cortisol, 203
Counseling and suicide, 230–233

Creative arts, 293–294
Csikszentmihalyi, Mihaly, 118
Culture of consent, 95
Cyberbullying, 117–118

Dabrowski, Kazimierz, 10–11, 14, 188, 326
Davis, J. L., 278
Dead Grass, 43
Death, modes of, 11
Deconstructing anxiety model, 143–148
Default mode network (DMN), 255
Depression, 3, 34–35, 133–134, 139–142
Deslauriers, Daniel, 39–40
Deterrence, 184–185
Diagnostic and Statistical Manual (DSM), 178–179
Dissociation, 127
Distress nightmare, 39–40
Dogs, therapy, 306–308
Domestic violence, 290–291
Dostie, Ryan Leigh, 106–107
Dow, Bruce, 282–283
Dream revision therapy, 282–283
Dreams and nightmares, 36–40, 275–280
Drouet, Emily, 116
Dumas, Catherine, 260
Durkheim, Émile: anomie, 222; exploration of suicide in *Suicide* (1897), 16–18, 326; influence on Lévy-Bruhl, 166; suicide as public health issue, 188; suicide in the military, 73; taxonomy, 192; tribal suicides, 174; types of suicide, 16–17, 167
Durkheim Project, 220
Dying City (Shinn), 294

Ecstasy, 312, 319
Educational neglect, 32
Egoistic suicide, 17
Eidelson, Ray, 242

Elderly and suicide, 177
Electroencephalography (EEG), 202, 203, 204
Ellis, Albert, 124, 134, 151, 207, 211, 234, 239
Ellis, Debbie Joffe, 211
Emotional expression, 276
Emotional neglect, 32
Emotional suicide, 192
Empathogen, 312
Engelman, Suzanne, 306–308
Entheogenic, 311
Epictetus, 208
Epigenetics, 203–204
Epstein, Jeffrey, 258
Euthanasia, 52–53
Evolutionary psychology and suicide, 183–185
Existential psychotherapy, 11–12
Exploitation, 32
Exposure, relaxation, and rescripting therapy (ERRT), 278
Exposure therapy (ET), 277, 278
Extreme present fatalism, 302
Eye movement desensitization and reprocessing (EMDR), 150, 152, 287–291

Faberow, Norman, 14–15
Fahrenheit 9/11, 19
Faith groups, sexual assault in, 98–102
Faria, João Teixeira de, 99–100
Farmers and suicide, 161–165
Farm-to-table, 164
Farrow, Dylan, 6
Fatalistic suicide, 17, 18, 259
Fear, 143–145
Ferguson, Christopher, 48–49
Fikretoglu, Deniz, 240
Flake, Jeff, 94
Foa, Edna, 151
For Colored Girls Who Have Considered Suicide/When the Rainbow Is Enuf (Shange), 294

Forbes, Susan, 240
Frank, Jerome, 197
Frankl, Viktor, 77, 271
Freud, Sigmund, 167, 197, 293
Friedman, Harris, 217
Fulfillment, 143–144, 145
Fundamentalist Church of Jesus Christ of Latter-Day Saints (FLDS), 99
Fungi, 313

Gallagher, Maria, 94
Galvin, Frank, 284
García, Alan, 259
Gardening, 306
Genital injury, 105–106
Global Assessment Tool (GAT), 241, 243
Golden Gate Bridge (San Francisco, CA), 198
Golding, William, 122
Grande, Ariana, 96
Graves, Glenn, 287–288
Greenberg, Gary, 81
Grey, Bobby, 156–157
Greyson, Bruce, 54
Grob, Charles, 311
Grof, Stanislav, 43–44, 215–216, 264, 326
Guarani (indigenous people), 171–174
Guarani, Dom João, 173–174
Guarani, Tonico Benites, 173

Hansen, Joey, 236–237
Harper, Robert, 236
Hartmann, Ernest, 37, 277, 284
Hayssen, Gail, 87–90
Healthy negative emotions, 209
Heath, Pamela Rae, 55
Heaven's Gate, 11, 199–200
Hedda Gabler (Ibsen), 294
Hemingway, Ernest, 18, 30–31
Hendrix, Jimi, 196
Hernandez, Aaron, 258–259
Heroin, 169

The Hidden Face of Suicide (Silverman), 293
High sensitivity and suicide, 30–31
Hillman, James, 192, 197, 222
Hippocratic oath, 52
Hispanics and suicide, 23–24
Holotropic psychotherapy, 215–216
Homosexuality, 4
Hong Kong suicide prevention program, 327–329
Horus, 195
Human Kindness Foundation, 259–260
Humanistic psychology, 213
Hypnosis, 80, 248

Ibsen, Henrik, 294
Imagery rehearsal therapy, 277–278
Implicit Association Test, 246
Indigenous peoples and suicide, 171–174
Intellectual suicide, 192–193
Internal Family Systems (IFS) therapy, 139–140
Iraq, 19, 69

Jacob, Kathleen, 40
Jacobs, Gilles, 219
James, William, 55
Jenkins, David, 279
Jesuits, 171–172
Jigaki, 192
Jilek, Wolfgang, 167
John, St., of the Cross, 264
Joiner, Thomas, 42, 177
Jones, Brian, 196
Jones, C. B., 118
Jones, Jim, 17
Joplin, Janis, 196
Journeyhawk, Fawn, 43, 168–170
Jung, Carl: analytical psychology, 213; archetypes, 191, 200; creative arts, 293; dreams, 37; mythology, 195, 197; transpersonal therapy, 326

Kabat-Zinn, Jon, 247
Kalu Rinpoche, 102
Kantor, Jodi, 330–331
Kavanaugh, Brett, 94
Ketamine, 312–313
Ketwig, John, 69
Kevorkian, Jack, 239
Klimo, Jon, 55
K9s for Warriors, 306
Kornfield, Jack, 102
Korten, David, 197
Krakow, Barry, 277
Krishnamurti, 102
Krueger, Alan, 8
Kuiken, Don, 290
Kyle, Chris, 81

Lack of attachment and suicide, 29–30
Lady Gaga, 96
Larson, Reed, 118
"Letting Go the Resistance to Resistance" technique, 147
Levin, Roger, 276
Lévy-Bruhl, Lucien, 166–167
LGBT (lesbian, gay, bisexual, transgender), 25
Liakata, Maria, 220
Lifeway Research, 101
Litman, R. E., 36–37
Lord of the Flies (Golding), 122
Loye, David, 238
Lozoff, Bo, 260
Lucid dreaming therapy (LDT), 284–285
The Lucifer Effect (Zimbardo), 124

MacKrell, Mike, 241
Macy, Joanna, 197
Marc Antony, 196
Marcus Aurelius, 208
Marijuana, 310–311
Markey, Patrick, 49
Mason, Karen, 100–101, 326

Master resilience trainers (MRTs), 241
Matlocks, Nikki, 116
Mattis, James, 78
May, Rollo, 197
McQueen, Alexander, 25
Meditation, 246–248
Memory element activation, 276
Memory element recombination, 276
Mendoza, Gonzalo de, 171
Mental illness and suicide, 42–46
Methylenedioxymethamphetamine (MDMA), 312, 319
#MeToo movement, 6, 95, 331
Milano, Alyssa, 95
Milgram, Stanley, 123
Military and suicide: Afghanistan war, 40; older veterans, 177; parking lots, 73–76; Paulson, Daryl, 61–66, 67–71; sexual assault, 104–107; suicide prevention programs, 329–330. *See also* Post-traumatic stress disorder (PTSD)
Miller, Alice, 31
Miller, Justin, 74
Milton, John, 34
Mindfulness, 246–248, 255
Mindfulness-Based Stress Reduction (MBSR), 247
Mindfulness meditation, 247
Minorities and suicide, 21–26
Mitchell, Aaron, 17
Mithoefer, Michael, 311, 312
Moore, Michael, 19
Moore, Ruth, 90–92
Moral injury, 18–20
Mormons, 99
Morrison, Jim, 196
Mous, Zahira Lieneke, 100
Muriello, Dan, 220
Mushrooms, 313
Muslim suicide bombers, 11
Myth, 166–167
Mythology, 196–201

Narrative exposure therapy (NET), 150, 152, 292–294
Narrative psychology, 200
Native Alaskans and suicide, 23
Native Americans and suicide, 23
Nature as healing method, 305–308
Near-death experiences (NDEs), 53–55, 265
Netflix, 48
Nettles, Bonnie, 199
Neurofeedback, 248
Neuroplasticity, 255–256
Neurotransmitters, 202–203
Neustadter, Sarah B., 216
Newsom, Jennifer Siebel, 50
Nielsen, Terri, 276
'Night Mother (Norman), 294
Night terrors, 38
Nightmares and dreams, 36–40, 275–280
Norcross, J. C., 178
Norman, Marsha, 294

Operation Enduring Freedom—Afghanistan, 6
Operation Iraqi Freedom, 6
Opioids, 3
Opportunistic rapist, 104
Osiris, 194
Osowobi, Oluwaseun Ayodrji, 96
OxyContin, 3
Oxytocin, 203

Pain and brain model, 184
Pargament, Kenneth, 263
Participation mystique, 166
Passive euthanasia, 53
Paulson, Daryl, 61–66, 67–71
People's Temple, 17
Personal mythology, 196–201
Physician-assisted suicide, 52–56, 239
Pitchford, Daniel, 280
Placebo effect, 166
Pompili, Maurizio, 203

Post-traumatic stress disorder (PTSD),
    135–137; Afghanistan war, 40;
    ayahuasca, 318–319; and *Diagnostic
    and Statistical Manual (DSM)*,
    178–179; evaluating treatments for,
    150–154; Grey, Bobby, 156–157;
    misuse of psychiatric medications
    for treating, 77–82; Vietnam War,
    5–6, 64, 67, 68, 69, 70; World War
    II, 4–5. *See also* Military and suicide
Post-traumatic stress disorder (PTSD)
    nightmares, 38, 275–280; dream
    revision therapy, 282–283; lucid
    dreaming therapy (LDT), 284–285
Poverty and suicide, 29
Prazosin, 277
Pressman, Todd, 143, 144, 147–148
Prisons and suicide, 258–261
Programmed cell death (PCD), 184
Progressive muscle relaxation (PMR),
    278–279
Prolonged exposure therapy (PET),
    150, 151–152
Prozac, 141
Psilocybin, 319
Psychache, 187
Psychedelics, 310–313
Psychological abuse, 31
Psychophysiology, 202–204
Psychospiritual crises, 43
Psychosynthesis, 214–215
Psychotherapy, 200, 311–313

Qiao, George, 24
Qigong, 80

Racial entitlement, 254
Rainforest Action Network (RAN), 174
Rape culture, 95
Rational emotive behavior therapy
    (REBT): and cognitive therapies,
    151; self-empowerment, 273;
    Shneidman, Edwin, 267–268; and
    suicide, 206–211, 224–225; and
    suicide prevention, 234–239

REACH-VET, 329
Red Tomahawk Halfmoon, 169
Religious and spiritual beliefs, 49–50
Religious Orienting System (ROS),
    262–263
Religious/spiritual struggles, 263–264
Resilience training, 240–244
Richman, Sandy, 50
Rogers, Sandra, 265
Roman Catholic Church, sexual
    assault in, 98–99
Rosa, Rich, 17
Rosmann, Michael, 162
Routh, Eddie Ray, 81
Roy, Conrad, III, 75
Rudgley, Richard, 317
Rudolf, Prince of Austria, 196
Ryan, Christopher, 332

Sacco, Frank, 121–122, 126–128
Sadistic rapist, 104
Safety Planning Intervention, 330
Sala, Luc, 214
Saleem, Haji, 219
Samaritan Befrienders Hong Kong,
    328
Schladale, Joann, 94
School violence and suicide, 50
Schwartz, Richard, 139
Schwarz, Jill, 290–291
*Seeds of Hope: An Arts-Based Approach
    to Suicide and Resilience*, 293
Selective serotonin-norepinephrine
    uptake inhibitors (SNRIs), 153
Selective serotonin reuptake inhibitors
    (SSRIs), 153
Self-empowerment, 271–274
Self-harm, 14
Self-regulation, 246–248
Seligman, Martin, 242, 243
Seppuku, 192
Serafini, Gianluca, 203
Serotonin, 202, 317
Set, 194
Sexual abuse, 31

Sexual assault: in churches and faith groups, 98–102; eye movement desensitization and reprocessing (EMDR), used by survivors of, 290–291; Hayssen, Gail, 87–90; in the military, 104–107; Moore, Ruth, 90–92; and suicide, 6–7, 93–96, 330–331

Sexual minorities and suicide, 25

Sexual trafficking, 31–32

Sexual trauma, 105

Sexual violence and bullying, 117

Shamans, 43, 44, 167–170

Shame, 121

Shange, Ntozake, 294

Shapiro, Francine, 152

Shauer, Maggie, 292

Shaw, George Bernard, 57

She Said, 331

Shermer, Michael, 122–123

Shinn, Christopher, 294

Shneidman, Edwin, 186–188, 198, 267–268, 326

SHORES, 231

Silverman, Yehudit, 293

Sinclair, Emily, 322

Sleep disorders, 177–178

Smartphones, 49

Smith, Channing, 115–116

Snyder, R. B., 128

Social integration, 16

Sommers, Marilyn Sawyer, 106

Soper, Cas, 184

Soros, George, 53

Soul retrieval, 168

South America, sexual abuse in, 99–100

Southern Baptist church, sexual assault in, 99

Sparrow, Scott, 38

Spirit sickness, soul loss, and suicide, 166–170

Spiritual emergencies, 43–44, 215–216

Spiritual fitness, 243–244

Spirituality and suicide, 262–266

Spruce, Richard, 316

Stauffler, Brian, 28, 30

Stellate ganglion, 136–137

Stewart, Jimmy, 84

Stormy Winds, 169

Study to Assess Risks and Resilience in Servicemembers (STARRS), 220

Styron, William, 34–35, 133

Sublimation, 111

Subpersonalities, 139–140

Suicide: allure of, 3–9; animal-assisted therapy (AAT), 306–308; anxiety, 135, 143–148; archetypes, 191–195; ayahuasca, 316–320, 322; bullying, 111–114, 120–124, 126–129, 331–332; bullying and the vulnerable, 115–118; and child abuse, 31–32; children, 176, 203–204; depression, 133–134, 139–142; dream revision therapy, 282–283; dreams and nightmares, 36–40; elderly, 177; evolutionary psychology, 183–185; eye movement desensitization and reprocessing (EMDR), 287–291; farmers, 161–165; five levels of, 10–11; and high sensitivity, 30–31; Hong Kong prevention program, 327–329; indigenous peoples, 171–174; lack of attachment and, 29–30; lucid dreaming therapy (LDT), 284–285; mental illness, 42–46; and military, 61–66, 67–71, 73–76, 77–82, 177, 329–330; and minorities, 21–26; misconceptions, 8; misunderstandings, 12–13; mythology, 196–201; narrative exposure therapy (NET), 292–294; nature as healing method, 305–308; in parking lots, 73–76; physician-assisted, 52–56; post-traumatic stress disorder (PTSD), 135–138, 150–154, 156–157, 177–178; post-traumatic stress disorder

Suicide (*cont.*)
(PTSD) nightmares, 275–280; and
poverty, 29; prevention, 229–233;
prevention and rational emotive
behavior therapy (REBT), 234–239;
prevention and resilience training,
240–244; in prisons, 258–261;
psychedelics, 310–313;
psychophysiology, 202–204; as
public health issue, 186–190;
rational emotive behavior therapy
(REBT), 206–211; school violence,
50; self-empowerment, 271–274;
self-regulation, 246–248; sexual
assault, 87–90, 93–96, 330–331;
sexual assault in churches and faith
groups, 98–102; sexual assault in
the military, 104–107; shamans,
167–170; sleep disorders, 177–178;
spirit sickness and soul loss,
166–170; spirituality as path away
from, 262–266; study of, 325–327,
332–333; systems theory, 219–223;
teenage, 48–51, 250–256; time
perspective therapy (TPT),
296–298, 300–303; transpersonal
psychology, 213; and trauma,
13–15; types of, 16–20; and
Western United States, 28
Suicide-prone, 5
Survivor's guilt, 68–69
Sword, Richard, 297–298, 301
Sword, Rosemary, 298, 301
Symbolic suicide, 192
Systems theory, 219–223

Tai Chi, 80
Talk therapy, 77
Tang, Luke, 24
Taylor, Robert, 14
Tchaikovsky, Pyotr, 25
Teenage suicides, 48–51, 250–256
Teresa, Mother, 264
Tetrahydrocannabinol (THC), 310

Therapy dogs, 306–308
Thich Quang Duc, 192–193
13 Reasons Why, 48–49
Tillier, William, 10, 14
Time perspective therapy (TPT),
296–298, 300–303
Tolstoy, Leo, 15
Toombs, John, 74–75
Toxic masculinity, 50
Traditional masculinity, 254
Transcendental negative/positive
future, 297
Transpersonal psychology, 213
Trauma and suicide, 13–15
Traumatic brain injury (TBI), 79
Tsypes, Aliona, 203–204
Turing, Alan, 4
Turner, Jim, 74
Twemlow, Stuart, 121–122, 126–128
Twohey, Megan, 330–331
Tyler, Daria, 163
Tyler, Dick, 162–163
Tyler, Lenore, 163
Tyler, Randall, 163

Ugaki, Matome, 17
Ullman, Montague, 282
Unconditional other acceptance
(UOA), 210–211
Unhealthy negative emotions, 209
U.S. Army "soldier fitness" program,
240–243

Vasquez, Debbie, 99
Vaughan, Alan G., 193–195
Vernon, Marcos, 172
Veterans. *See* Military and suicide;
Post-traumatic stress disorder
(PTSD)
Vetsera, Baroness Mary, 196
Video games, 49
Vietnam War, 5–6, 61–66, 67–69
Vine of the spirits, 316–320, 322
Virtual Hope Box, 330

Wampold, B. E., 178
War combat, 5–6
"Warrior's Stance" technique, 146, 148
Watkins, Paula, 247
Watts, Alan, 213
Weinstein, Harvey, 94, 330–331
We're All Doing Time (Lozoff), 259–261
West, Ellen, 12
Western United States and suicide, 28
White Owl, 169

Whitson, Signe, 129
Wilber, Ken, 221
Wilber Quadrant, 221–222
Williams, Robin, 18
Wilson, Colin, 57–58, 135
Winfrey, Oprah, 96
Winkelman, Michael, 313
"Witness" technique, 146, 148
Witt, Joshua, 263
Wright, Bobby, 22
Wurtzel, Elizabeth, 134, 141

Zimbardo, Philip, 123–124, 296, 298

About the Authors

Stanley Krippner, PhD, is a member of the American Association of Suicidology and the International Society for the Study of Trauma and Dissociation. He has coedited or coauthored five books on trauma, including *Integrated Care for the Traumatized: A Whole-Person Approach.* He is a fellow of the Society for the Study of Peace, Conflict and Violence, and the 2002 recipient of the American Psychological Association Award for Distinguished Contributions to the Advancement of International Psychology.

Linda Riebel, PhD, is on the faculty of Saybrook University. She conducted a psychotherapy practice in San Francisco and Berkeley for twenty-five years, specializing in eating disorders, anxiety, and depression. She is the author of many professional journal articles and six books and is a contributor to the third edition of the *Encyclopedia of Creativity* (2020). She also lost a nephew to suicide.

Debbie Joffe Ellis, PhD, is on the adjunct faculty at Columbia University Teachers College, where she teaches Rational Emotive Behavior Therapy and Comparative Psychotherapies. Her most recent book is the second edition of *Rational Emotive Behavior Therapy* (2019).

Daryl S. Paulson, PhD, is a decorated Vietnam combat veteran, a counselor specializing in trauma-associated disorders, and the president/CEO of BioScience Laboratories, Inc. He has advanced degrees in microbiology, statistics, counseling, human science, and psychology. Dr. Paulson is the author of numerous articles and fourteen books and is the coauthor of *Haunted by Combat.*